PRINCIPLES & LABS

FOR PHYSICAL FITNESS AND WELLNESS

WERNER W.K. HOEGER
Boise State University

SHARON A. HOEGER

THIRD EDITION

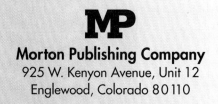

Morton Publishing Company
925 W. Kenyon Avenue, Unit 12
Englewood, Colorado 80110

DEDICATION

In memory of my mother.

True love never dies.

Heavenly Father is love. Heavenly Father is eternal. Love and life are also eternal. As my love for you is eternal, I look to the day when once again I can be in your arms to tell you:
I love you Mom.

Werner

Cover Design by Bob Schram, Bookends.

Interior book design by Gloria Brown.

Printed in the United States of America

10   9   8   7   6   5   4   3   2

ISBN: 0–89582–260–1

PREFACE

The current American way of life does not provide the human body with sufficient physical activity to maintain adequate health and improve the quality of life. Many present lifestyle patterns are such a serious threat to our health that they actually increase the deterioration rate of the human body and often lead to premature illness and mortality.

People in the United States are firm believers in the benefits of physical activity, good nutrition, and positive lifestyle habits as a means to promote a healthier, happier, and more productive life. Nevertheless, the great majority do not enjoy a better quality of life because they are either led astray by a multi-billion dollar "quick fix — fad" industry, or simply do not know how to implement a sound fitness and wellness program that will yield positive results.

Principles and Labs for Physical Fitness and Wellness contains seventeen chapters and thirty-nine laboratories (eleven new labs) that serve as a guide to implement a complete lifetime fitness and wellness program. Book contents point out the need to go beyond the basic components of fitness to achieve total well-being. In addition to a thorough discussion on physical fitness, including all health- and skill-related components; extensive and up to date information is provided on nutrition, weight management, cardiovascular and cancer risk reduction, exercise and aging, stress management, prevention of sexually transmitted diseases, and substance abuse control (including tobacco, alcohol, and other psychoactive drugs).

As students work through the various chapters and laboratories in this book, they will develop and regularly update their own lifetime program to improve fitness components and personal wellness. *The emphasis throughout the book is on teaching students how to take control of their own personal health and lifestyle habits so that they can make a constant and deliberate effort to stay healthy and achieve the highest potential for well-being.*

The chapters in the **third edition** of *Principles and Labs for Physical Fitness and Wellness* have been revised and updated to include new information reported in the literature and at professional health, physical education, and sportsmedicine meetings. A questionnaire was given to almost all users of the second edition to evaluate the book. The recommendations made proved extremely valuable in the preparation of this new edition. While it was difficult to include all of the suggestions, the great majority were addressed.

The most significant changes of the third edition are:

- The book now contains seventeen chapters instead of sixteen. Because of the importance of AIDS and substance abuse prevention programs, this information is presented separately in Chapter 16. This change allows for a greater discussion of these topics.
- Chapter 17 (Relevant Fitness and Wellness Issues) contains the rest of the information previously provided in Chapter 16. Further, the information on spiritual wellness has been enhanced. Guidelines for the prevention of consumer fraud, factors to consider when selecting a health/fitness club, and reliable sources for updated wellness (health, fitness, and nutrition) information are also discussed.
- A discussion on the U.S. Health Objectives for the Year 2000 are included in Chapter 1. These health objectives clearly emphasize the need for health promotion and disease prevention, personal responsibility, and health benefits for all people in the United States.
- An update on current health care costs in the United States and throughout most developed countries around the world is included.
- The order of the first few chapters was changed. The nutrition, body composition, and weight control chapters are grouped together as Chapters 2, 3, and 4, respectively.
- The nutrition chapter (Chapter 2) now contains information on the Food Guide Pyramid, the role of glycogen in the body, nutrition for athletes, and the antioxidant effect of some vitamins and minerals in the prevention of disease.
- Hydrostatic weighing to determine percent body fat and the Body Mass Index (BMI) to assess risk for disease were added to the body composition chapter.
- A broader discussion of the terms obesity, overweight, recommended weight, and "tolerable" weight is included in Chapter 4. Such information helps students make an informed decision as to what constitutes a realistic target weight.
- A 1.0-Mile Walk Test and a Twelve-Minute Swim Test were added to the cardiovascular endurance assessment chapter. These protocols are useful for individuals, who, because of personal or facility limitations, are unable to use any of the other three assessment techniques previously included in the book.
- A new *Exercise Readiness* questionnaire (given in Lab

6B) is discussed in the cardiovascular exercise prescription chapter. The questionnaire helps to assess a person's readiness for exercise based on four categories of evaluation: mastery (self-control), attitude, health, and commitment. A new *Fitness Ratings of Aerobic Activities* chart is also presented in Chapter 6.

- New Grip and Abdominal Crunch Strength Tests and information on anabolic steroids and plyometrics were added to the strength chapters.
- Modifications have been made to the cardiovascular disease risk management chapter. Major updates include new information on diabetes and exercise, blood lipid recommendations by the National Cholesterol Education Program (NCEP), cholesterol lowering drugs, antioxidant effects of vitamins and minerals, and the effects of low fat diets on cholesterol levels.
- The cancer prevention chapter contains more information on the effects of a healthy lifestyle on cancer mortality, the ever expanding role of nutrition in cancer prevention, and additional data on skin cancer.
- Enhancements to the stress management chapter include concepts on stress vulnerability and time management.
- Eleven new labs have been added to enhance fitness and wellness experiences and point to the need of behavior modification to improve health and quality of life.
- A comprehensive glossary that includes key terms used in the text has been added at the end of the book.
- New color photography and many outstanding new graphs are included throughout the book.

SUPPLEMENTS

The following ancillaries are provided free of charge to all qualified *Principles and Labs for Physical Fitness and Wellness* adopters:

- Two of the most **comprehensive computer software packages** available with any fitness/wellness textbook. Both packages include a *Fitness and Wellness Profile*, a *Personalized Cardiovascular Exercise Prescription*, a *Nutrient Analysis*, and a weekly and monthly *Exercise Log*. Software package one also provides a pre- and post-test comparison, including percent change for each fitness and wellness item on the profile. The second software package offers several individual program options for use with different wellness items contained in the book. Both software packages help provide a more meaningful experience to all participants.
- A new feature of the third edition is the *Nutrient Analysis Data Base Enhancer* software. This software allows course instructors to add food items to the already existing data base available with the book.
- A **video** containing a detailed explanation of many of the fitness assessment test items used in the book. Instructors can use this video to help familiarize themselves with the proper test protocols for each fitness test. This audio-visual aid contains the following test items: 1.5-Mile Run Test, Step Test, Astrand-Ryhming Test, Muscular Strength and Endurance Test, Muscular Endurance Test, Strength-to-Body Weight Ratio Test, Modified Sit-and-Reach Test, Body Rotation Test, Shoulder Rotation Test, Skinfold Thickness Test, and Girth Measurements Test.
- The Morton Test II Fitness and Wellness **Computerized Testbank** with the following options: (a) over 600 multiple choice questions, (b) additional multiple choice, true-false or essay test questions can be added by the course instructors, (c) previously generated tests can be recalled — creating new exam versions — since all multiple choice answers rotate with each new test generated, (d) capability to generate tests using a LaserJet printer, and (e) answer sheets can be formatted to be read by a scanner.
- Sixty color **overhead transparency acetates** of the book's most important illustrations and figures to facilitate class instruction and help explain key fitness and wellness concepts.
- An **instructor's manual** to aid with the implementation of your physical fitness and wellness course.

ACKNOWLEDGMENTS

We wish to express gratitude to Doug Morton for his total commitment to fitness and wellness; Ruth Horton for her constant encouragement and support; and Joanne Saliger for her patience, creativity, and hard work. Special thanks to our colleagues throughout the country who evaluated the second edition of *Principles and Labs for Physical Fitness and Wellness*. Your feedback greatly enhanced the preparation of this edition. We also thank Charles Scheer for his time, efforts, and expertise; Amy Stoneman and John Shaffer for their valuable assistance; and Julie Wagner, Jennifer Blackman, Scott Whiles, Eric Heinz, Neil Edwards, Julie Hammons, Brad Thompson, Michelle Chupurdia, Amy Gibson, and Michelle Puetz who helped with the photography in this edition.

CONTENTS

v

L A B S

PHYSICAL FITNESS AND WELLNESS

1

L A B S

KEY CONCEPTS

Wellness
Physical fitness
Health-related fitness
Skill-related fitness
Chronic diseases
Epidemiology
Health care costs
Heart rate
Blood pressure

OBJECTIVES

- Define wellness and list its components.

- Define physical fitness and list the components of health-related and skill-related fitness.

- Become familiar with health-fitness standards and physical-fitness standards.

- Identify the major health problems in the United States.

- Understand the benefits and the significance of participating in a lifetime fitness and wellness program.

- Identify risk factors that may interfere with safe participation in exercise.

- Learn to assess heart rate and blood pressure.

Widespread interest in health and preventive medicine over the last two decades has led to a tremendous increase in the number of people participating in fitness and wellness programs. From an initial fitness fad in the early 1970s, physical fitness and wellness programs became a trend that now is very much a part of the American way of life. The growing number of participants is attributed primarily to scientific evidence linking regular exercise and positive lifestyle habits to better health, quality of life, and total well-being.

Research findings in the last few years have shown that physical inactivity and negative lifestyle habits pose a serious threat to the health of the nation. Movement and activity are functions the human organism needs to grow, develop, and maintain health. However, advances in modern technology have almost completely eliminated the necessity of physical exertion in daily life. The automated society in which we live no longer provides us with enough activity to ensure adequate health. Instead, it hastens the deterioration rate of the human body.

At the beginning of the 20th century, the most common health problems in the United States were infectious diseases such as tuberculosis, diphtheria, influenza, kidney disease, polio, and other diseases of infancy. Progress in the field of medicine has largely eliminated these diseases. As the American people started to enjoy the so-called good life (sedentary living, alcohol, fatty foods, excessive sweets, tobacco, drugs), though, we saw a parallel increase in the incidence of chronic diseases such as hypertension, coronary heart disease, atherosclerosis, strokes, diabetes, cancer, emphysema, and cirrhosis of the liver (see Figure 1.1).

As the incidence of chronic diseases climbed, we came to recognize prevention as the best medicine. Consequently, a new fitness and wellness movement developed gradually over the last two decades. People began to realize that good health is mostly self-controlled and that the leading causes of premature death and illness in the United States could be prevented by adhering to positive lifestyle habits.

WELLNESS: A COMPREHENSIVE, HEALTHY LIFESTYLE

Most people recognize that people who participate in fitness programs improve their quality of life. In recent years, however, we came to realize that improving physical fitness alone was not always sufficient to lower the risk for disease and ensure better health.

For example, individuals who run 3 miles a day, lift weights regularly, participate in stretching exercises, and watch their body weight easily can be classified as being in good or excellent fitness. If these same people, however, have high blood pressure, smoke, are under constant stress, consume alcohol excessively, and eat too many fatty foods, they are at risk for cardiovascular disease and may not be aware of it. These characteristics that predict which people may develop a certain disease are called *risk factors*.

One of the best examples that good fitness does not always provide a risk-free guarantee of a healthy

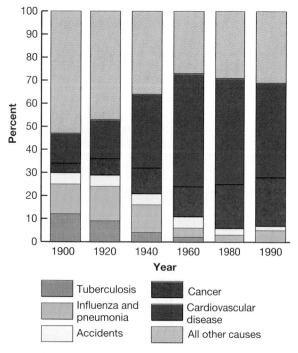

Source: National Center for Health Statistics, Division of Vital Statistics.

FIGURE 1.1

Deaths for selected causes as a percent of all deaths: United States, selected years, 1900 to 1990.

and productive life was the tragic death in 1984 of Jim Fixx, author of *The Complete Book of Running*. At the time of his death by heart attack, Fixx was 52 years old. He had been running between 60 and 80 miles a week and had believed that people at his high level of fitness could not die from heart disease.

At age 36, Jim Fixx smoked two packs of cigarettes per day, weighed about 215 pounds, did not participate in regular cardiovascular exercise, and had a family history of heart disease. His father, having had a first heart attack at age 35, later died at age 43.

Perhaps in an effort to lessen his risk for heart disease, Fixx began to raise his level of fitness. He started to jog, lost 50 pounds, and quit cigarette smoking. On several occasions, though, Fixx declined to have an exercise electrocardiogram (ECG) test, which most likely would have revealed his cardiovascular problem. His unfortunate death is a tragic example that exercise programs by themselves will not make high-risk people immune to heart disease, though they may delay the onset of a serious or fatal problem.

Good health, therefore, no longer is viewed as simply the absence of illness. The notion of good health has evolved notably in the last few years and continues to change as scientists learn more about lifestyle factors that bring on illness and affect wellness. Once the idea took hold that fitness by itself would not always decrease the risk for disease and ensure better health, a new wellness concept developed in the 1980s.

Wellness is defined as *the constant and deliberate effort to stay healthy and achieve the highest potential for well-being.* The term *wellness* implies an all-inclusive umbrella covering a variety of activities aimed at helping individuals recognize components of lifestyle that are detrimental to their health. Wellness living requires implementing positive programs to change behavior to improve health and quality of life, prolong life, and achieve total well-being.

The wellness concept goes well beyond the absence of disease and optimal fitness. Wellness incorporates factors such as adequate fitness, proper nutrition, stress management, disease prevention, spirituality, smoking cessation, personal safety, substance abuse control, regular physical examinations, health education, and environmental support (Figure 1.2).

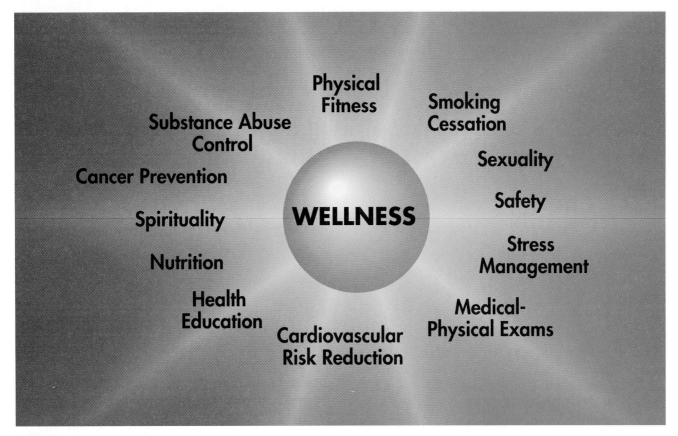

FIGURE 1.2
Components of wellness.

For a wellness way of life, not only must individuals be physically fit and manifest no signs of disease, but they also must have no risk factors for disease (such as hypertension, hyperlipidemia, cigarette smoking, negative stress, faulty nutrition, careless sex). The relationship between adequate fitness and wellness is illustrated in the wellness continuum in Figure 1.3 Even though an individual tested in a fitness center may demonstrate adequate or even excellent fitness, indulgence in unhealthy lifestyle behaviors still will increase the risk for chronic diseases and decrease the person's well-being.

PHYSICAL FITNESS

The most comprehensive definition of physical fitness is that of the American Medical Association, which has defined physical fitness as the general capacity to adapt and respond favorably to physical effort. Individuals are physically fit when they can meet the ordinary as well as the unusual demands of daily life safely and effectively without being overly fatigued, and still have energy left for leisure and recreational activities.

FIGURE 1.3
Wellness continuum.

HEALTH RELATED

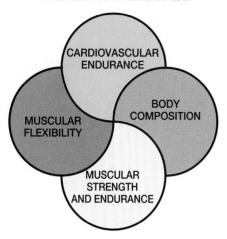

FITNESS COMPONENTS

FIGURE 1.4
Health-related components of physical fitness.

As the fitness concept grew during the 1970s, it became clear that no single test was sufficient to assess overall fitness. A battery of tests was necessary because several specific components have to be established to determine an individual's overall level of fitness.

Physical fitness can be classified into health-related and motor skill-related fitness. As shown in Figure 1.4, the four **health-related fitness** components are: cardiovascular (aerobic) endurance, muscular strength and endurance, muscular flexibility, and body composition. **Skill-related fitness** components consist of agility, balance, coordination, power, reaction time, and speed (Figure 1.5). The

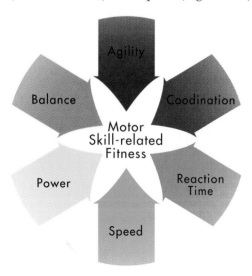

FIGURE 1.5
Skill-related components of physical fitness.

latter are aimed primarily at succeeding in athletics and may not be as crucial in developing better health.

In terms of preventive medicine, the main emphasis of fitness programs should be on the health-related components. Nevertheless, total fitness is achieved by taking part in specific programs to improve both health-related and skill-related components.

WELLNESS, FITNESS, AND LONGEVITY

During the late 1960s and in the 1970s, we began to realize that good fitness is important in the fight against chronic diseases, particularly those of the cardiovascular system. Because of more participation in fitness programs in the last few years, cardiovascular mortality rates have dropped. The rate started to decline in about 1963, and by 1982 had dropped by 37%. In 1983 alone, cardiovascular deaths were an estimated 165,000 fewer than had been expected. This decrease is credited to higher levels of wellness and better health care in the country. More than half of the decline is attributed to improvements in diet and fewer people smoking.

Furthermore, several studies have shown an inverse relationship between exercise and premature cardiovascular mortality rates. In a study[15] conducted among 16,936 Harvard alumni linking physical activity habits and mortality rates, as the amount of weekly physical activity increased, the risk of cardiovascular deaths decreased. The largest decrease in cardiovascular deaths was observed among alumni who used up more than 2,000 calories per week through physical activity (Figure 1.6).

A major study[6] published in the *Journal of the American Medical Association*, based on data from 13,344 people followed over an average of 8 years, substantiated the findings of the Harvard alumni study. Conducted by Dr. Steven N. Blair and co-researchers at the Institute of Aerobics Research in Dallas, Texas, study results confirm that the level of cardiovascular fitness is related to mortality from all causes. The study revealed a graded and consistent inverse relationship between cardiovascular fitness and mortality, regardless of age and other risk

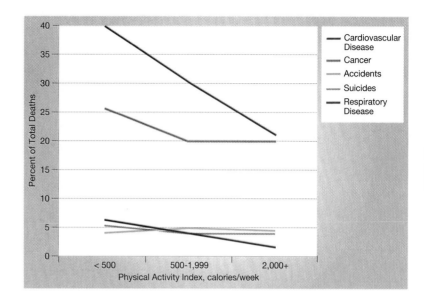

From Paffenbarger, R. S., R. T. Hyde, A. L. Wing, and C. H. Steinmetz. "A Natural History of Athleticism an Cardiovascular Health. *JAMA* 252:491–495, 1984.

FIGURE 1.6
Cause-specific death rates per 10,000 man-years of observation among 16,936 Harvard alumni, 1962-1978, by physical activity index. Adjusted for differences in age, cigarette smoking, and hypertension.

factors (see Figure 1.7). The higher the level of cardiovascular fitness, the longer mortality was delayed. Death rates from all causes for the least fit (group 1) men were 3.4 times higher than the most fit men. For the least fit women, the death rates were 4.6 times higher than the most fit women.

This study also reported a greatly reduced rate of premature death, even at moderate fitness levels that most adults can achieve easily. Even greater protection is attained when increased fitness levels are combined with reduction in other risk factors such as hypertension, serum cholesterol, cigarette smoking, and excessive body fat.

In another major research study[8] conducted in the 1980s, a healthy lifestyle was shown to contribute to some of the lowest mortality rates ever reported in the literature. Compared with the general White population, a group of 5,231 men and 4,631 women (wives) from the Church of Jesus Christ of Latter Day Saints (LDS or Mormon Church) had much lower cancer, cardiovascular, and overall death rates.

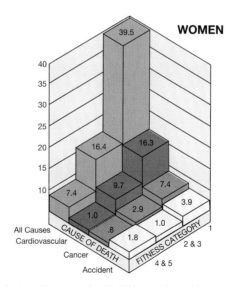

Based on data from Blair, S. N., H. W. Kohl III, R. S. Paffenbarger, Jr., D. G. Clark, K. H. Cooper, and L. W. Gibbons. "Physical Fitness and All-Cause Mortality: A Prospective Study of Healthy Men and Women" *JAMA* 262:2395–2401, 1989.

FIGURE 1.7
Age-adjusted cause-specific death rates per 10,000 person-years of follow-up (1970 to 1985) by physical fitness groups in men and women in the aerobics center longitudinal study in Dallas, Texas. Fitness group 1 is the least fit group, fitness group 5 is the most fit group. (One person-year indicates one person followed up 1 year later.)

Healthy lifestyle habits include abstaining from tobacco, alcohol, caffeine, and drugs, and adhering to a well-balanced diet, based on grains, fruits, and vegetables, and moderate consumption of poultry and red meat. The investigators (non-LDS) in this study looked at three general health habits among the participants: lifetime abstinence from smoking, regular physical activity, and sleep.

The results indicated that men in this study had one-third the death rate from cancer, one-seventh the death rate from cardiovascular disease, and one-fifth the rate of overall mortality. The wives had about half the rate of cancer and overall mortality and a third the death rate from cardiovascular disease. Life expectancy for 25-year-olds who adhered to the three health habits were 85 and 86 years, respectively, as compared to 74 and 80 for the average U.S. White man and woman (see Figure 1.8).

We can conclude from this study that people who adhere to a lifetime healthy lifestyle indeed will reap healthy rewards. Better health leads to improvements in quality of life. The additional 6 to 11 years of "golden" life are precious to those who maintain a lifetime wellness program. As discussed in Chapter 17, most people who maintain this type of program will indeed live a healthier, active, and independent life throughout the golden years.

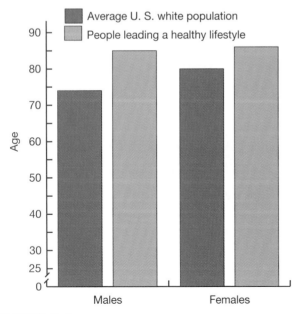

FIGURE 1.8
Life expectancy for 25-year-old individuals who adhere to a lifetime healthy lifestyle program as compared to the average U.S. white population.

FITNESS STANDARDS: HEALTH VERSUS PHYSICAL FITNESS

Throughout the discussion of health-related fitness assessment in Chapters 3, 5, 7, and 9, several tests are identified to assess fitness. A meaningful debate regarding age- and gender-related fitness standards for the general population has resulted in the two standards: A health fitness standard and a physical fitness standard.

HEALTH-FITNESS STANDARDS

The proposed health fitness standards are based on epidemiological* data linking minimum fitness values to disease prevention and health. These standards seem to be the lowest fitness requirements for maintaining good health, decreasing the risk for chronic diseases, and lowering the incidence of muscular-skeletal injuries.

For instance, cardiovascular endurance is measured in terms of the maximal amount of oxygen the body is able to utilize per minute of physical activity (see Chapter 5). Maximal oxygen uptake commonly is expressed in milliliters of oxygen per kilogram of body weight per minute (ml/kg/min). Individual values can range from about 10 ml/kg/min in cardiac patients to approximately 80 to 90 ml/kg/min in world-class runners and cross-country skiers.

Data from the research study presented in Figure 1.7 indicate that maximal oxygen uptake values of 35 and 32.5 ml/kg/min for men and women, respectively, may be sufficient to lower the risk for all-cause mortality significantly. Although greater improvements in fitness yield a slightly lower risk for premature death, the largest drop is seen between the least fit (group 1) and the moderately fit (groups 2 and 3). Therefore, the 35 and 32.5 ml/kg/min values could be selected as the health fitness standards.

Attaining the health fitness standards requires only moderate amounts of physical activity. For example, a 2-mile walk in less than 30 minutes, five to six times per week, seems to be sufficient to achieve the health fitness standard for cardiovascular endurance.

---

*Epidemiology is the study of diseases that affect many individuals within a population.

PHYSICAL-FITNESS STANDARDS

Physical fitness standards are set higher than the health fitness norms and require a more vigorous exercise program. Many experts believe that people who meet the criteria of "good" physical fitness should be able to do moderate to vigorous physical activity without undue fatigue and to maintain this capability throughout life. In this context, physically fit people of all ages will have the freedom to enjoy most of life's daily and recreational activities to their fullest potential. Current health fitness standards may not be enough to achieve these objectives.

Sound physical fitness gives the individual a degree of independence throughout life that many people in the United States no longer enjoy. Most older people should be able to carry out activities similar to those conducted in their youth, though not with the same intensity.

Although a person does not have to be an elite athlete, activities such as changing a tire, chopping wood, climbing several flights of stairs, playing a vigorous game of basketball, mountain biking, playing soccer with grandchildren, walking several miles around a lake, and hiking through a national park require more than the current "average fitness" level of the American people.

If the main objective of the fitness program is to lower the risk for disease, attaining the health fitness standards may be enough to ensure better health. On the other hand, if the individual wants to participate in moderate to vigorous fitness activities, achieving a high physical fitness standard is recommended. For the purposes of this book, therefore, both health fitness and physical fitness standards are given for each fitness test. The individual then needs to decide the personal objectives for the fitness program.

MAJOR HEALTH PROBLEMS IN THE UNITED STATES

The most prominent causes of death in the United States today are basically lifestyle-related (see Table 1.1). According to research, more than 50% of all disease is self-controlled, 64% of the factors contributing to mortality are caused by lifestyle (48%) and environmental (16%) factors, and 83% of deaths prior to age 65 are preventable. Most Americans are threatened by the very lives they lead today.

TABLE 1.1
Leading Causes of Death in the United States: 1991

Cause	Total Number of Deaths	Percent of Total Deaths
1. Major cardiovascular diseases	916,342	42.2
2. Cancer	514,657	23.7
3. Chronic and obstructive pulmonary disease	90,650	4.2
4. Accidents	89,347	4.1
5. All other causes	558,522	25.7

Source: Advance Report of Final Mortality Statistics, 1991. Monthly Vital Statistics Report, National Center for Health Statistics, U.S. Department of Health and Human Services: 42(2):36-37, 1993.

Current statistics indicate that approximately 70% of all deaths in the United States are caused by cardiovascular disease and cancer. Nearly 80% of these deaths could be prevented through a healthy lifestyle program. The third cause of death, chronic and obstructive pulmonary disease, is related largely to tobacco use. Accidents are the fourth leading cause of death. Even though not all accidents are preventable, many are. Fatal accidents are often related to abusing drugs and not wearing seat belts.

CARDIOVASCULAR DISEASE

The most prevalent degenerative diseases in the United States are those of the cardiovascular system. As shown in Table 1.1, almost half of all deaths in this country are attributed to heart and blood vessel disease.

In 1990, according to estimates by the American Heart Association, more than 70 million Americans were afflicted with diseases of the cardiovascular system, including 63.6 million with hypertension and 6.2 million with coronary heart disease. Many of these people have more than one type of cardiovascular disease.

In addition, the 1993 estimated cost of heart and blood vessel disease exceeded $117 billion. Heart attacks alone cost American industry approximately 132 million workdays annually, including $15 billion in lost productivity because of physical and emotional disability.

About a million and a half people have heart attacks each year. Half a million of them die as a consequence. About half the time, the first symptom of coronary heart disease is the heart attack itself, and 40% of those who have a first heart attack die within the first 24 hours. In one of every five cardiovascular deaths, sudden death is the initial symptom.

About half of those people who die are men in their most productive years, between ages 40 and 65. Furthermore, the American Heart Association estimates that more than $700 million a year is spent in replacing employees who have had heart attacks. Most coronary heart disease risk factors, however, are reversible and preventable and can be controlled through lifestyle modifications (see Chapter 12).

CANCER

The second leading cause of death in the United States is cancer. Unlike cardiovascular disease, the mortality rate for cancer has increased steadily over the last few decades (see Figure 1.1). Even though cancer is not the number-one killer, it certainly is the number-one health fear of the American people.

Cancer is defined as *an uncontrolled growth and spread of abnormal cells in the body*. Some cells grow into a mass of tissue called a tumor, which can be either benign or malignant. A malignant tumor is

considered a cancer. If the spread of cells is not controlled or checked, death is the inevitable result.

Approximately 23% of all deaths in the United States are from cancer. Almost 526,000 people died from this disease in 1993, and an estimated 1,170,000 new cases were reported the same year. The overall medical costs for cancer were estimated to be in excess of $104 billion for 1990. Table 1.2 shows the 1993 estimated new cases and deaths for major sites of cancer, excluding nonmelanoma skin cancer and carcinoma in situ.

Testing procedures for early detection of cancer, as well as treatment modalities, are changing and improving continuously. More than 8 million Americans with a history of cancer now are alive, and close to 5 million of them can be considered cured. The American Cancer Society maintains that the most influential factor in fighting cancer today is prevention through health education programs. Evidence indicates that as much as 80% of all human cancer can be prevented through positive lifestyle behaviors.

The basic recommendations for cancer prevention include a diet high in cabbage-family vegetables, high in fiber, high in vitamins A and C, and low in fat. Alcohol and salt-cured, smoked, and nitrite-cured foods should be consumed in moderation. Cigarette smoking and tobacco use in general should be eliminated, and obesity should be avoided.

TABLE 1.2
Estimated Deaths and New Cases for Major Sites of Cancer: 1993

	Estimated New Cases			Estimated Deaths		
	Total	Male	Female	Total	Male	Female
Lung	170,000	100,000	70,000	149,000	93,000	56,000
Colon-Rectum	152,000	77,000	75,000	57,000	28,800	28,200
Breast*	183,000	1,000	182,000	46,300	300	46,000
Prostate	165,000	165,000	—	35,000	35,000	—
Pancreas	27,700	13,500	14,200	25,000	12,000	13,000
Urinary	79,500	55,800	23,700	20,800	13,000	7,800
Leukemia	29,300	16,700	12,600	18,600	10,100	8,500
Ovary	22,000	—	22,000	13,300	—	13,300
Uterus**	44,500	—	44,500	10,100	—	10,100
Oral	29,800	20,300	8,500	7,750	4,975	2,725
Skin***	32,600	17,000	15,000	6,800	4,200	2,600

* Invasive cancer only
** New cases total over 55,000 if carcinoma in situ is included
*** Estimates are over 600,000 if new cases of nonmelanoma are included

Source: 1993 Cancer Facts and Figures. American Cancer Society.

BENEFITS OF PHYSICAL FITNESS AND WELLNESS PROGRAMS

A most inspiring story illustrating what fitness can do for a person's health and well-being is that of George Snell from Sandy, Utah. At age of 45, Snell weighed approximately 400 pounds, his blood pressure was 220/180, he was blind because of diabetes he did not know he had, and his blood glucose level was 487.

Snell had determined to do something about his physical and medical condition, so he started a walking/jogging program. After about eight months of conditioning, Snell had lost almost 200 pounds, his eyesight had returned, his glucose level was down to 67, and he was taken off medication. Two months later, less than 10 months after beginning his personal exercise program, he completed his first marathon, a running course of 26.2 miles.

Most people exercise because it improves their personal appearance and makes them feel good about themselves. Although many benefits accrue from participation in a regular fitness and wellness program and active people generally live longer (Figure 1.8), the greatest benefit of all is that physically fit individuals enjoy a better quality of life (Figure 1.9). These people live life to its fullest, with fewer health problems than inactive individuals who also may indulge in negative lifestyle patterns.

Although compiling an all-inclusive list of the benefits reaped through fitness and wellness program participation is difficult, the following list summarizes many of these benefits:

1. Improves and strengthens the cardiovascular system (by facilitating oxygen supply to all parts of the body, including the heart, muscles, and brain).
2. Maintains better muscle tone, muscular strength and endurance.
3. Improves muscular flexibility.
4. Helps maintain recommended body weight.
5. Improves posture and physical appearance.
6. Lowers the risk for chronic diseases and illness (such as coronary heart disease, cancer, and strokes).

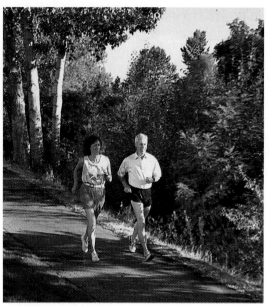

FIGURE 1.9
Regular participation in a lifetime exercise program increases quality of life and longevity.

7. Decreases the mortality rate from chronic diseases.
8. Thins the blood so it is less likely to clot (decreasing the risk for coronary heart disease and strokes).
9. Lowers blood pressure.
10. Helps prevent diabetes.
11. Helps people sleep better.
12. Helps prevent chronic back pain.
13. Relieves tension and helps in coping with life stresses.
14. Raises levels of energy and job productivity.
15. Extends longevity and slows down the aging process.
16. Improves self-image and morale and helps fight depression.
17. Motivates toward positive changes in lifestyle (better nutrition, stopping smoking, alcohol and drug abuse control).
18. Speeds recovery time following physical exertion.
19. Speeds recovery following injury and disease.
20. Regulates and improves overall body functions.
21. Improves physical stamina and counteracts chronic fatigue.
22. Improves quality of life; makes people feel better and live a healthier and happier life.

In addition to the many health benefits, the economic impact of sedentary living has left a strong impression on the nation's economy. As the need for physical exertion steadily decreased during the last century, the nation's health care expenditures increased dramatically.

Health care costs in the United States rose from $12 billion in 1950 to approximately $738 billion in 1992 (Figure 1.10). If the rate of escalation continues, health care expenditures will reach $1.6 trillion by the year 2002. The 1992 figure represents over 12% of the gross national product (GNP). It is projected to reach about 18% by the year 2002 and 37% by 2030. Furthermore, and as illustrated in Figure 1.11, the 1989 average health care cost per person in the United States ($2,354) was almost twice as high as for most other industrialized nations.

Strong scientific evidence now links fitness and wellness program participation not only to better health but also to lower medical costs and higher job productivity. Most of this research is being conducted and reported by organizations that already have implemented fitness or wellness programs. Approximately half of the health care expenditures in the United States are being absorbed by American business and industry.

In 1989 business spending on health insurance premiums and health care for employees and former employees was more than 100% of after-tax profits by all U.S. companies combined. As a result of the recent staggering rise in medical costs, many organizations are beginning to realize that keeping employees healthy costs less than treating them once they are sick.

Containing the costs of health care through fitness and wellness programs has become a major issue for many organizations around the country. Let's examine the evidence.

The backache syndrome, usually the result of physical degeneration (inelastic and weak muscles), costs American industry more than $1 billion a year in lost productivity and services. An additional $250 million is spent in workers compensation. The Adolph Coors Company in Golden, Colorado, which offers a wellness program for employees and their families, reported savings of more than $319,000 in 1983 alone through a preventive and rehabilitative back injury program.

The Prudential Insurance Company of Houston, Texas, released the findings of a study conducted on its 1,386 employees. Those who participated for at least one year in the company's fitness program averaged 3.5 days of disability, compared to 8.6 days for nonparticipants. A further breakdown by level of fitness showed no disability days for those in the high fitness group, 1.6 days for the good fitness group, and 4.1 days for the fair fitness group.

Since 1979 the Mesa Petroleum Company in Amarillo, Texas, has offered an on-site fitness program to its employees and their family members. A 1982 survey showed an average of $434 per person in medical costs for the nonparticipating group in the company and an average of only $173 per person per year for the participating group. This represented a yearly reduction of $200,000 in medical expenses. Sick leave time also was significantly less for the physically active group — 27 hours per year, compared to 44 for the inactive group.

Data analysis conducted in 1982 and 1983 by Tenneco Incorporated in Houston, Texas, showed a significant reduction in medical care costs for men and women who participated in an exercise program (see Figure 1.12). Annual medical care costs for male and female exercisers were $562 and $639, respectively. For the nonexercising group, the costs were reported at $1,004 for the men and $1,536 for the women. Sick leave also was reduced in the men and women participants.

Furthermore, a survey of the more than 3,000 employees at Tenneco found that job productivity is

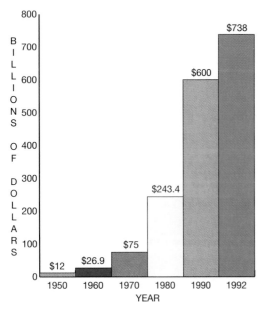

FIGURE 1.10
U.S. health care cost increments since 1950.

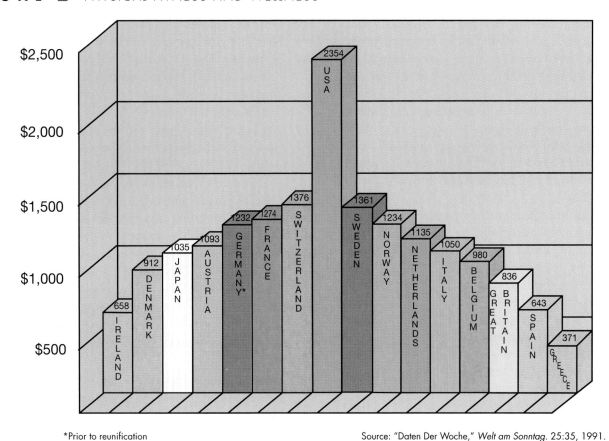

*Prior to reunification

Source: "Daten Der Woche," *Welt am Sonntag.* 25:35, 1991.

FIGURE 1.11
1989 average health care costs per person for selected countries in the world.

related to fitness. The company reported that individuals with high job performance ratings also rated high in exercise participation.

Strong data also are coming in from Europe. Research in Germany reported 68.6% less absenteeism by workers with cardiovascular symptoms

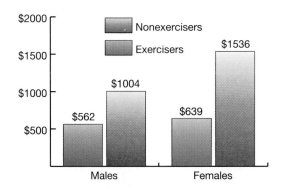

From "New Fitness Data Verifies: Employees Who Exercise Are Also More Productive." *Athletic Business* 8(12):24-30, 1984.

FIGURE 1.12
Annual medical care costs for Tenneco Incorporated, Houston, Texas: 1982-83.

who participated in a fitness program. The law also mandates that corporations employing workers for sedentary jobs must provide an in-house facility for physical exercise.

The Goodyear Company in Norrkoping, Sweden, indicated a 50% reduction in absenteeism following implementation of a fitness program. Studies in the former Soviet Union report expanded physical work capacity and motor coordination, lower incidence of disease, shorter duration of illness, and fewer relapses among individuals participating in industrial fitness programs.

Another reason some organizations are offering wellness programs to their employees — overlooked by many because it does not seem to affect the bottom line directly — is simply concern by top management for the physical well-being of employees. Whether the program lowers medical costs is not the main issue. The only reason that really matters to top management is that wellness programs help individuals feel better about themselves and improve quality of life.

Such is the case of Mannington Mills Corporation, which invested $1.8 million in an on-site fitness center. The return on investment is secondary to the company's interest in happier and healthier employees. The center also is open to dependents and retirees. As a result of this program, Mannington Mills believes the participants — about half of the 1,600 people who are eligible — can enjoy life to its fullest potential, and the employees most likely will be more productive simply because of the company's caring attitude.

In addition to the financial and physical benefits, some corporations are offering wellness programs as an incentive to attract, hire, and retain employees. Many companies are taking a hard look at the fitness and health level of potential employees and are seriously using this information in their screening process. Some organizations refuse to hire smokers or overweight individuals.

Other executives believe that an on-site health promotion program is the best fringe benefit they can offer at their corporation. Young executives are looking for such organizations as these, not only for the added health benefits but also because the head corporate officers are showing an attitude of concern and care.

THE WELLNESS CHALLENGE FOR THE TURN OF THE CENTURY

Because a better and healthier life is something every person needs to strive to attain, our biggest challenge as we look to the turn of the century is to teach people how to take control of their personal health habits by adhering to a positive lifestyle. Considering the wealth of information available on the benefits of fitness and wellness programs, improving the quality and possible length of our lives is a matter of personal choice.

To significantly improve health and extend life, a person should:

1. **Participate in a lifetime exercise program.** Exercise regularly three to six times a week. The exercise program should consist of 20 to 30 minutes of aerobic exercise, along with some strengthening and stretching exercises.

2. **Do not smoke cigarettes.** Cigarette smoking is the largest preventable cause of illness and premature death in the United States. When considering all related deaths, *smoking is responsible for more than 450,000 unnecessary deaths each year.*

3. **Eat right.** Eat a good breakfast and two additional well-balanced meals every day. Unless snacks consist of healthy foods, refrain from snacking between meals. Avoid eating too many calories and foods with a lot of sugar, fat, and sodium (salt). Increase your daily consumption of fruits, vegetables, and whole-grain products.

4. **Maintain recommended body weight.** Maintain proper body weight through adequate nutrition and exercise. This is important in preventing chronic diseases and in developing a higher level of fitness.

5. **Get sufficient rest.** Sleep 7 to 8 hours each night.

6. **Decrease stress.** Reduce your vulnerability to stress and practice stress management techniques as needed.

7. **Be wary of alcohol.** Drink only moderate amounts of alcohol or none at all. Alcohol abuse leads to mental, emotional, physical, and social problems.

8. **Surround yourself with healthy friendships.** Unhealthy friendships contribute to destructive behaviors and low self-esteem. Associating with people who strive to maintain good fitness and health reinforces a positive outlook in life and encourage positive behaviors. Constructive social interactions enhance well-being.

9. **Be informed about the environment.** Seek clean air, clean water, and a clean environment. Be aware of pollutants and occupational hazards: asbestos fibers, nickel dust, chromate, uranium dust, and so on. Be cautious when using pesticides and insecticides.

10. **Take personal safety measures.** Although not all accidents are preventable, many are. Failing to take simple precautionary measures, such as using seat belts and keeping electrical appliances away from water (see Lab 17A), increases the risk for avoidable accidents.

Thanks to current scientific data and the fitness and wellness movement of the past two decades, most Americans now see a need to participate in programs to improve and maintain health. Many people still are not taking part, though, because they are unaware of the basic principles for safe and effective participation in exercise. Others are exercising incorrectly and therefore are not reaping the full benefits of their program.

Although almost half the adult population in the United States claims to participate in some sort of physical activity, slightly more than 10% report daily aerobic activity lasting more than 30 minutes. Aerobic activities are the most popular form of exercise, so even a lower percentage of the population probably engages in and derives benefits from strength and flexibility programs. In addition, at least half of the adults in the United States is estimated to have a weight problem.

GENERAL OBJECTIVES

Because fitness and wellness needs vary significantly from one individual to the other, all exercise and wellness prescriptions must be personalized to obtain best results. The information in the following chapters and the laboratory experiences in the back of the book set forth all of the necessary guidelines to develop a personal lifetime program to improve fitness and promote preventive health care and personal wellness.

The laboratory experiences have been prepared on tear-out sheets so they can be turned in to class instructors. The corresponding labs for each chapter and any other information necessary to prepare for the labs are given at the end of the chapters. As you study this book and complete the respective laboratory experiences you will learn to:

■ Determine whether you need medical clearance to safely participate in exercise.

■ Conduct nutritional analyses and follow the recommendations for adequate nutrition.

■ Write sound diet and weight control programs.

■ Assess and improve the health-related components of fitness (cardiovascular endurance, muscular strength and endurance, muscular flexibility, and body composition).

■ Assess the various skill-related components of fitness (agility, balance, coordination, power, reaction time, and speed).

■ Determine potential risk for cardiovascular disease, and implement a risk reduction program.

■ Follow a cancer risk reduction program.

■ Determine your levels of tension and stress, reduce stress vulnerability, and implement stress management programs.

■ Implement a smoking cessation program if applicable.

■ Avoid chemical dependency and know where to find assistance if needed.

■ Learn the health consequences of sexually transmitted diseases, including AIDS, and guidelines for preventing STDs.

■ Discover the relationship between fitness and aging.

■ Write objectives to improve your fitness and wellness, and learn how to chart a wellness program for the future.

■ Discern between myths and facts of exercise and health-related concepts.

U.S. HEALTH OBJECTIVES FOR THE YEAR 2000

Every ten years the U.S. Department of Health and Human Services releases a list of objectives for disease prevention and health promotion. From its onset in 1980, this ten-year plan has helped develop a new sense of purpose and focus for public health and preventive medicine.

The Year 2000 objectives, published in the document *Healthy People 2000: National Health Promotion and Disease Prevention Objectives* address three important points:

1. **Personal responsibility.** The need for individuals to become increasingly health-conscious: Responsible and informed behaviors are the key to good health.

2. **Health benefits for all people.** Lower socio-economic conditions and poor health are often interrelated. Extending the benefits of good health to all people is crucial to the health of our Nation.

3. **Health promotion and disease prevention.** A shift from treatment to preventive techniques to drastically cut health care costs and help all Americans achieve a higher quality of life.

The development of the Year 2000 Health Objectives involved over 10,000 people representing 300 national organizations, including the Institute of Medicine of the National Academy of Sciences, all state health departments, and the federal Office of Disease Prevention and Health Promotion. A summary of key objectives is provided in Figure 1.16 at the end of this chapter. Living the fitness and wellness principles provided in this book will not only enhance the quality of your life, but will allow you to be an active participant in the achievement of the *Healthy People 2000 Objectives*.

SAFETY OF EXERCISE PARTICIPATION

In recent years, several prominent national figures died while participating in an exercise program. These unfortunate deaths raised some questions as to the safety of exercise participation.

Even though exercise testing and participation is relatively safe for most apparently healthy individuals under age 45, the reaction of the cardiovascular system to higher levels of physical activity cannot be totally predicted. Consequently, a person takes a small but real risk of certain bodily changes occurring during exercise testing or participation. These include abnormal blood pressure, irregular heart rhythm, fainting, and, in rare instances, a heart attack or cardiac arrest.

HEALTH HISTORY QUESTIONNAIRE

Before you start to engage in an exercise program or participate in any exercise testing, you should fill out the questionnaire in Lab 1A. If your answer to any of the questions is yes, you should see a physician before participating in a fitness program. Exercise testing and participation is not wise under some of the conditions listed in Lab 1A and may require a stress electrocardiogram (ECG) test (see Figure 1.13). If you have any questions regarding your current health status, consult your doctor before initiating, continuing, or increasing your level of physical activity.

HEART RATE AND BLOOD PRESSURE ASSESSMENT

You will learn, in Lab 1B, how to determine your heart rate and blood pressure. Heart rate can be obtained by counting your pulse either on the wrist, by placing two fingers over the radial artery (inside of the wrist on the side of the thumb), or over the carotid artery in the neck, just below the jaw next to the voice box (see Figures 5.5 and 5.6 in Chapter 5).

You may count your pulse for 30 seconds and multiply by two or take it for a full minute. The heart rate usually is at its lowest point (resting heart rate) late in the evening after you have been sitting quietly for about half an hour watching a relaxing TV show or reading in bed, or early in the morning just before you get out of bed.

Unless you have a pathological condition, a lower resting heart rate indicates a stronger heart. To adapt to cardiovascular or aerobic exercise, the heart enlarges and the muscle gets stronger. A bigger and stronger heart can pump more blood with fewer strokes.

Resting heart rate ratings are given in Table 1.3. Although resting heart rate decreases with training, the extent of bradycardia (slow heart rate) depends not only on the amount of training but also on genetic factors. Although most highly trained athletes have a resting heart rate around 40 beats per minute, Jim Ryan, world record holder for the

FIGURE 1.13
Exercise electrocardiogram. An exercise tolerance test with twelve-lead electrocardiographic monitoring may be required of some individuals prior to initiating an exercise program.

TABLE 1.3
Resting Heart Rate Ratings

Heart Rate (beats/minute)	Rating
≤59	Excellent
60-69	Good
70-79	Average
80-89	Fair
≥90	Poor

1-mile run in the 1960s, had a consistent resting heart rate in the 70s even during peak training months during his athletic career. For most individuals, however, the resting heart rate decreases as the level of cardiovascular endurance increases.

Blood pressure is assessed using a sphygmomanometer and a stethoscope. The sphygmomanometer consists of an inflatable bladder contained within a cuff and a mercury gravity manometer or an aneroid manometer from which the pressure is read (see Figures 1.14 and 1.15). The appropriate size cuff must be used to get accurate readings. Size is determined by the width of the inflatable bladder, which should be about 40% of the circumference of the midpoint of the arm.

Blood pressure usually is measured while the person is in the sitting position, with the forearm and the manometer at the same level as the heart. At first, the pressure is recorded from each arm, and after that from the arm with the highest reading.

If in doubt, consult your doctor before initiating, continuing, or increasing your level of physical activity.

The cuff should be applied approximately an inch above the antecubital space (natural crease of the elbow), with the center of the bladder directly over the medial (inner) surface of the arm. The stethoscope head should be applied firmly, but with little pressure, over the brachial artery in the antecubital space. The arm should be slightly flexed and placed on a flat surface.

The bladder can be inflated while feeling the radial pulse to about 30 to 40 mmHg above the point at which the pulse disappears. The cuff should

FIGURE 1.14
Aneroid blood pressure gauge and stethoscope.

not be overinflated, as this may cause blood vessel spasm, resulting in higher blood pressure readings. The pressure should be released at a rate of 2 mmHg per second.

As the pressure is released, systolic blood pressure is determined at the point where the initial pulse sound is heard. The diastolic pressure is determined at the point where the sound disappears. The recordings should be made to the nearest 2 mmHg (even numbers) and expressed as systolic over diastolic pressure — for example, 124/80.

When taking more than one reading, the bladder should be completely deflated, and at least one minute should be allowed before making the next recording. The person measuring the pressure also should note whether the pressure was recorded from the left or the right arm. Resting blood pressure ratings are given in Table 1.4.

FIGURE 1.15
Blood pressure assessment using a mercury gravity manometer.

TABLE 1.4
Blood Pressure Ratings in mmHg*

Systolic	Diastolic	Rating
≤120	≤80	Very Low Risk
121-130	81-89	Low Risk
131-140	90-99	Moderate Risk
141-150	100-105	High Risk
≥151	≥106	Very High Risk

*Ratings expressed in terms of cardiovascular disease risk.

In some cases the pulse sounds become less intense (point of muffling sounds) and can still be heard at a lower pressure (50 or 40 mmHg) or even all the way down to zero. In this situation the diastolic pressure is recorded at the point of a clear, definite change in the loudness of the sound (also referred to as fourth phase), and at complete disappearance of the sound (fifth phase) (e.g., 120/78/60 or 120/82/0.

When measuring resting heart rate and blood pressure, several readings should be taken by different people or at different times of the day, to establish the real values. A single reading may not be an accurate value because of the various factors that can affect blood pressure.

WELLNESS LIFESTYLE QUESTIONNAIRE

Most people go to college to learn how to make a living, but a fitness and wellness course will teach you how to live — that is, how to truly live life to its fullest potential. Don't even think for a moment that "success in life is measured by how much you make." Making a good living will not help you unless you live a wellness lifestyle that will allow you to enjoy what you have.

Everyone would like to enjoy good health and wellness, but most people don't know how to reach this objective. Lifestyle is the most important factor affecting our personal well-being. While some people live long because of genetic factors, the quality of life during middle age and the "golden" years is basically related to wise choices initiated during youth and continued throughout life.

In a few short years, lack of wellness leads to a loss of vitality and gusto for life, as well as premature morbidity and mortality. The Wellness Lifestyle Questionnaire given in Lab 1C will provide an initial rating of your current efforts to stay healthy and well, and the components of a wellness lifestyle are discussed in subsequent chapters of this book.

Upon completion of the questionnaire, select the areas where you think you will need the most improvement. While you need to pay attention to all aspects of wellness, initially work on those lifestyle factors in which definite improvements are required. *Lifestyle choices that you make now will have an impact on how well you live the rest of your life.*

COMPUTER SOFTWARE OPTIONS

Qualified course instructors can obtain computer software for use with this book. If the instructor has the software, students may be able to obtain a computerized fitness and wellness profile. Two software packages are available:

1. The *options* software allows the user to enter each fitness/wellness component separately. As you gather selected data (e.g., cardiovascular endurance or body composition), you may enter the data for that component and generate a printout for that component. You also may obtain a comprehensive fitness and wellness profile with all the information entered into the computer to that point.

2. The *pre- and post-test software* requires the user to enter the data for all components at once. The computer then generates the fitness and wellness profile. The printout includes your current test results and fitness rating. A unique feature of this software package is that if a second set of data is entered, the program will print out both the pre- and post-tests, the current fitness rating, and a percent change from pre- to post-test (see Figure 1.17).

LABORATORY EXPERIENCE

LAB 1A
Clearance for Exercise Participation

Lab Preparation
None required.

LAB 1B
Heart Rate and Blood Pressure Assessment

Lab Preparation
Wear exercise clothing, including a shirt with short or loose-fitting sleeves to allow for placement of the blood pressure cuff around the upper arm. Do not engage in any form of exercise several hours prior to this lab.

LAB 1C
Wellness Lifestyle Questionnaire

Lab Preparation
None required.

REFERENCES

1. Allsen, P. E., J. M. Harrison, and B. Vance. *Fitness for Life: An Individualized Approach.* Dubuque, IA: Wm. C. Brown, 1993.

2. American Cancer Society. 1993 *Cancer Facts and Figures.* New York: The Society, 1993.

3. American College of Sports Medicine. "The Recommended Quantity and Quality of Exercise for Developing and Maintaining Cardiorespiratory and Muscular Fitness in Healthy Adults." *Medicine and Science in Sports and Exercise* 22:265-274, 1990.

4. American Heart Association. *1993 Heart and Stroke Facts Statistics.* Dallas, TX: The Association, 1992.

5. Blair, S., D. Jacobs, and K. Powell. "Relationships Between Exercise or Physical Activity and Other Health Behaviors." *Public Health Reports* 100:172-180, 1985.

6. Blair, S. N., H. W. Kohl III, R. S. Paffenbarger, Jr, D. G. Clark, K. H. Cooper, and L. W. Gibbons. "Physical Fitness and All-Cause Mortality: A Prospective Study of Healthy Men and Women." *Journal of the American Medical Association* 262:2395-2401, 1989.

7. Davies, N. E., and L. H. Felder. "Applying Brakes to the Runaway American Health Care System." *Journal of the American Medical Association* 263:73-76, 1990.

8. Enstrom, J. E. "Health Practices and Cancer Mortality Among Active California Mormons." *Journal of the National Cancer Institute* 81:1807-1814, 1989.

9. Gettman, L. R. "Cost/Benefit Analysis of a Corporate Fitness Program." *Fitness in Business* 1(1):11-17, 1986.

10. Hatziandreu, E. L., J. P. Koplan, M. C. Weinstein, C. J. Caspersen, K. E. Warner. "A Cost-effectiveness Analysis of Exercise as a Health Promotion Activity." *American Journal of Public Health* 78:1417-1421, 1988.

11. Hoeger, W. W. K., and S. A. Hoeger. *Lifetime Physical Fitness & Wellness: A Personalized Program.* Englewood, CO: Morton Publishing Company, 1992.

12. Kaufman, J. E. "State of the Art: Physical Fitness in Corporations." *Employee Services Management* 26(1):8-9, 26-27, 1983.

13. Koplan, J. P., C. J. Caspersen, and K. E. Powell. "Physical Activity, Physical Fitness, and Health: Time to Act." *Journal of the American Medical Association* 262:2437, 1989.

14. Marcotte, B., and J. H. Price. "The Status of Health Promotion Programs at the Worksite, A Review." *Health Education* 4-8, July/August, 1983.

15. Paffenbarger, R. S., Jr, R. T. Hyde, A. L. Wing, and C. H. Steinmetz. "A Natural History of Athleticism and Cardiovascular Health." *Journal of the American Medical Association* 252:491-495, 1984.

16. Smith, L.K. "Cost-Effectiveness of Health Promotion Programs." *Fitness Management* 2(3):12-15, 1986.

17. Staff. "New Fitness Data Verifies: Employees Who Exercise Are Also More Productive." Athletic Business 8(12):24-30, 1984.

18. Van Camp, S. P. "The Fixx Tragedy: A Cardiologist's Perspective." *Physician and Sportsmedicine* 12(9): 153-155, 1984.

19. Wilmore, J. H. "Design Issues and Alternatives in Assessing Physical Fitness Among Apparently Healthy Adults in a Health Examination Survey of the General Population." In Drury, F. (Editor). *Assessing Physical Fitness and Activity in General Population Studies.* Washington, D.C.: U.S. Public Health Service. National Center for Health Statistics, 1988.

20. Wright, C. C. "Cost Containment Through Health Promotion Programs." *Journal of Occupational Medicine* 22:36-39, 1980.

HEALTHY PEOPLE 2000:*
SELECTED HEALTH OBJECTIVES FOR THE YEAR 2000

I. Physical Activity and Fitness

1. Increase the proportion of people who engage regularly, preferably daily, in *light* to *moderate* physical activity for at least 30 minutes per day.
2. Increase the proportion of people who engage in *vigorous* physical activity that promotes the development and maintenance of cardiorespiratory fitness 3 or more days per week for 20 or more minutes per occasion.
3. Increase the proportion of people who regularly perform physical activities that enhance and maintain muscular strength, muscular endurance, and flexibility.
4. Reduce the proportion of people who engage in no leisure-time physical activity.
5. Reduce overweight to a prevalence of no more than 20% among people aged 20 and older and no more than 15% among adolescents aged 12 through 19.
6. Increase to at least 50% the proportion of overweight people aged 12 and older who have adopted sound dietary practices combined with regular physical activity to attain an appropriate body weight.

II. Nutrition

1. Reduce dietary fat intake to an average of 30% of calories or less and average saturated fat intake to less than 10% of calories among people aged 2 and older.
2. Increase complex carbohydrate and fiber-containing foods in the diets of adults to 5 or more daily servings for vegetables and fruits, and to 6 or more daily servings for grain products.
3. Increase calcium consumption in the diet.
4. Reduce iron deficiency among children 1 through 4 and women of childbearing age.
5. Decrease salt and sodium intake in the diet.
6. Increase to at least 85% the proportion of people aged 18 and older who use food labels to make nutritious selections.

III. Chronic Diseases

1. Increase years of healthy life to at least 65 years.
2. Reduce coronary heart disease deaths.
3. Reduce the mean serum cholesterol level among adults to no more than 200 mg/dL.
4. Increase the proportion of adults with high blood cholesterol who are aware of their condition and are taking action to reduce their blood cholesterol to recommended levels.
5. Increase the proportion of people with high blood pressure whose blood pressure is under control.
6. Increase the proportion of people with high blood presssure who are taking action to help control their blood pressure.
7. Reverse the rise in cancer deaths.
8. Slow the rise in lung cancer deaths.
9. Reduce the rate of breast cancer deaths.
10. Reduce colorectal cancer deaths.
11. Reduce diabetes-related deaths.
12. Reduce the proportion of people with asthma who experience activity limitation.
13. Reduce deaths from cirrhosis of the liver.
14. Reduce hip fractures among older adults.
15. Reduce activity limitation due to chronic back conditions.
16. Reduce the proportion of people who experience a limitation in major activity due to chronic conditions.

IV. Mental Health and Disorders

1. Reduce the prevalence of mental disorders.
2. Reduce the suicide rate.

3. Reduce the proportion of people who experience adverse health effects from stress.
4. Decrease the proportion of people who experience stress who do not take steps to reduce or control their stress.

V. Tobacco

1. Reduce the incidence of cigarette smoking.
2. Reduce the initiation of cigarette smoking by children and youth.
3. Reduce the proportion of children who are regularly exposed to tobacco smoke at home.
4. Reduce smokeless tobacco use.
5. Increase the proportion of worksites with a formal smoking policy that prohibits or severely restricts smoking at the workplace.

VI. Alcohol and Other Drugs

1. Reduce the proportion of young people who have used alcohol, marijuana, and cocaine.
2. Reduce the proportion of high school seniors and college students engaging in recent occasions of heavy drinking of alcoholic beverages.
3. Reduce alcohol consumption by people aged 14 and older to an annual average of no more than 2 gallons of ethanol per person.
4. Increase the proportion of high school seniors who associate risk of physical or psychological harm with the heavy use of alcohol, occasional use of marijuana, and experimentation with cocaine.
5. Reduce the proportion of male high school seniors who use anabolic steroids.
6. Reduce deaths caused by alcohol-related motor vehicle crashes.
7. Reduce drug-related deaths.
8. Increase the proportion of all intravenous drug abusers who are in drug abuse treatment programs.
9. Increase the proportion of intravenous drug abusers not in treatment who use only uncontaminated drug paraphernalia ("works").

VII. AIDS, HIV Infection, and Sexually Transmitted Diseases

1. Confine annual incidence of diagnosed AIDS cases to no more than 98,000 cases.
2. Confine the prevalence of HIV infection to no more than 800 per 100,000 people.
3. Increase the proportion of sexually active, unmarried people who used a condom at last sexual intercourse.
4. Reduce the incidence of gonorrhea.
5. Reduce the incidence of Chlamydia.
6. Reduce the incidence of primary and secondary syphilis.
7. Reduce the incidence of genital herpes and genital warts.
8. Reduce the incidence of pelvic inflammatory disease.
9. Reduce the incidence of sexually transmitted hepatitis B infection.

VIII. Family Planning

1. Reduce the number of pregnancies that are unintended.
2. Reduce the proportion of adolescents who have engaged in sexual intercourse.
3. Increase the proportion of sexually active, unmarried people aged 19 and younger who use contraception, especially combined method contraception that both effectively prevents pregnancy and provides barrier protection against disease.

IX. Unintentional Injuries

1. Reduce deaths caused by unintentional injuries.
2. Increase use of occupant protection systems, such as safety belts, inflatable safety restraints, and child safety seats among motor vehicle occupants.
3. Increase use of helmets among motorcyclists and bicyclists.

* Adapted from the U.S. Department of Health and Human Services, Public Health Service. *Healthy People 2000: National Health Promotion and Disease Prevention Objectives*. Boston, Jones and Bartlett Publishers, 1992. Refer to this publication for further information on these objectives.

FIGURE 1.16
National health objectives for the year 2000.

FITNESS AND WELLNESS PROFILE
by Werner W.K. Hoeger and Sharon A. Hoeger
PRINCIPLES AND LABS FOR PHYSICAL FITNESS AND WELLNESS
Morton Publishing Company

James Doe
Age: 19
Course: Foundations of Wellness
Section: 08
Instructor: Werner Hoeger

Test Item	Previous Test 01-12-1994	Current Test 04-30-1994	Current Fitness Rating	Percent Change
Cardiovascular Endurance (Astrand-Ryhming test)	40.2 ml/kg/min	52.1 ml/kg/min	Good	+30
Muscular Endurance	17 %tile	53 %tile	Average	
Bench jumps	42 reps - 10 %tile	52 reps - 40 %tile	Fair	+24
Chair dips	14 reps - 10 %tile	26 reps - 50 %tile	Average	+86
Abdominal curl-ups	22 reps - 30 %tile	46 reps - 70 %tile	Good	+109
Muscular Flexibility	23 %tile	40 %tile	Fair	
Sit and reach	11.5 in - 10 %tile	12.5 in - 20 %tile	Poor	+9
Right body rotation	18.5 in - 40 %tile	19.0 in - 60 %tile	Average	+3
Shoulder rotation	30.0 in - 20 %tile	25.0 in - 40 %tile	Fair	+17
Body Composition				
Percent body fat	22.9 %	14.7 %	Good	+36
Body weight	188.0 lbs	170.5 lbs		
Lean body mass	144.9 lbs	145.4 lbs		+0
Recommended percent body fat		12 to 22 %		
Recommended body weight		165.3 to 186.5 lbs		
Skill-Related Fitness				
Agility	13.5 sec- 10 %tile	12.1 sec- 40 %tile	Fair	+10
Balance	5.9 sec- 30 %tile	12.1 sec- 60 %tile	Average	+105
Coordination	9.0 sec- 60 %tile	8.6 sec- 70 %tile	Good	+4
Power	6' 9" - 30 %tile	7' 2" - 50 %tile	Average	+6
Reaction time	5.0 in - 70 %tile	4.9 in - 80 %tile	Good	+2
Speed	6.9 sec- 30 %tile	6.4 sec- 70 %tile	Good	+7
Cardiovascular System				
Coronary heart disease risk	18 points	14 points	Low risk	+22
Resting heart rate	82 bpm	66 bpm	Good	+20
Systolic blood pressure	124 mmHg	120 mmHg	Very low risk	+3
Diastolic blood pressure	86 mmHg	82 mmHg	Low risk	+5

FIGURE 1.17
Computerized Fitness and Wellness Profile.

FITNESS AND WELLNESS PROFILE
by Werner W.K. Hoeger and Sharon A. Hoeger
PRINCIPLES AND LABS FOR PHYSICAL FITNESS AND WELLNESS
Morton Publishing Company

James Doe

Test Item	Previous Test 01-12-1994	Current Test 04-30-1994	Current Fitness Rating	Percent Change
Cancer Risk				
Skin and lymph nodes	2 point(s)	1 point(s)	Low risk	+50
Head and neck	1 point(s)	1 point(s)	Low risk	+0
Respiratory system	3 point(s)	2 point(s)	Moderate risk	+33
Urinary tract	1 point(s)	1 point(s)	Low risk	+0
Gastrointestinal tract	2 point(s)	2 point(s)	Moderate risk	+0
Male reproductive system	2 point(s)	1 point(s)	Low risk	+50
Pancreatic cancer	1 point(s)	1 point(s)	Low risk	+0
Oral cancer	2 point(s)	1 point(s)	Low risk	+50
Thyroid cancer	1 point(s)	1 point(s)	Low risk	+0
Liver cancer	2 point(s)	1 point(s)	Low risk	+50
Leukemia	1 point(s)	1 point(s)	Low risk	+0
Stress				
Life Experiences Survey	12 points	7 points	Fair	+42
Type A Personality Assessment	11 points	14 points	Low	+27
Smoking	Cigarette smoker	Quit smoking	Low risk	

Please note that for cardiovascular endurance, muscular strength and endurance, sit-and-reach flexibility, body rotation flexibility, lean body mass, balance, power, and type A personality assessment; the higher the score, the higher the level of fitness. In the case of shoulder rotation flexibility, percent body fat (within reasonable limits), agility, coordination, reaction time, speed, coronary heart disease risk, resting heart rate and blood pressure (within reasonable limits), all cancer sites risk, and the Life Experiences Survey; the lower the score, the better the fitness rating. While in some cases the higher the score the better, and in others, the lower the better; IN ALL INSTANCES, improvements in any fitness and wellness component are denoted with a positive (+) percent change, while a negative (-) percent change indicates a decrement in fitness and wellness.

FIGURE 1.17 *(Continued)*
Computerized Fitness and Wellness Profile.

PRINCIPLES OF NUTRITION FOR WELLNESS

2

The science of nutrition studies the relationship of foods to optimal health and performance. Although all the answers are not in yet, scientific evidence has long linked good nutrition to overall health and well-being.

Proper nutrition means that a person's diet supplies all the essential nutrients to carry out normal tissue growth, repair, and maintenance. These nutrients should be obtained from a wide variety of sources (see Figure 2.1). The diet also should provide enough substrates* to produce the energy necessary for work, physical activity, and relaxation.

Too much or too little of any nutrient can precipitate serious health problems. The typical American diet is too high in calories, sugar, fat, saturated fat, and sodium and not high enough in fiber — factors that undermine good health. Today's American diet has almost no deficiencies. Overconsumption is the major problem.

Diseases of dietary excess and imbalance are among the leading causes of death in the United States.

According to a 1988 report on nutrition and health issued by the United States Surgeon General — the first ever of its kind — diseases of dietary excess and imbalance are among the leading causes of death in the country. Of the total 2.1 million deaths in the U.S. in 1987, an estimated 1.5 million people died of diseases associated with faulty nutrition. In the report, based on more than 2,000 scientific studies, the U.S. Surgeon General said dietary changes can bring a substantial measure of better health to all Americans. Other surveys reveal that on a given day nearly half of the American people eat no fruit and almost a fourth eat no vegetables.

*Substrates are the bases on which an organism lives, or substances that are acted upon in the body.

KEY CONCEPTS

Nutrition
Carbohydrates
Dietary fiber
Fats
Saturated fat
Protein
Amino acid
Vitamins
Minerals
Eating disorders
Lipoproteins
RDA
Daily values
Glycogen
Osteoporosis

OBJECTIVES

- Define nutrition and describe its relationship to health and well-being.

- Describe the functions of carbohydrates, fats, proteins, vitamins, and minerals in the human body.

- Describe the role and health benefits of adequate fiber in the diet.

- Be able to differentiate and characterize saturated, monounsaturated, and polyunsaturated fats.

- Recognize eating disorders and their health consequences.

- Identify myths and fallacies regarding nutrition supplementation.

- Learn how to conduct a comprehensive nutrient analysis.

- Become acquainted with the five food groups and learn how to achieve a balanced diet within that framework.

Studies also indicate that diet and nutrition often play a crucial role in the development and progression of chronic diseases. A diet high in saturated fat and cholesterol increases the risk for atherosclerosis and coronary heart disease. In sodium-sensitive individuals, high salt intake has been linked to high blood pressure.

Some researchers believe that 30% to 50% of all cancers are diet-related (see Chapter 13). Obesity, diabetes mellitus, and osteoporosis also have been associated with faulty nutrition.

An effective wellness program must incorporate current dietary recommendations to lower the risk for chronic disease. A summary of guidelines for a healthful diet include:

- Eating a variety of foods.
- Avoiding too much fat, saturated fat, and cholesterol.
- Eating foods with adequate starch and fiber.
- Avoiding too much sugar and sodium.
- Maintaining adequate calcium intake.
- Maintaining recommended body weight.
- If you drink alcoholic beverages, do so in moderation.

These guidelines will be discussed throughout this chapter and later chapters (4, 12, and 13) of this book.

NUTRIENTS

The essential nutrients the human body requires are carbohydrates, fat, protein, vitamins, minerals, and water. The first three are called fuel nutrients because they are the only substances the body uses to supply the energy (commonly measured in calories) needed for work and normal body functions. Vitamins, minerals, and water have no caloric value but are still necessary for a person to function normally and maintain good health. Many nutritionists add a seventh nutrient to this list, one that has received a great deal of attention recently: dietary fiber.

Carbohydrates, fats, proteins, and water are termed *macronutrients* because proportionately large amounts are needed daily. Vitamins and minerals are required only in small amounts. Therefore, nutritionists refer to them as *micronutrients*.

Depending on the amount of nutrients and calories, foods can be classified according to high nutrient density and low nutrient density. High nutrient density refers to foods that contain few or moderate calories but are packed with nutrients. Foods that have a lot of calories but few nutrients are of low nutrient density and commonly are called "junk food."

Food Guide Pyramid
A Guide to Daily Food Choices

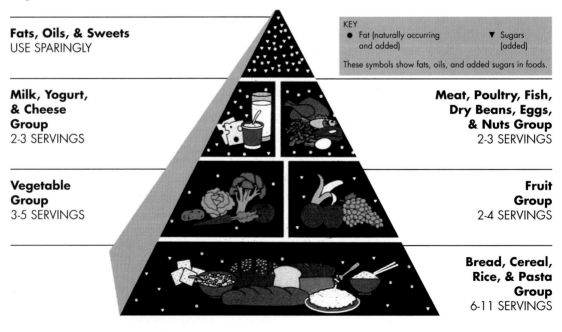

FIGURE 2.1

Calorie is the unit of measure indicating the energy value of food and cost of physical activity. Technically, a kilocalorie (kcal) or large calorie is the amount of heat necessary to raise the temperature of 1 kilogram of water 1° Centigrade, but for simplification people call it a calorie rather than kcal. For example, if the caloric value of a food is 100 calories (kcal), the energy in this food could raise the temperature of 100 kilograms of water by 1° Centigrade.

CARBOHYDRATES

Carbohydrates constitute the major source of calories the body uses to provide energy for work, maintain cells, and generate heat. They also help digest and regulate fat and metabolize protein. Each gram of carbohydrates provides the human body with four calories.

The major sources of carbohydrates are breads, cereals, fruits, vegetables, and milk and other dairy products. Carbohydrates are classified into *simple carbohydrates* and *complex carbohydrates* (Figure 2.2).

SIMPLE CARBOHYDRATES
(simple sugars)

Monosaccharides
Glucose
Fructose
Galactose

Disaccharides
Sucrose
(glucose + fructose)
Lactose
(glucose + galactose)
Maltose
(glucose + glucose)

COMPLEX CARBOHYDRATES

Polysaccharides
Starches
Dextrins

Fiber
Cellulose
Hemicellulose
Pectins
Gums

FIGURE 2.2
Major types of carbohydrates.

Simple carbohydrates

Often called sugars, simple carbohydrates are formed by simple or double sugar units with little nutritive value (for example, candy, soda, cakes). Simple carbohydrates are divided into monosaccharides and disaccharides. These carbohydrates — with *-ose* endings — often take the place of more nutritive foods in the diet.

Monosaccharides, the simplest sugars, are formed by five- or six-carbon skeletons. The three most common monosaccharides are glucose, fructose, and galactose.

1. *Glucose* is a natural sugar found in food, but it also is produced in the body from other simple and complex carbohydrates.
2. *Fructose,* or fruit sugar, occurs naturally in fruits and honey.
3. *Galactose* is produced from milk sugar in the mammary glands of lactating animals.

Both fructose and galactose are readily converted to glucose in the body. Glucose is used as a source of energy, or it may be stored in the muscles and liver in the form of *glycogen* (a long chain of glucose molecules hooked together). Excess glucose in the blood is converted to fat and stored in adipose (fat) tissue. Some of it is eliminated by the kidneys through the urine.

Disaccharides are formed by the linkage of two monosaccharide units, one of which is glucose. The three major disaccharides are:

1. *Sucrose* or table sugar (glucose + fructose).
2. *Lactose* (glucose + galactose).
3. *Maltose* (glucose + glucose).

Complex Carbohydrates

Complex carbohydrates are formed when three or more simple sugar molecules bind together. Therefore, they also are called **polysaccharides**. Anywhere from about 10 to thousands of monosaccharide molecules can unite to form a single polysaccharide. Examples of complex carbohydrates are starches, dextrins, and glycogen.

1. **Starch** is the storage form of glucose in plants, needed to promote initial growth. Starch is found commonly in grains, seeds, corn, nuts, roots, potatoes, and legumes. Grains, the richest source of starch, should supply most of the energy in a healthful diet. Once eaten, starch is converted to glucose for the body's own energy use.

2. **Dextrins** are formed from the breakdown of large starch molecules exposed to dry heat, such as in baking bread or producing cold cereals. Complex carbohydrates of plant origin provide many valuable nutrients and can be an excellent source of fiber, or roughage.

3. **Glycogen** is the animal polysaccharide synthesized from glucose and found only in slight amounts in meats. Although it serves a function in humans similar to that of starch in plants, glycogen is not found in plants. Glycogen constitutes the body's reservoirs of glucose. Many hundreds to thousands of glucose molecules are linked together to be stored as glycogen in liver and muscle.

When a surge of energy is needed, enzymes in the muscle and the liver break down glycogen and thus make glucose readily available for energy transformation. This is discussed later in the chapter, under Nutrition for Athletes.

DIETARY FIBER

Dietary fiber is a type of complex carbohydrate made up of plant material the human body cannot digest. It is present mainly in leaves, skins, roots, and seeds. Processing and refining foods removes almost all of the natural fiber. In our daily diets the main sources of dietary fiber are whole-grain cereals and breads, fruits, and vegetables.

The most common types of fiber are:

1. *Cellulose* and *hemicellulose*, found in plant cell walls.
2. *Pectins*, found in fruits.
3. *Gums*, also found in small amounts in foods of plant origin.

Cellulose and hemicellulose are water-insoluble fibers; pectins and gums are water-soluble fibers.

Fiber is important in the diet because it binds water, causing a softer and bulkier stool that increases peristalsis (involuntary muscle contraction of intestinal walls that force the stool onward) and allows food residues to pass through the intestinal tract more quickly. Many researchers believe that speeding up passage of food residues through the intestines lowers the risk for colon cancer, mainly because cancer-causing agents are not in contact as long with the intestinal wall. Fiber also is thought to bind with carcinogens (cancer-producing substances), and more water in the stool may dilute the cancer-causing agents, lessening their potency.

Increased fiber intake also may lower the risk for coronary heart disease because: (a) saturated fats often take the place of fiber in the diet, increasing cholesterol formation or absorption, and (b) specific water-soluble fibers such as pectin and guar gum, found in beans, oat bran, corn, and fruits, seem to bind cholesterol in the intestines, preventing its absorption. In addition to heart disease, several health disorders, including constipation, diverticulitis, hemorrhoids, gallbladder disease, and obesity have been linked to low fiber intake.

Determining the amount of fiber in your diet can be confusing at times because it can be measured either as crude fiber or as dietary fiber. *Crude fiber* is the smaller portion of the dietary fiber, which actually remains after chemical extraction in the digestive tract. The recommended amount of *dietary fiber* is 20 to 35 grams per day, the equivalent of 7 grams of crude fiber. Because most nutrition labels list the fiber content in terms of dietary fiber, the 20 to 35 gram guideline should be used (see Table 2.1).

This may be surprising, but too much fiber also can be detrimental to health. It can produce loss of calcium, phosphorus, and iron, not to mention gastrointestinal discomfort. When eating more fiber, a person also should drink more water, as too little fluid can cause constipation and even dehydration.

FAT

Fats, or *lipids*, are also used by the human body as a source of energy. They are the most concentrated energy source. Each gram of fat supplies nine calories to the body. Fats are a part of the cell structure. They are used as stored energy and as an insulator to preserve body heat. They absorb shock, supply essential fatty acids, and carry the fat-soluble vitamins A, D, E, and K. Fats can be classified into three main groups: simple, compound, and derived (Figure 2.3). The basic sources of fat are milk and other dairy products, and meats and alternates.

Simple Fats

A simple fat consists of a glyceride molecule linked to one, two, or three units of fatty acids. According to the number of fatty acids attached, simple fats are divided into **monoglycerides** (one fatty acid), **diglycerides** (two fatty acids), and **triglycerides** (three fatty

TABLE 2.1
Dietary Fiber Content of Selected Foods

Food	Serving Size	Dietary Fiber (gm)
Almonds	1 oz.	3.0
Apple	1 medium	4.3
Banana	1 medium	3.3
Beans — red, kidney	.5 cup	10.2
Blackberries	.5 cup	4.9
Beets (cooked)	.5 cup	2.0
Brazil nuts	1 oz.	2.5
Broccoli (cooked)	.5 cup	3.3
Brown rice (cooked)	.5 cup	2.0
Carrots (cooked)	.5 cup	2.9
Cauliflower (cooked)	.5 cup	1.7
Cereal		
All Bran	1 oz.	8.5
Cheerios	1 oz.	1.1
Cornflakes	1 oz.	0.5
Fruit and Fibre	1 oz.	4.0
Fruit Wheats	1 oz.	2.0
Just Right	1 oz.	2.0
Wheaties	1 oz.	2.0
Corn (cooked)	.5 cup	3.9
Eggplant (cooked)	.5 cup	3.0
Lettuce (chopped)	.5 cup	0.4
Orange	1 medium	3.0
Parsnips (cooked)	.5 cup	2.1
Pear	1 medium	5.0
Peas (cooked)	.5 cup	3.7
Popcorn (plain)	1 cup	1.5
Potato (baked)	1 medium	3.9
Strawberries	.5 cup	1.6
Summer squash (cooked)	.5 cup	1.6
Watermelon	1 cup	0.8

SIMPLE FATS

Monoglyceride (glyceride + one fatty acid*)
Diglycerides (glyceride + two fatty acids)
Triglycerides (glyceride + three fatty acids)

COMPOUND FATS

Phospholipids
Glucolipids
Lipoproteins

DERIVED FATS

Sterols
(cholesterol)

*Fatty acids can be saturated or unsaturated.

FIGURE 2.3
Major types of fats (lipids).

Saturated Fatty Acid

Monounsaturated Fatty Acid

Polyunsaturated Fatty Acid

*Glyceride component

FIGURE 2.4
Chemical structure of saturated and unsaturated fats.

acids). More than 90% of the weight of fat in foods and more than 95% of the stored fat in the human body are in the form of triglycerides.

The length of the carbon atom chain and the amount of hydrogen saturation in fatty acids vary. Based on the extent of saturation, fatty acids are said to be **saturated** or **unsaturated**. Unsaturated fatty acids are classified further into **monounsaturated** and **polyunsaturated**. Saturated fatty acids are mainly of animal origin. Unsaturated fats are found mostly in plant products.

In **saturated fatty acids** the carbon atoms are fully saturated with hydrogens; only single bonds link the carbon atoms on the chain (see Figure 2.4). These saturated fatty acids often are called saturated fats. Examples of foods high in saturated fatty acids are meats, meat fat, lard, whole milk, cream, butter, cheese, ice cream, hydrogenated oils (a process that makes oils saturated), coconut oil, and palm oils.

In **unsaturated fatty acids** (unsaturated fats), double bonds form between the unsaturated carbons. In **monounsaturated fatty acids** (MUFA) only one double bond is found along the chain. Olive, canola, rapeseed, peanut and sesame oils, and avocado are examples of monounsaturated fatty acids. **Polyunsaturated fatty acids** (PUFA) contain two or more double bonds between unsaturated carbon atoms along the chain. Corn, cottonseed, safflower, walnut, sunflower, and soybean oils are high in polyunsaturated fatty acids.

Saturated fats typically do not melt at room temperature. Unsaturated fats usually are liquid at room temperature. Coconut and palm oils are exceptions, as they are high in saturated fats. Shorter fatty acid chains also tend to be liquid at room temperature.

In general, saturated fats raise the blood cholesterol level, whereas polyunsaturated and monounsaturated fats tend to lower blood cholesterol (the role of cholesterol in health and disease is discussed in Chapter 12). Polyunsaturated fats, nonetheless, also seem to cause reduction of the "good" (HDL) cholesterol, which may not really improve the cholesterol profile (see compound fats, below, and also the discussion of cholesterol in Chapter 12). Monounsaturated fats, on the other hand, seem to lower only the "bad" (LDL) cholesterol and not the good (HDL) cholesterol.

One type of polyunsaturated fatty acids that has gained attention in recent years are **omega-3 fatty acids**. These fatty acids seem to be effective in lowering blood cholesterol and triglycerides. Fish, especially fresh or frozen mackerel, herring, tuna, salmon, and lake trout, have omega-3 fatty acids. Canned fish is not recommended because the canning process destroys most of the omega-3 oil. These fatty acids also are found, but to a lesser extent, in canola oil, walnuts, soybeans, and wheat germ.

Limited data suggest that eating one or two servings of fish weekly lessens the risk for coronary heart disease. People with diabetes, a history of hemorrhaging or strokes, on aspirin and blood-thinning therapy, and pre-surgical patients should not consume fish oil except under their physician's instruction.

Compound Fats

Compound fats are a combination of simple fats and other chemicals. Examples are:

1. *Phospholipids,* similar to triglycerides except that phosphoric acid takes the place of one of the fatty acid units.
2. *Glucolipids,* a combination of carbohydrates, fatty acids, and nitrogen.
3. *Lipoproteins,* water-soluble aggregates of protein with triglycerides, phospholipids, or cholesterol.

Because lipids do not dissolve in water, lipoproteins transport fats in the blood. As the name indicates, lipoproteins are a combination of lipids covered by proteins (known as apoproteins).

The major forms of lipoproteins are **high density (HDL), low density (LDL), and very low density (VLDL) lipoproteins**. Lipoproteins play a large role in developing or in preventing heart disease. HDL is more than half protein and contains little cholesterol. High HDL levels have been associated with a lower risk for coronary heart disease. LDL is approximately a fourth protein and nearly half cholesterol. High LDL levels have been linked to increased risk for coronary heart disease. VLDL contains mostly triglycerides (about half) and only about 10% protein and 20% cholesterol. Chapter 12 provides more information on the role these lipoproteins play in coronary heart disease.

Derived Fats

Derived fats combine simple and compound fats. Sterols are an example. Although sterols contain no fatty acids, they are considered fats because they do not dissolve in water. The most often mentioned sterol is cholesterol, which is found in many foods or can be manufactured from saturated fats in the body.

PROTEIN

Proteins are the main substances the body uses to build and repair tissues such as muscles, blood, internal organs, skin, hair, nails, and bones. They are a part of hormones, antibodies, and enzymes. Enzymes play a key role in all of the body's processes. Because all enzymes are formed by proteins, this nutrient is necessary for normal functioning. Proteins also help maintain the normal balance of body fluids.

Proteins can be used as a source of energy, too, but only if not enough carbohydrates are available. Each gram of protein yields four calories of energy. The main sources of protein are meats and alternates, and milk and other dairy products. Excess proteins may be converted to glucose or fat or even excreted in the urine.

The human body uses 20 **amino acids,** the basic building blocks to form different types of protein. Amino acids contain nitrogen, carbon, hydrogen, and oxygen. Nine of the 20 amino acids are called *essential amino acids* because the body cannot produce them. The other 11, termed *nonessential amino acids,* can be manufactured in the body if food proteins in the diet provide enough nitrogen. For normal body function all amino acids must be present at the same time.

Proteins that contain all the essential amino acids are known as **complete or higher-quality protein.** These types of proteins usually are of animal source. If one or more of the essential amino acids is missing, the proteins are termed **incomplete or lower-quality protein.** Individuals have to take in enough protein to ensure nitrogen for adequate amino acid production and also to get enough high-quality protein to obtain the essential amino acids.

> *Two glasses of skim milk combined with about 4 ounces of poultry or fish meet the daily protein requirement.*

Protein deficiency is not a problem in the usual American diet. Two glasses of skim milk combined with about 4 ounces of poultry or fish meet the daily protein requirement. Protein deficiency, however, could be a concern in some vegetarian diets. Vegetarians rely primarily on foods from the bread and cereal and fruit and vegetable groups and avoid most foods from animal sources found in the milk and meat groups. The four basic types of vegetarians are:

1. Vegans, who eat no animal products at all.
2. Ovovegetarians, who allow eggs in the diet.
3. Lactovegetarians, who eat foods from the milk group.
4. Ovolactovegetarians, who include egg and milk products in the diet.

Vegans, in particular, must be careful to eat protein foods that provide a balanced distribution of essential amino acids, such as grain products and beans. Strict vegans also need a supplement of vitamin B_{12}. This vitamin is not found in plant foods and its deficiency may lead to anemia.

Vegetarians who do not select their food combinations properly may develop nutritional deficiencies of protein, vitamins, minerals, and even calories. Vegetarian diets can be balanced, but this is a complicated issue that cannot be covered adequately in a few paragraphs. Those who are interested in vegetarian diets should consult other resources.

Too much animal protein can cause serious health problems as well. Many people eat twice as much protein as they need. Protein foods from animal sources often are high in fat, saturated fat, and cholesterol, which can lead to cardiovascular disease and cancer. Too much animal protein also decreases blood enzymes that prevent precancerous cells from developing into tumors.

As discussed later in this chapter, a well-balanced diet contains a variety of foods from all five basic food groups, including wise selection of foods from animal sources. Based on current nutrition data, meat (poultry and fish included) should be replaced by grains, legumes, vegetables, and fruits as main courses. Meats should be used more for flavoring than substance. Daily consumption of beef, poultry, or fish should be limited to 3 to 6 ounces (about the size of a deck of cards).

VITAMINS

Vitamins are organic substances necessary for normal bodily metabolism, growth, and development. Vitamins function as antioxidants, as coenzymes (primarily the B complex), which regulate the work of the enzymes; and vitamin D even functions as a hormone.

Vitamins C, E, beta-carotene (a precursor to vitamin A) and the mineral selenium serve as **antioxidants,** preventing oxygen from combining with other substances that it may damage. During metabolism oxygen changes carbohydrates and fats into energy. In this process oxygen is transformed into stable forms of water and carbon dioxide. A small amount of oxygen, however, ends up in an unstable form, referred to as *oxygen free radicals.* Solar radiation, cigarette smoke, radiation, and other environmental factors also seem to encourage the formation of free radicals.

TABLE 2.2
Antioxidant Nutrients, Sources, and Functions

Nutrient	Good Sources	Antioxidant Effect
Vitamin C	Citrus fruit, kiwi fruit, cantaloupe, strawberries, broccoli, green or red peppers, cauliflower, cabbage	Appears to inactivate oxygen-free radicals
Vitamin E	Vegetable oils, yellow and green leafy vegetables, margarine, wheat germ, oatmeal, almonds, and whole grain breads, cereals	Protects lipids from oxidation.
Beta-carotene	Carrots, squash, pumpkin, sweet potatoes, broccoli, green leafy vegetables	Soaks up oxygen-free radicals
Selenium	Seafood, meat, whole grains	Helps prevent damage to cell structures

A free radical molecule has a normal proton nucleus with a single unpaired electron. Having only one electron makes the free radical extremely reactive, and it constantly looks to pair the electron up with one from another molecule. When it steals the second electron from another molecule, that other molecule in turn becomes a free radical. This chain reaction goes on until two free radicals meet to form a stable molecule. Antioxidants help stabilize free radicals so they will not be as reactive until a match can be found.

Free radicals attack and damage proteins and lipids, in particular the cell membrane and DNA. This damage is thought to play a key role in the development of conditions such as heart disease, cancer, and emphysema (also see Chapters 12 and 13). The beneficial effects of antioxidants are given in Table 2.2.

Researchers believe that antioxidants offer protection by absorbing free radicals before they can cause damage and also by interrupting the sequence of reactions once damage has begun (Figure 2.5), thwarting certain chronic diseases.[8]

Vitamins are classified into two types based on their solubility: *fat-soluble* vitamins (A, D, E, and K), and *water-soluble* vitamins (B complex and C). In general, the body does not manufacture vitamins. Vitamins can be obtained only through a well-balanced diet. To decrease vitamin losses during cooking, natural foods should be microwaved or steamed rather than boiled in water that later is thrown out.

A few exceptions, such as A, D, and K, are formed in the body. Vitamin A is produced from beta-carotene, found in foods such as carrots, pumpkin, and sweet potatoes. Ultraviolet light from the sun changes a compound in the skin called 7-dehydrocholesterol into vitamin D. Vitamin K is created in the body by intestinal bacteria. A description of the major functions of vitamins is presented in Table 2.3.

FIGURE 2.5
The antioxidant effect of beta-carotene, vitamins C and E, and the mineral selenium appear to protect against certain diseases (including heart disease and cancer) by preventing oxygen-free radicals from damaging cells and by stopping the sequence of reactions once damage has begun.

TABLE 2.3
Major Functions of Vitamins

Nutrient	Good Sources	Major Functions	Deficiency Symptoms
Vitamin A	Milk, cheese, eggs, liver, and yellow/dark green fruits and vegetables	Required for healthy bones, teeth, skin, gums, and hair. Maintenance of inner mucous membranes, thus increasing resistance to infection. Adequate vision in dim light.	Night blindness, decreased growth, decreased resistance to infection, rough-dry skin.
Vitamin D	Fortified milk, cod liver oil, salmon, tuna, egg yolk	Necessary for bones and teeth. Needed for calcium and phosphorus absorption	Rickets (bone softening), fractures, and muscle spasms
Vitamin E	Vegetable oils, yellow and green leafy vegetables, margarine, wheat germ, whole grain breads and cereals	Related to oxidation and normal muscle and red blood cell chemistry	Leg cramps, red blood cell breakdown
Vitamin K	Green leafy vegetables, cauliflower, cabbage, eggs, peas, and potatoes	Essential for normal blood clotting	Hemorrhaging
Vitamin B$_1$ (Thiamine)	Whole grain or enriched bread, lean meats and poultry, organ fish, liver, pork, poultry, organ meats, legumes, nuts, and dried yeast	Assists in proper use of carbohydrates. Normal functioning of nervous system. Maintenance of good appetite.	Loss of appetite, nausea, confusion, cardiac abnormalities, muscle spasms
Vitamin B$_2$ (Riboflavin)	Eggs, milk, leafy green vegetables, whole grains, lean meats, dried beans and peas	Contributes to energy release from carbohydrates, fats, and proteins. Needed for normal growth and development, good vision, and healthy skin	Cracking of the corners of the mouth, inflammation of the skin, impaired vision.
Vitamin B$_6$ (Pyridoxine)	Vegetables, meats, whole grain cereals, soybeans, peanuts, and potatoes	Necessary for protein and fatty acids metabolism, and normal red blood cell formation	Depression, irritability, muscle spasms, nausea
Vitamin B$_{12}$	Meat, poultry, fish, liver, organ meats, eggs, shellfish, milk, and cheese	Required for normal growth, red blood cell formation, nervous system and digestive tract functioning	Impaired balance, weakness, drop in red blood cell count
Niacin	Liver and organ meats, meat, fish, poultry, whole grains, enriched breads, nuts, green leafy vegetables, and dried beans and peas	Contributes to energy release from carbohydrates, fats, and proteins. Normal growth and development, and formation of hormones and nerve-regulating substances	Confusion, depression, weakness, weight loss
Biotin	Liver, kidney, eggs, yeast, legumes, milk, nuts, dark green vegetables	Essential for carbohydrate metabolism and fatty acid synthesis	Inflamed skin, muscle pain, depression, weight loss
Folic Acid	Leafy green vegetables, organ meats, whole grains and cereals, and dried beans	Needed for cell growth and reproduction and red blood cell formation	Decreased resistance to infection
Pantothenic Acid	All natural foods, especially liver, kidney, eggs, nuts, yeast, milk, dried peas and beans, and green leafy vegetables	Related to carbohydrate and fat metabolism	Depression, low blood sugar, leg cramps, nausea, headaches
Vitamin C (Ascorbic Acid)	Fruits and vegetables	Helps protect against infection; formation of collagenous tissue. Normal blood vessels, teeth, and bones	Slow healing wounds, loose teeth, hemorrhaging, rough-scaly skin, irritability

MINERALS

Minerals are inorganic elements found in the body and in food. Approximately 25 minerals have important roles in body functioning. Minerals are contained in all cells, especially those in hard parts of the body (bones, nails, teeth).

Minerals are crucial in maintaining water balance and the acid-base balance. They are essential components of respiratory pigments, enzymes, and enzyme systems, and they regulate muscular and nervous tissue excitability, blood clotting, and normal heart rhythm.

The three minerals most commonly mentioned are calcium, iron, and sodium. As pointed out later in this chapter, calcium deficiency may result in osteoporosis, and low iron intake in iron-deficiency anemia. High sodium intake may lead to

hypertension (also see blood pressure in Chapter 12). The specific functions of some of the most important minerals are given in Table 2.4.

WATER

Approximately 70% of total body weight is water. Water is the most important nutrient, involved in almost every vital body process: in digesting and absorbing food, in the circulatory process, in removing waste products, in building and rebuilding cells, and in transporting other nutrients.

Water is contained in almost all foods but primarily in liquid foods, fruits, and vegetables. Besides the natural content in foods, every person should drink about eight glasses of fluids a day.

TABLE 2.4
Major Functions of Minerals

Nutrient	Good Sources	Major Functions	Deficiency Symptoms
Calcium	Milk, yogurt, cheese, green leafy vegetables, dried beans, sardines, and salmon	Required for strong teeth and bone formation. Maintenance of good muscle tone, heart beat, and nerve function	Bone pain and fractures, periodontal disease, muscle cramps
Iron	Organ meats, lean meats, seafoods, eggs, dried peas and beans, nuts, whole and enriched grains, and green leafy vegetables	Major component of hemoglobin. Aids in energy utilization	Nutritional anemia, and overall weakness
Phosphorus	Meats, fish, milk, eggs, dried beans and peas, whole grains, and processed foods	Required for bone and teeth formation. Energy release regulation	Bone pain and fracture, weight loss, and weakness
Zinc	Milk, meat, seafood, whole grains, nuts, eggs, and dried beans	Essential component of hormones, insulin, and enzymes. Used in normal growth and development	Loss of appetite, slow healing wounds, and skin problems
Magnesium	Green leavy vegetables, whole grains, nuts, soybeans, seafood, and legumes	Needed for bone growth and maintenance. Carbohydrate and protein utilization. Nerve function. Temperature regulation	Irregular heartbeat, weakness, muscle spasms, and sleeplessness
Sodium	Table salt, processed foods, and meat	Body fluid regulation. Transmission of nerve impulse. Heart action	Rarely seen
Potassium	Legumes, whole grains, bananas, orange juice, dried fruits, and potatoes	Heart action. Bone formation and maintenance. Regulation of energy release. Acid-base regulation	Irregular heartbeat, nausea, weakness
Selenium	Seafood, meat, whole grains	Component of enzyme; functions in close association with vitamin E	Muscle pain, possible heart muscle deterioration; possible hair and nail loss

ENERGY (ATP) PRODUCTION

The energy derived from food is not used directly by the cells. It is transferred to form an energy-rich compound called **adenosine triphosphate**, or **ATP**. The subsequent breakdown of this compound provides the energy used by all energy-requiring processes of the body. ATP must be recycled continually to sustain life and work.

ATP can be resynthesized in three ways: (also see Figure 2.6):

1. **ATP and ATP-CP system.** The body stores small amounts of ATP and creatine phosphate (CP). These stores are used during all-out activities up to 10 seconds in duration, such as sprinting, long jumping, and power (weight) lifting. The amount of stored ATP provides energy for just a few seconds. With all-out efforts, ATP is resynthesized from CP, another high-energy phosphate compound. This is referred to as the ATP-CP or phosphagen system.

   Depending on the amount of physical training, the concentration of CP stored in cells is sufficient to allow maximal exertion for up to 10 seconds. Once the CP stores are depleted, the person is forced to slow down or rest to allow ATP to form through anaerobic and aerobic pathways.

2. **Anaerobic or lactic acid system.** During high intensity (anaerobic) exercise that is sustained between 10 and 180 seconds maximum, ATP is replenished from the breakdown of glucose through a series of chemical reactions that do not require oxygen. In the process, though, lactic acid is produced, which causes muscular fatigue.

   Because of the accumulation of lactic acid with high intensity exercise, the formation of ATP is limited to about 3 minutes. A recovery period then is necessary to allow for the elimination of lactic acid. Formation of ATP through the anaerobic system is possible from glucose (carbohydrates) only.

3. **Aerobic system.** The production of energy during slow-sustained exercise is derived primarily through aerobic metabolism. Both glucose (carbohydrates) and fatty acids (fat) are used in this process. Oxygen is required to form ATP, and under steady state exercise conditions lactic acid accumulation is minimal.

   Because oxygen is required, a person's capacity to utilize oxygen (maximal oxygen uptake, or Max VO_2 (see Chapter 5) is critical for successful athletic performance in aerobic events. The higher the Max VO_2, the greater is the capacity to generate ATP through the aerobic system.

BALANCING THE DIET

Most people would like to live life to its fullest, have good health, and lead a productive life. One of the fundamental ways to accomplish this goal is through a well-balanced diet. As illustrated in Figure 2.7, the recommended guidelines state that daily caloric intake should be distributed so about *58% of the total calories come from carbohydrates* (48% complex carbohydrates and 10% sugar), *less than 30% of the total calories from fat* (equally divided [10% each] among saturated, monounsaturated, and polyunsaturated fats), and *12% of the total calories from protein* (0.8 grams of protein per kilogram [2.2 pounds] of body weight). The diet also must include all of the essential vitamins, minerals, and water. To accurately rate a diet is difficult without a complete nutrient analysis.

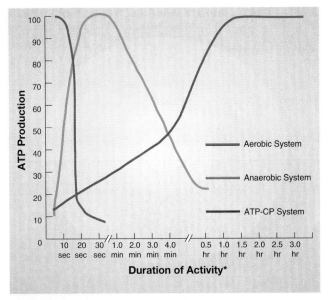

FIGURE 2.6
Contributions of the energy formation mechanisms during various forms of physical activity.

The American diet has changed significantly since the turn of the century. People in the 1990s eat more fat, less carbohydrates, and about the same amount of protein, but fewer calories. At the same time, we weigh more than we did in 1900, an indication that we are not as physically active as our grandparents were.

> *People in the 1990s weigh more than in 1900 even though they consume fewer calories.*

Diets also were much healthier at the turn of the century. In 1909, carbohydrates accounted for 57% of the total daily caloric intake, 67% of which were complex carbohydrates. Today, carbohydrate intake has decreased to 51%, and complex carbohydrates account for only 47% of the daily carbohydrate intake. The proportion of fat has risen from 32% to 37%. Protein intake has remained unchanged at about 12% of the total caloric intake.

NUTRIENT ANALYSIS

The first step in evaluating your diet is to conduct a nutrient analysis. This can be quite an educational experience because most people do not realize how harmful and non-nutritious many common foods are. The analysis covers calories, carbohydrates, fats,

cholesterol, and sodium, as well as eight crucial nutrients: protein, calcium, iron, vitamin A, thiamin, riboflavin, niacin, and vitamin C. If the diet has enough of these eight nutrients, the foods consumed in natural form to provide these nutrients typically contain all the other nutrients the human body needs.

To do the nutrient analysis, keep a 3-day record of everything you eat, using the forms in Lab 2A, Figure 2A.1. At the end of each day, look up the nutrient content for those foods in the list of Nutritive Value of Selected Foods, in Appendix A. Record this information on your 3-day listing of foods in Figure 2A.1 (Lab 2A). If you do not find a food in the list given in Appendix A, the information often is stated on the food container itself, or you might refer to the references at the end of the list.

When you have recorded the nutritive values for each day, add up each column and write the totals at the bottom of the chart. After the third day, use Figure 2A.2 and compute an average for the 3 days. To rate your diet, compare your figures with those in the recommended dietary allowances (RDA) (Figure 2.8). The results give a good indication of areas of strength and deficiency in your current diet.

Every ten years or so, the National Academy of Sciences issues a new RDA based on a review of the most current research on nutrient needs for healthy people. The RDA provides daily nutrient intake recommendations, usually set high enough to encompass 97.5% of the healthy population in the United States. Stated another way, the RDA recommendation for any nutrient is well above almost everyone's actual requirement.

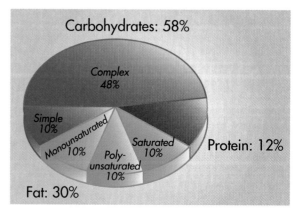

FIGURE 2.7.
Current and recommended distribution of fat, carbohydrate, and protein intake expressed in percentages of total daily caloric consumption.

	Calories	Protein	Fat	Sat. Fat	Choles-terol (mg)	Carbo-hydrates	Calcium (mg)	Iron (mg)	Sodium (mg)	Vit. A (I. U.)	Thiamin (Vit. B$_1$) (mg)	Riboflavin (Vit. B$_2$) (mg)	Niacin (mg)	Vit. C (mg)
Men 15–18 years	See below[a]	See below[b]	< 30%[c]	< 10%[c]	< 300	50% >[c]	1,200	12	2,400	5,000	1.5	1.8	20	60
Men 19–24 years			< 30%[c]	< 10%[c]	< 300	50% >[c]	1,200	10	2,400	5,000	1.5	1.7	19	60
Men 25–50 years			< 30%[c]	< 10%[c]	< 300	50% >[c]	800	10	2,400	5,000	1.5	1.7	19	60
Men 51 +			< 30%[c]	< 10%[c]	< 300	50% >[c]	800	10	2,400	5,000	1.2	1.4	15	60
Women 15–18 years			< 30%[c]	< 10%[c]	< 300	50% >[c]	1,200	15	2,400	4,000	1.1	1.3	15	60
Women 19–24 years			< 30%[c]	< 10%[c]	< 300	50% >[c]	1,200	15	2,400	4,000	1.1	1.3	15	60
Women 25–50 years			< 30%[c]	< 10%[c]	< 300	50% >[c]	800	15	2,400	4,000	1.1	1.3	15	60
Women 51 +			< 30%[c]	< 10%[c]	< 300	50% >[c]	800	10	2,400	4,000	1.0	1.2	13	60
Pregnant			< 30%[c]	< 10%[c]	< 300	50% >[c]	1,200	30	2,400	4,000	1.5	1.6	17	70
Lactating	↓	↓	< 30%[c]	< 10%[c]	< 300	50% >[c]	1,200	15	2,400	6,000	1.6	1.8	20	95

[a] Use Table 4.1 for all categories.
[b] Protein intake should be .8 grams per kilogram of body weight. Pregnant women should consume an additional 15 grams of daily protein, while lactating women should have an extra 20 grams.
[c] Percentage of total calories based on recommendations by nutrition experts.
* Adapted from *Recommended Dietary Allowances*, © 1989, by the National Academy of Sciences, National Academy Press, Washington D.C.

FIGURE 2.8
Recommended Dietary Allowances (RDA).

Between the late 1960s and the early 1990s, nutrient information on labels was expressed in terms of the U. S. RDA — a set of standard values for the average consumer — derived from the 1968 edition of the RDA. In 1993, the Food and Drug Administration (FDA) revised food labeling regulations and has replaced the U. S. RDA with *Daily Values* (see Figure 2.9). These daily values are based on a 2,000 calorie diet and may require adjustments by the individual depending on daily caloric needs.

In setting the Daily Values, the FDA first created two sets of standards: Reference Daily Intakes (RDI) and Daily Reference Values (DRV). For FDA purposes, these two sets of standards serve different functions. To avoid consumer confusion in food labeling, however, the FDA combined the RDI and DRV into the Daily Values.

The RDI are reference values for protein, vitamins, and minerals. These are similar in purpose to the old U. S. RDA, but reflecting average allowances based on the 1989 RDA.

The DRV are standards for nutrients and food components that do not have an established RDA. The DRV include carbohydrate, fat, saturated fat, fiber, cholesterol, and sodium. These standards (computed in grams and milligrams based on a 2,000 calorie diet) represent dietary intakes to attain or restrict based on a consensus of critical values that are associated with health. For example, carbohydrate intake should be 60% of total daily calories (300 grams), while fat intake should be limited to less than 30% (65 grams).

Both the RDA and the Daily Values apply only to healthy people. They are not intended for

Better by Design
How to recognize the new food labels

The new food labels feature a revamped nutrition panel titled "Nutrition Facts," with nutrient listings that reflect current health concerns. Now you'll be able to find information on fat, fiber and other food components fundamental to lowering your risk of cancer and other chronic diseases. Listings for nutrients like thiamin and riboflavin will no longer be required, because Americans generally eat enough of them these days.

Size Up the Situation
All serving sizes are created equal

Now you can compare similar products and know that their serving sizes are basically identical. So when you realize how much fat is packed into that carton of double-dutch-chocolate-caramel-chew ice cream you're eyeing, you might opt for lowfat frozen yogurt instead. Serving sizes will also be standardized, so manufacturers can't make nutrition claims for unrealistically small portions. That means a chocolate cake, for example, must be divided into 8 servings sized to satisfy the average person — not 16 servings sized to satisfy the average munchkin.

Look Before You Leap
Use the Daily Values

You will find the Daily Values on the bottom half of the "Nutrition Facts" panel. Some represent maximum levels of nutrients that should be consumed each day for a healthful diet (as with fat) while others refer to minimum levels that can be exceeded (as with carbohydrates). They are based on both a 2,000 and 2,500 calorie diet. Your own needs may be more or less, but these figures give you a point from which to compare. For example, the sample label indicates that someone with a 2,000 calorie diet should eat no more than 65 grams of fat per day. This is based on a diet getting 30% of calories as fat. If you normally eat less calories, or want to eat less than 30% of calories as fat, your daily fat consumption will be lower.

Rate It Right
Scan the % Daily Values

The % Daily Values make judging the nutritional quality of a food a snap. For instance, you can look at the % Daily Value column and find that a food has 25% of the Daily Value for fiber. This means the product will give you a substantial portion of the recommended amount of fiber for the day. You can also use this column to compare nutrients in similar products. The % Daily Values are based on a 2,000 calorie diet.

Trust Adjectives
Descriptors have legal definitions

Terms like "low," "high" and "free" have long been used on food labels. What these words actually mean, however, could vary. Thanks to the new labeling laws, such descriptions must now meet legal definitions. For example, you may be shopping for foods high in vitamin A, which has been linked to lower risk of certain cancers. Under the new label laws, a food described as "high" in a particular nutrient must contain 20% or more of the Daily Value for that nutrient. So if the bottle of juice you're thinking of buying says "high in vitamin A,'" you can now feel confident that it really is a good source of the vitamin.

Read Health Claims with Confidence
The nutrient link to disease prevention

You can also expect to see food packages with health claims linking certain nutrients to reduced risk of cancer and other diseases. The federal government has approved three health claims dealing with cancer prevention: a low fat diet may reduce your risk for cancer; high fiber foods may reduce your risk for cancer; and fruits and vegetables may reduce your risk for cancer. A food may not make such a health claim for one nutrient if it contains other nutrients that undermine its health benefits. A high fiber, but high fat, jelly doughnut cannot carry a health claim!

Many factors affect cancer risk. Eating a diet low in fat and high in fiber may lower risk of this disease.

- GOOD SOURCE OF FIBER
- LOWFAT

Reprinted with permission from the American Institute for Cancer Research.

FIGURE 2.9
Food label and the U.S. RDA (U.S. Recommended Daily Allowance): A standard for nutrition labeling derived from the RDA.

people who are ill and may require additional nutrients.

If you are using the software available with this book, you need only record the foods by code and the number of servings based on the standard amounts given in the list of selected foods in Appendix A (the form provided in Figure 2A.3 of Lab 2A). A sample nutrient analysis printout is shown in Figures 2.16 and 2.17 at the end of this chapter.

Some of the most revealing information learned in a nutrient analysis is the source of fat intake in the diet. The average daily fat consumption in the American diet is about 37% of the total caloric intake, which greatly increases the risk for chronic diseases such as cardiovascular disease, cancer, diabetes, and obesity. Less than 30% of total calories should come from fat (see Figures 2.7 and 2.10).

As illustrated in Figure 2.11, each gram of carbohydrates and protein supplies the body with four calories, and fat provides nine calories per gram consumed (alcohol yields seven calories per gram). In this regard, just looking at the total grams consumed for each type of food can be misleading.

For example, a person who eats 160 grams of carbohydrates, 100 grams of fat, and 70 grams of protein has a total intake of 330 grams of food. This indicates that 33% of the total grams of food is in the form of fat (100 grams of fat ÷ 330 grams of total food × 100). In reality, almost half of that diet is fat calories.

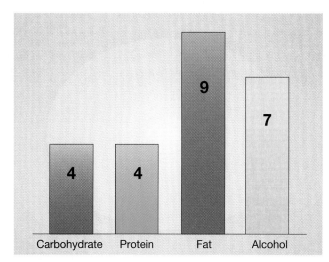

FIGURE 2.11
Caloric value of food (fuel nutrients).

In the sample diet, 640 calories are derived from carbohydrates (160 grams × 4 calories/gram), 280 calories from protein (70 grams × 4 calories/gram), and 900 calories from fat (100 grams × 9 calories/gram), for a total of 1,820 calories. If 900 calories are derived from fat, almost half of the total caloric intake is in the form of fat (900 ÷ 1,820 × 100 = 49.5%).

Beware of products labeled 97% fat-free. These products use weight and not percent of total calories as a measure of fat.

Each gram of fat provides nine calories. A useful guideline when figuring out the fat content of individual foods is: As shown in Figure 2.12, all you have to do is multiply the grams of fat by 9 and divide by the total calories in that particular food. You then multiply that number by 100 to get the percentage. For example, if a food label lists a total of 100 calories and 7 grams of fat, the fat content is 63% of total calories. This simple guideline can help you decrease the fat in your diet. The fat content of selected foods, given in grams and as a percent of total calories, is presented in Table 2.5.

Beware also of products labeled 97% fat-free. These products use weight and not percent of total calories as a measure of fat. As illustrated in Figure 2.12, many of these foods are still in the range of 30% fat calories.

FIGURE 2.10
An apple a day will not keep the doctor away if most meals are high in fat content.

TABLE 2.5
Fat Content of Selected Foods (Expressed in Grams and as a Percent of Total Calories)

Food	Amount	Calories	Fat (g)	Percent of Calories
Avocado	.5 medium	185	19	92
Bacon	2 slc.	86	8	84
Beef, ground (lean)	3 oz.	186	10	48
Beef, round steak	3 oz.	222	13	53
Beef, sirloin	3 oz.	329	27	74
Butter	1 tsp.	36	4	100
Cheese, American	1 oz.	100	8	72
Cheese, cheddar	1 oz.	114	9	71
Cheese, cottage (1% fat)	.5 cup	82	1	11
Cheese, cottage (4% fat)	.5 cup	112	5	40
Cheese, cream	1 oz.	99	8	73
Cheese, muenster	2 oz.	208	17	74
Cheese, parmesan	2 oz.	261	17	61
Cheese, swiss	2 oz.	214	16	67
Chicken, light meat, no skin	3 oz.	141	3	17
Chicken, dark meat, no skin	3 oz.	149	5	30
Egg (hard cooked)	1	72	5	63
Frankfurter	1	176	16	82
Halibut	3 oz.	144	6	38
Ice Cream (vanilla)	.5 cup	135	7	47
Ice Milk (vanilla)	.5 cup	100	3	27
Lamb leg, roast, trimmed	3 oz.	237	16	61
Margarine	1 tsp.	34	4	100
Mayonnaise	1 tsp.	36	4	100
Milk, skim	1 cup	88	0	3
Milk, low fat (2%)	1 cup	145	5	31
Milk, whole	1 cup	159	9	51
Nuts (brazil)	1 oz.	186	19	92
Salmon, broiled with butter	3 oz.	156	6	35
Sherbet	.5 cup	135	2	12
Shrimp, boiled	3 oz.	99	1	9
Tuna (canned, oil, drained)	3 oz.	167	7	38
Tuna (canned, water, drained)	3 oz.	126	1	1
Turkey, light and dark	3 oz.	162	5	28

ACHIEVING A BALANCED DIET

Anyone who has completed a nutrient analysis and has given careful attention to Tables 2.3 (vitamins) and 2.4 (minerals) probably will realize that a well-balanced diet entails eating a variety of foods and reducing daily intake of fats and sweets. The Healthy Eating Pyramid contained in Figure 2.13, recently published by the U.S. Department of Agri-culture, provides simple and sound instructions for nutrition. The pyramid contains five major food groups, along with fats, oils, and sweets, which are to be used sparingly. The daily recommended number of servings of the five major food groups are:

1. Six to eleven servings of the bread, cereal, rice, and pasta group.
2. Three to five servings of the vegetable group.
3. Two to four servings of the fruit group.

Nutrition Facts

Serving Size 1 cup (240 ml)
Servings Per Container 4

Amount Per Serving

Calories 120   Calories from Fat 45

	% Daily Value*
Total Fat 5g	**8%**
Saturated Fat 3g	**15%**
Cholesterol 20mg	**7%**
Sodium 120mg	**5%**
Total Carbohydrate 12g	**4%**
Dietary Fiber 0g	**0%**
Sugars 12g	
Protein 8g	

Vitamin A 10%	•	Vitamin C	4%
Calcium 30%	•	Iron	0%

*Percent Daily Values are based on a 2,000 calorie diet. Your daily values may be higher or lower depending on your calorie needs:

		Calories	2,000	2,500
Total Fat	Less than		65g	80g
Sat Fat	Less than		20g	25g
Cholesterol	Less than		300mg	300mg
Sodium	Less than		2,400mg	2,400mg
Total Carbohydrate			300g	375g
Fiber			25g	30g

Calories per gram:
Fat 9 • Carbohydrate 4 • Protein 4

Percent Fat Calories = (gr of fat × 9)
÷ calories per serving × 100

5 g of fat × 9 calories per g of fat =
45 calories from fat

45 calories from fat ÷ 120 calories per serving
× 100 = 38% fat

FIGURE 2.12
Computation for fat content in food.

4. Two to three servings of the milk, yogurt, and cheese group.
5. Two to three servings of the meat, poultry, fish, dry beans, eggs, and nuts group.

As illustrated in the Healthy Eating Pyramid, grains, vegetables, and fruits provide the nutritional base for a healthy diet. Daily fruits and vegetables should include as a minimum, one good source of vitamin A (apricots, cantaloupe, broccoli, carrots, pumpkin, dark leafy vegetables) and one good source of vitamin C (citrus fruit, kiwi fruit, cantaloupe, strawberries, broccoli, cabbage, cauliflower, green pepper).

Milk, poultry, fish, and meats are to be consumed in moderation. Milk should be skim, and milk products should be low-fat. Three ounces of poultry, fish, or meat daily is the recommendation and not to exceed 6 ounces per day. All visible fat and skin should be trimmed off meats and poultry before cooking. Egg consumption should be limited to no more than three eggs per week.

Learning how to calculate percent fat calories in food can help you make better food selections.

As an aid in balancing your diet, the form given in Figure 2B.1 in Lab 2B enables you to record your daily food intake. This record is much easier to keep than the complete dietary analysis. Make as many copies of this lab as the number of days you wish to record. Whenever you have something to eat, record, in Figure 2B.1, the food and the amount eaten. Record this information immediately after each meal so you will be able to keep track of your actual food intake more easily.

If you eat twice the amount of a standard serving, double the number of servings. Evaluate your diet by checking whether you ate the minimum required servings for each food group. If you meet the minimum required servings at the end of each day, you are doing quite well in balancing your diet.

Restructure your meals on the plate so rice, pasta, beans, breads, and vegetables are in the center, meats are on the side and are added primarily for flavoring, and desserts consist of fruits. Substitute low or nonfat milk and milk products (Figure 2.14). This is another strategy to help you enjoy a healthy diet, prevent disease, and improve your overall quality of life.

FIGURE 2.13
Healthy Eating Pyramid: A guide to daily food choices.

FIGURE 2.13 (continued)
Healthy Eating Pyramid: A guide to daily food choices.

FIGURE 2.14
Contemporary Nutrition Concept: Restructuring your meals so that rice, pasta, beans, breads, and vegetables are in the center of the plate; meats are on the side and added primarily for flavoring; fruits are used for desserts; and low or nonfat milk products are used.

NUTRIENT SUPPLEMENTATION

According to the Food and Drug Administration, four of every 10 adults in the United States take nutrient supplements daily, and one in every seven has a nutrient intake almost eight times the RDA. In reality, vitamin and mineral requirements for the body can be met by consuming as few as 1,200 calories per day, as long as the diet contains the recommended servings from the five food groups.

Water-soluble vitamins cannot be stored as long as fat-soluble vitamins. The body readily excretes excessive intakes. Small amounts, however, can be retained for weeks or months in various organs and tissues of the body. Fat-soluble vitamins, on the other hand, are stored in fatty tissue. Therefore, daily intake of these vitamins is not as crucial. Too much vitamin A and vitamin D actually can be detrimental to health.

People should not take megadoses of vitamins. For most vitamins, a megadose is 10 times the RDA or more. For vitamins A and D, it is respectively five and two times the RDA. Mineral doses should not exceed three times the RDA.

No standard percentage above the RDA is established to guide us in determining the level at which a high dose of a given nutrient may cause health problems. For some nutrients, a dose of five times the RDA taken over several months may create problems. For others, it may not pose any threat to human health.

Iron supplementation frequently is recommended for women who have heavy menstrual flow. Iron deficiency (determined through blood testing) is common in these women. Some pregnant and lactating women also may require supplements. According to 1990 guidelines by the National Academy of Science, the average pregnant woman who eats an adequate amount of a variety of foods needs only to take a low dose of daily iron supplement. Women who are pregnant with more than one baby may need additional supplements. In the above instances, supplements should be taken under a physician's supervision.

Other people who may benefit from supplementation are alcoholics and street-drug users who do not have a balanced diet, smokers, strict vegetarians, individuals on extremely low-calorie diets, elderly people who don't eat balanced meals regularly, and newborn infants (usually given a single dose of vitamin K to prevent abnormal bleeding).

For healthy people with a balanced diet, most supplements do not seem to provide additional benefits. They do not help people run faster, jump higher, relieve stress, improve sexual prowess, cure a common cold, or boost energy levels.

Supplements do not help healthy people run faster, jump higher, relieve stress, improve sexual prowess, cure a common cold, or boost energy levels.

Much research currently is being done to study the effects of antioxidant supplements (vitamins C, E, beta-carotene, and the mineral selenium) in thwarting several chronic diseases (see the discussion earlier in this chapter on vitamins). Antioxidants are believed to offer protection, but the effects of supplements have not yet been clearly established.

The benefits of antioxidants have been researched primarily through diet alone, by studying people who eat foods high in antioxidants and not through supplements. Researchers do not know if the protective effects are caused by the antioxidants themselves, in combination with other nutrients, or actually by some other nutrients in food that have not yet been investigated. In the case of selenium, excessive amounts may be toxic. A diet with substantial fruits, vegetables, and grains is the best means to obtain ample amounts of antioxidants.

Many people who regularly eat fast foods high in fat content or too many sweets think they need vitamin and mineral supplementation to balance their diet. This is another fallacy about nutrition. The problem in these cases is not a lack of vitamins and minerals but, instead, a diet too high in calories, fat, and sodium. Supplementation will not offset these poor eating habits.

If you think your diet is not balanced, you first need to determine which nutrients are missing (see nutrient analysis). Then use the Healthy Eating Pyramid and the vitamin and mineral charts in this chapter, and eat more of the foods high in antioxidants and those with nutrients that are deficient in your diet.

NUTRITION FOR ATHLETES

The two main fuels that supply energy for physical activity are glucose and fat (fatty acids). The body uses amino acids, derived from proteins, as an energy substrate when glucose is low, such as during fasting or on a low carbohydrate diet.

Glucose is derived from foods high in carbohydrates such as breads, cereals, grains, pasta, beans, fruits, vegetables, and sweets in general. Glucose is stored in the form of glycogen in muscles and the liver. As noted earlier in the chapter, fatty acids are derived from the breakdown of fats. Unlike glucose, an almost unlimited supply of fatty acids, stored as fat in the body, can be used during exercise.

During resting conditions fat supplies about two-thirds of the energy to sustain the vital processes. During exercise the body uses both glucose and fat in combination to supply the energy demands. The proportion of fat to glucose changes with the intensity of exercise. When exercising below 70% of the individual's maximal work capacity, fat is used as the primary energy substrate. As the intensity of exercise increases, so does the percentage of glucose utilization, up to 100% during maximal work sustained for 2 to 3 minutes.

In general, athletes do not require special supplementation or any other special type of diet. Unless the diet is deficient in basic nutrients, no special, secret, or magic diet will help people perform better or develop faster as a result of what they eat. As long as the diet is balanced, based on a large variety of nutrients from the basic food groups, athletes do not require supplements. Even in strength training and body building, no additional protein in excess of 20% of total daily caloric intake is necessary.

The main differences between a sedentary person and a highly active individual is in the total number of calories required daily and the amount of carbohydrate intake during bouts of prolonged physical activity. During training, people consume more calories because of the greater energy expenditure required as a result of intense physical training.

CARBOHYDRATE SUPPLEMENTATION

The regular diet also should be altered during several days of heavy aerobic training or when a person is going to participate in a long-distance event of more than 90 minutes (for example, marathon, triathlon, road cycling). As an average, people store between 1,500 and 2,000 calories in the form of glycogen. About 75% of the glycogen is stored in muscle tissue. During prolonged exercise glycogen is broken down into glucose, which then is readily available to the muscle for energy production. In comparison to fat, glucose frequently is referred to as the "high octane fuel" because it provides about 6% more energy per unit of oxygen consumed. Heavy training over several consecutive days leads to glycogen depletion at a faster rate than it can be replaced through the diet. Glycogen depletion with heavy training is common in athletes. Signs of depletion include chronic fatigue, difficulty in maintaining accustomed exercise intensity, and lower performance.

During consecutive days of exhaustive physical training, a carbohydrate-rich diet, 70% of total daily caloric intake, is recommended. This diet often restores glycogen levels in 24 hours. Along with the high-carbohydrate diet, a day of rest often is needed to allow the muscles to recover from glycogen depletion following days of intense training.

By following a special diet/exercise regimen five days before a long-distance event, highly trained (aerobically) individuals are capable of storing two to three times the amount of glycogen found in the average person. Athletic performance is enhanced for long distance events of more than 90 minutes by eating a regular balanced diet along with intensive physical training the fifth and fourth days before the event, followed by a diet high in carbohydrates (about 70%) and a gradual decrease in training intensity the three days before the event.

The amount of glycogen stored as a result of a carbohydrate-rich diet does not seem to be related to the proportion of complex and simple carbohydrates. Intake of simple carbohydrate (sugar) can be raised while on a 70% carbohydrate diet, as long as 48% of the total calories still are derived from complex carbohydrates. The latter, however, provide more nutrients and fiber, making them a better choice for a healthier diet.

AMINO ACID SUPPLEMENTS

A myth regarding athletic performance is the unnecessary use of protein (amino acid) supplements to increase muscle mass. The claims and safety of these products have not been proven scientifically. The RDA for protein is .8 grams per kilogram of body weight.

Most athletes, including weight lifters and body builders, automatically will increase their caloric intake during periods of intense training. As caloric intake increases, so does the intake of protein, approaching in many instances 2 or more grams per kilogram of body weight. This amount is more than enough to build and repair muscle tissue. Strength-training athletes typically consume between 3 and 4 grams per kilogram of body weight.

People who take costly free-amino acid supplements are led to believe that this contributes to the development of muscle mass. The human body cannot distinguish between amino acids obtained from food or through supplements. Excess protein either is used for energy or is turned into fat.

With amino acid supplements, each capsule provides up to 500 milligrams of amino acids and no additional nutrients. Three ounces of meat or fish provide more than 20,000 milligrams of amino acids along with other essential nutrients such as iron, niacin, and thiamin.

Proponents of free-amino acid supplements further claim that only a small amount of amino acids in food are absorbed and that free-amino acids are more readily absorbed than protein food. Neither claim is correct. The human body absorbs and utilizes between 85% and 99% of all protein from food intake. The body handles whole proteins better than single amino acids predigested in the laboratory setting.

Amino acid supplementation even can be dangerous to the body. Supplementation of a group of chemically similar amino acids often prevents the absorption of other amino acids, potentially causing critical imbalances and toxicities. Long-term risks associated with amino acid supplementation have not been determined.

The rate of absorption provides no additional benefit because building muscle takes hours and not minutes. Muscle overload through heavy training, not supplementation, builds muscle. Expensive protein supplements benefit only those who stand to gain financial benefits from selling them.

SPECIAL NUTRITION CONSIDERATIONS FOR WOMEN

BONE HEALTH AND OSTEOPOROSIS

Osteoporosis has been defined as the *softening, deterioration, or loss of total body bone.* Bones, primarily of the hip, wrist, and spine, become so weak and brittle that they fracture readily.

Osteoporosis is a preventable condition. The process begins slowly in the third and fourth decade of life. Women are especially susceptible after menopause because of the accompanying estrogen loss, which increases the rate at which bone mass is broken down.

Approximately 15 to 20 million women in the United States have osteoporosis, and about 1.5 million fractures are attributed to this condition each year. An estimated 30,000 to 60,000 of the 200,000 women with hip fractures die of complications resulting from these fractures. According to Dr. Barbara Drinkwater, a leading researcher in this area, "Shocking as these figures are, they cannot adequately convey the pain and deterioration in the quality of life of women who suffer the crippling effects of osteoporotic fractures."[5]

In maximizing bone density in young women and decreasing the rate of bone loss later in life, the importance of normal estrogen levels, adequate calcium intake, and physical activity cannot be overemphasized. All three factors are crucial in preventing osteoporosis (Figure 2.15). The absence of any one

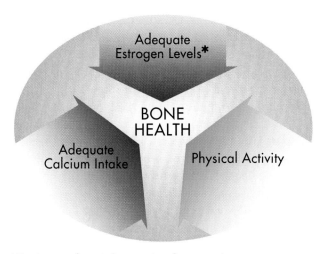

Adequate
Estrogen Levels*

BONE
HEALTH

Adequate
Calcium Intake

Physical Activity

*Most important factor in the prevention of osteoporosis.

FIGURE 2.15
Variables that impact the prevention of osteoporosis.

of these three factors leads to bone loss for which the other two factors never completely compensate.

Prevention of osteoporosis begins early in life by having enough calcium in the diet (the RDA is 800 to 1,200 mg per day) and by participating in exercise. The calcium RDA can be met easily through diet alone.

Along with adequate calcium intake, an additional amount of vitamin D may be needed for optimal calcium absorption. Table 2.6 provides a list of selected foods and their respective calcium content. Many experts recommend that women after age 45

should get 1,500 mg of calcium per day and men, 1,000 mg.

Also, high protein intake may affect calcium absorption by the body. The more protein eaten, the higher the calcium content in the urine. This might be the reason why countries with a high protein intake, like the U.S., also have the highest rates of osteoporosis.

Weight-bearing types of exercise such as walking, jogging, and weight training are especially helpful. Not only do they tone up muscles, but they also produce stronger and thicker bones.

Current studies indicate that people who are active have denser bone mineral than inactive people do. Similar to other benefits of participation in exercise, there is no such thing as "bone in the bank." To have good bone health, people need to participate in a regular lifetime exercise program.

Prevailing research also tells us that estrogen is the most important factor in preventing bone loss. In one study, lumbar bone density in women who had always had regular menstrual cycles exceeded that of women with a history of oligomenorrhea (irregular cycles) and amenorrhea (cessation of menstruation) interspaced with regular cycles. Furthermore, the lumbar density of these two groups of women was higher than that of women who had never had regular menstrual cycles.

Following menopause, every woman should consider hormone replacement therapy and discuss it

TABLE 2.6
Low-Fat Calcium-Rich Foods

Food	Amount	Calcium (mg)	Calories	Calories From Fat
Beans, red kidney, cooked	1 cup	70	218	4%
Beet, greens, cooked	1/2 cup	72	13	—
Broccoli, cooked, drained	1 sm stalk	123	36	—
Burrito, bean	1	173	307	28%
Cottage cheese, 2% lowfat	1/2 cup	78	103	18%
Milk, nonfat, powdered	1 tbsp	52	27	1%
Milk, skim	1 cup	296	88	3%
Ice milk (vanilla)	1/2 cup	102	100	27%
Instant breakfast, whole milk	1 cup	301	280	26%
Kale, cooked, drained	1/2 cup	103	22	—
Okra, cooked, drained	1/2 cup	74	23	—
Shrimp, boiled	3 oz.	99	99	9%
Spinach, raw	1 cup	51	14	—
Yogurt, fruit	1 cup	345	231	8%
Yogurt, lowfat, plain	1 cup	271	160	20%

with her physician. Women who have estrogen therapy do not lose bone mineral density at the rate of women who do not have estrogen therapy. Neither exercise nor calcium supplementation will offset the damaging effects of lower estrogen levels.

For instance, amenorrheic athletes (who have lower estrogen levels) have lower bone mineral density than even non-athletes with normal estrogen levels. One study[6] showed that amenorrheic athletes at age 25 have the bones of 52-year-old women. Furthermore, a sedentary woman with normal estrogen levels has better bone mineral density than an active amenorrheic athlete. Many experts believe the best predictor of bone mineral content is the history of menstrual regularity.

IRON DEFICIENCY

Iron is a key element of hemoglobin in blood, which carries oxygen from the lungs to all tissues of the body. The RDA of iron for adult women is 15 mg per day (10 mg for men).

According to a survey by the U.S. Department of Agriculture, 19- to 50-year-old women in the United States consumed only 60% of the RDA for iron. People who do not have enough iron in the body can develop iron deficiency anemia, in which the concentration of hemoglobin in the red blood cells is less than it should be.

Physically active women also may have a greater than average need for iron. Heavy training creates a demand for iron that is higher than the recommended intake because small amounts of iron are lost through sweat, urine, and stools. Mechanical trauma, caused by pounding the feet on pavement during extensive jogging, also may lead to the destruction of iron-containing red blood cells.

A large percentage of female endurance athletes is reported to have iron deficiency. Blood ferritin levels, a measure of stored iron in the human body, should be checked frequently in women who participate in intense physical training.

Individuals vary in their rates of iron absorption and iron loss. In most cases, though, people can get enough iron by eating more iron-rich foods such as beans, peas, green leafy vegetables, enriched grain products, egg yolk, fish, and lean meats. Although organ meats, such as liver, are especially good sources, they also are high in cholesterol. A list of foods high in iron content is given in Table 2.7.

NATIONAL ACADEMY OF SCIENCE'S DIETARY RECOMMENDATIONS

Based on the available scientific research on nutrition and health and the current dietary habits of the American people, the National Academy of Science's

TABLE 2.7
Iron-Rich Foods

Food	Amount	Iron (mg)	Calories	Cholesterol	Calories From Fat
Beans, red kidney, cooked	1 cup	4.4	218	0	4%
Beef, ground lean	3 oz.	3.0	186	81	48%
Beef, sirloin	3 oz.	2.5	329	77	74%
Beef, liver, fried	3 oz.	7.5	195	345	42%
Beet, greens, cooked	1/2 cup	1.4	13	0	—
Broccoli, cooked, drained	1 sm stalk	1.1	36	0	—
Burrito, bean	1	2.4	307	14	28%
Egg, hard, cooked	1	1.0	72	250	63%
Farina (Cream of Wheat), cooked	1/2 cup	6.0	51	0	—
Instant breakfast, whole milk	1 cup	8.0	280	33	26%
Peas, frozen, cooked, drained	1/2 cup	1.5	55	0	—
Shrimp, boiled	3 oz.	2.7	99	128	9%
Spinach, raw	1 cup	1.7	14	0	—
Vegetables, mixed, cooked	1 cup	2.4	116	0	—

Committee on Diet and Health in 1989 issued dietary recommendations for healthy North American adults and children. These guidelines potentially can reduce the risk of developing certain chronic diseases. The committee's recommendations are:[17]

■ Reduce fat intake to 30% or less of total calories. Reduce saturated fatty acid intake to less than 10% of total calories and the intake of cholesterol to no more than 300 mg daily. Intake of fat and cholesterol can be lowered by substituting fish, poultry without skin, lean meats, and low or non-fat dairy products for fatty meats and whole-milk dairy products; by choosing more vegetables, fruits, cereals, and legumes; and by limiting oils, fats, egg yolks, and fried and other fatty foods.

■ Every day eat five or more servings of a combination of vegetables and fruits, especially green and yellow vegetables and citrus fruits. Also, increase intake of starches and other complex carbohydrates by eating six or more servings daily of a combination of breads, cereals, and legumes.

   An average serving is equal to a half cup for most fresh or cooked vegetables, fruits, dry or cooked cereals and legumes, one medium piece of fresh fruit, one slice of bread, or one roll or muffin. The committee also recommends increasing the intake of carbohydrates to more than 55% of total calories.

■ Maintain protein intake at moderate levels (not to exceed 1.6 grams per kilogram of body weight or twice the RDA).

■ Balance food intake and physical activity to maintain appropriate body weight (see Chapter 4 for a comprehensive weight control program).

■ If you drink alcoholic beverages, limit consumption to the equivalent of less than an ounce of pure alcohol in a single day. This translates into two cans of beer, two small glasses of wine, or two average cocktails. If pregnant, avoid alcoholic beverages altogether.

■ Limit total daily intake of salt to 6 grams or less. Limit the use of salt in cooking, and do not add it to food at the table. Sparingly consume salty, highly processed salty, salt-preserved, and salt-pickled foods.

■ Maintain adequate calcium intake.

■ Do not take supplements in excess of the RDA in any one day.

■ Maintain an optimal intake of fluoride, particularly during the years of primary and secondary tooth formation and growth.

PROPER NUTRITION: A LIFETIME PRESCRIPTION FOR HEALTHY LIVING

Proper nutrition, a sound exercise program, and quitting smoking (for those who smoke) are the three factors that do the most for health, longevity, and quality of life. Achieving and maintaining a balanced diet is not as difficult as most people think. If parents were to do a better job of teaching and reinforcing proper nutrition habits in early youth, we would not have the magnitude of nutrition-related health problems we do.

Children tend to eat the way their parents do. If parents adopt a healthy diet, children most likely will follow. The difficult part for most people is retraining themselves to follow a lifetime healthy nutrition plan — a diet that includes lots of grains, legumes, fruits, vegetables, and low-fat dairy products, with moderate use of animal protein, junk food, sodium, and alcohol.

In spite of the ample scientific evidence linking poor dietary habits to early disease and mortality rates, most people are not willing to change their eating patterns. Even when faced with obesity, elevated blood lipids, hypertension, and other nutrition-related conditions, people do not change. The motivating factor to change one's eating habits seems to be a major health breakdown, such as a heart attack, a stroke, or cancer. By this time the damage already has been done. In many cases it is irreversible, and for some, fatal.

An ounce of prevention is worth a pound of cure. The sooner you implement the dietary guidelines presented in this chapter, the better will be your chances of preventing chronic diseases and reaching a higher state of wellness.

L A B O R A T O R Y   E X P E R I E N C E

LAB 2A
Nutrient Analysis

Lab Preparation
Prior to your lab, keep a 3-day record of all food consumed, using Figure 2A.1 from Lab 2. You also should record all of the nutrients from the list of Nutritive Values of Selected Foods (Appendix A). Note that if your serving is twice the standard amount, you should double all of the nutrient contents. If you have only half a serving, record only half of the contents, and so forth. You also should total your nutrient intake for each day before the lab session. If you are using the computer software available with this book, you will need only record the codes and the number of servings eaten (use Figure 2A.3) prior to your lab session.

LAB 2B
Balancing Your Diet

Lab Preparation
None required. This lab will be given as homework to follow up the nutrient analysis (see Lab 2B).

R E F E R E N C E S

1. American Medical Association: Council on Scientific Affairs. "Dietary Fiber and Health." *Journal of the American Medical Association* 262:542–546, 1989.

2. Brownell, K. and J. P. Forey. *Handbook of Eating Disorders* (New York: Basic Books, 1986).

3. Cristian, J. L. and J. L. Greger. *Nutrition for Living* (Menlo Park, CA: Benjamin/Cummings Publishing, 1991).

4. Coleman, E. L. *Eating for Endurance* (Palo Alto, CA: Bull Publishing, 1992).

5. Drinkwater, B. L. *Nutrition, Exercise, and Bone Health.* (Seattle: Pacific Medical Center, 1990).

6. Drinkwater, B. L. "Osteoporosis and the Female Masters Athlete." In *Sports Medicine for the Mature Athlete.* edited by J. R. Sutton, and R. M. Brock (Benchmark Press, 1986: pp. 353–359).

7. Drinkwater, B. L., B. Bruemner, and C. H. Chestnut III. "Menstrual History as a Determinant of Current Bone Density in Young Athletes," *Journal of the American Medical Association* 263 (1990): 545–548.

8. Gaziano, J. M. and C. H. Hennekens. "A New Look at What Can Unclog Your Arteries," *Executive Health Report* 27(8) 1991:16.

9. Girdano, D. A., D. Dusek, and G. S. Everly. *Experiencing Health* (Englewood Cliffs, NJ: Prentice Hall, 1985).

10. "How to Balance Your Diet." *Fit,* April 1983, pp. 46, 47.

11. Hoeger, W. W. K. and S. A. Hoeger. *Lifetime Physical Fitness and Wellness* (Englewood, CO: Morton Publishing, 1992).

12. Hoeger, W. W. K. *The Complete Guide for the Development & Implementation of Health Promotion Programs* (Englewood, CO: Morton Publishing Co., 1987).

13. Kanders, B., D. W. Demster, and R. Lindsay. "Interaction of Calcium Nutrition and Physical Activity on Bone Mass in Young Women," *Journal of Bone Mineral Research* 3 (1988):145–149.

14. Kirschmann, J. D. *Nutrition Almanac* (New York: McGraw-Hill Book Company, 1990).

15. S. M. Kleiner, S. M. "Seafood and Your Heart," *Physician and Sportsmedicine* 18(4) 1990:19–20.

16. Morgan, B. L. G. *The Lifelong Nutrition Guide* (Englewood Cliffs, NJ: Prentice-Hall, 1983).

17. National Academy of Sciences, *Diet and Health: Implications for Reducing Chronic Disease Risk.* (Washington, DC: National Academy Press, 1989).

18. National Academy of Sciences, Institute of Medicine. *Eat for Life: the Food and Nutrition Board's Guide to Reducing Your Risk of Chronic Disease.* edited by C. E. Woteki and P. R. Thomas (Washington, DC: National Academy Press, 1992).

19. "The Fallacies of Taking Supplementation," *Tufts University Diet & Nutrition Letter,* July 1987.

20. Thornton, J. S. "Feast or Famine: Eating Disorders in Athletes." *Physician and Sportsmedicine* 18(4) (1990):116–122.

21. "Use a Variety of Fibers," *Health Letter,* March 1982.

22. Whitney, E. N. and S. R. Rolfes. *Understanding Nutrition* (St. Paul, MN: West Publishing, 1993).

NUTRIENT ANALYSIS
FITNESS & WELLNESS SERIES
by Werner W.K. Hoeger & Sharon A. Hoeger
Morton Publishing Company -- Englewood, Colorado

Jane R. Moore   Date: 02-12-1992
Age: 20
Body Weight: 141 lbs (64.0 kg)
Activity Rating: Moderate

Food Intake Day One

Food	Amount	Calo-ries	Pro-tein gm	Fat gm	Sat Fat gm	Cho-les-terol mg	Car-bohy-drate gm	Cal-cium mg	Iron mg	Sodium mg	Vit A I.U.	Thi-amin mg	Ribo-fla-vin mg	Nia-cin mg	Vit C mg
Cocoa/hot/with whole milk	1 cup	218	9.1	9	6.1	33	26	298	0.8	123	318	0.10	0.44	0.4	2
Egg/scrambled w/milk butter	1 egg(s)	95	6.0	7	3.0	282	1	54	0.9	176	510	0.04	0.18	0.0	0
Bread/white	2 slice(s)	136	4.4	2	0.4	0	26	42	1.2	254	0	0.12	0.10	1.2	0
Butter	2 tsp	72	0.0	8	0.8	24	0	2	0.0	92	320	0.00	0.00	0.0	0
Milk/whole	1 c	159	9.0	9	5.1	34	12	288	0.1	120	350	0.07	0.40	0.2	2
Bread/whole wheat	2 slice(s)	122	5.2	2	1.2	0	24	50	1.6	264	0	0.12	0.06	1.4	0
Tuna/canned/oil/drained	1.5 oz.	84	12.5	4	0.9	30	0	4	0.8	69	35	0.02	0.05	5.1	0
Mayonnaise	2 tsp.	72	0.0	8	1.4	6	0	2	0.0	56	26	0.00	0.00	0.0	0
Pickles/dill	1 large	15	0.9	0	0.0	0	3	35	1.4	1,928	140	0.00	0.03	0.0	8
Potato/French fried	20 strips	428	6.8	20	3.4	0	56	24	2.0	10	0	0.20	0.12	4.8	32
Tomato sauce (catsup)	1 tbsp.	16	0.3	0	0.0	0	4	3	0.1	156	105	0.01	0.01	0.2	2
Apple/raw	1 med	80	0.3	1	0.0	0	20	10	0.4	1	120	0.04	0.03	0.1	6
Soda pop/root beer	12 oz.	140	0.0	0	0.0	0	36	17	0.2	45	0	0.00	0.00	0.0	0
Coleslaw	1 c	173	1.6	17	1.0	5	6	53	0.5	144	190	0.06	0.06	0.4	35
Spaghetti/meat balls/sauce	1 c	332	18.6	12	3.0	75	39	124	3.7	1,009	1,590	0.25	0.30	4.0	22
Pie/apple	1 pc. (3.5 in.)	302	2.6	13	3.5	120	45	9	0.4	355	40	0.02	0.02	0.5	1
Totals Day One		2,444	77.3	111	29.8	609	298	1,015	14.1	4,802	3,744	1.0	1.8	18.3	110

FIGURE 2.16
Computerized Nutritional Analysis: Sample food list.

NUTRITIONAL ANALYSIS: DAILY ANALYSIS, AVERAGE, AND
RECOMMENDED DIETARY ALLOWANCE (RDA) COMPARISON

	Calo-ries	Pro-tein gm	Fat %	Sat Fat %	Cho-les-terol mg	Car-bohy-drate %	Cal-cium mg	Iron mg	Sodium mg	Vit A I.U.	Thi-amin mg	Ribo-fla-vin mg	Nia-cin mg	Vit C mg
Day One	2,444	77.3	40	11	609	48	1,015	14.1	4,802	3,744	1.0	1.8	18.3	110
Day Two	2,234	105.1	44	12	536	37	639	20.6	5,719	1,902	1.1	1.7	21.6	60
Day Three	2,491	92.0	43	19	603	43	1,787	14.7	3,919	6,351	1.6	3.5	18.2	55
Three Day Average	2,390	91.5	42	14	583	43	1,147	16.5	4,813	3,999	1.3	2.3	19.4	75
RDA	1,904*	51.2	<30	<10	<300	50>	1,200	15.0	1,904	4,000	1.1	1.3	15.0	60

*Estimated caloric value based on gender, current body weight, and activity rating (does not include
additional calories burned through a physical exercise program).

OBSERVATIONS

Daily caloric intake should be distributed in such a way that 50 to 60 percent of the total calories come from carbohydrates and
less than 30 percent of the total calories from fat. Protein intake should be about .8 to 1.5 grams per kilogram of body weight or
about 15 to 20 percent of the total calories. Pregnant women need to consume an additional 15 grams of daily protein, while lactating women should have an extra 20 grams of daily protein (these additional grams of protein are already included in the RDA values
for pregnant and lactating women). Saturated fats should constitute less than 10 percent of the total daily caloric intake.
Please note that the daily listings of food intake express the amount of carbohydrates, fat, saturated fat, and protein in grams.
However, on the daily analysis and the RDA, only the amount of protein is given in grams. The amount of carbohydrates, fat, and saturated fat are expressed in percent of total calories. The final percentages are based on the total grams and total calories for all
days analyzed, not from the average of the daily percentages.

If your average intake for protein, fat, saturated fat, cholesterol, or sodium is high, refer to the daily listings and decrease the
intake of foods that are high in those nutrients. If your diet is deficient in carbohydrates, calcium, iron, vitamin A, thiamin, riboflavin, niacin, or vitamin C, refer to the statements below and increase your intake of the indicated foods or consult the list of
selected foods in your textbook.

Caloric intake may be too high.

Total fat intake is too high.

Saturated fat intake is too high, which increases your risk for coronary heart disease.

Dietary cholesterol intake is too high. An average consumption of dietary cholesterol above 300 mg/day increases the risk for coronary heart disease. Do you know your blood cholesterol level?

Carbohydrate intake is low. Good sources of carbohydrates are whole grain breads and cereals, pasta, rice, fruits, and vegetables
such as potatoes and peas.

Calcium intake is low. Good sources of calcium are milk, yogurt, cheese, green leafy vegetables, dried beans, sardines, and salmon.

Sodium intake is high.

Vitamin A intake is low. Foods high in vitamin A include skim milk fortified with vit. A, cheese, butter, fortified margarine, eggs
(yolk), liver, and dark green/yellow fruits and vegetables.

FIGURE 2.17
Computerized Nutritional Analysis: Sample daily analysis, average, and recommended dietary allowance comparison.

BODY COMPOSITION ASSESSMENT

KEY CONCEPTS

Body composition
Recommended body weight
Healthy weight
Percent body fat

LABS

Lean body mass
Essential fat
Storage fat
Hydrostatic weighing
Skinfold thickness
Girth measurements
Bioelectrical impedance
Waist-to-hip ratio
Body mass index

OBJECTIVES

■ Define body composition and its relationship to recommended body weight assessment.

■ Learn the difference between essential fat and storage fat.

■ Understand the methodology used to assess body composition according to hydrostatic weighing, skinfold thickness, and girth measurements.

■ Understand the importance of waist-to-hip ratio and body mass index.

■ Be able to determine recommended weight according to recommended percent body fat values.

Body composition is used in reference to the *fat and nonfat components of the human body.* The fat component usually is called fat mass or percent body fat. The nonfat component is termed lean body mass.

For many years people relied on height/weight charts to determine recommended body weight. We now know, however, that these tables can be highly inaccurate for many people and they fail to identify critical fat values associated with higher risk for disease. The proper way to determine **recommended weight** is through body composition by finding out what percent of total body weight is fat and what amount is lean tissue.

Once the fat percentage is known, recommended body weight can be calculated from recommended body fat. Recommended body weight, also called "**healthy weight**," is defined as the *body weight at which there seems to be no harm to human health.* This includes the absence of any medical condition that would improve with weight loss and a fat distribution pattern that is not associated with increased risk for illness.

Although various techniques for determining percent body fat were developed several years ago, many people still are unaware of these procedures and continue to depend on height/weight charts to find out their recommended body weight. The standard height/weight tables were first published in 1912. They were based on average weights (including shoes and clothing) for men and women who obtained life insurance policies between 1888 and 1905. The recommended body weight on these tables is obtained according to gender, height, and frame size. Because no scientific guidelines are given to determine frame size, most people choose their frame size based on the column in which the weight comes closest to their own!

To determine whether people are truly obese or falsely at recommended body weight, body composition must be established. Obesity is related to an excess of body fat. If body weight is the only criterion, an individual easily can be overweight, according to height/weight charts, yet not have any excess body fat. Football players, body builders, weight lifters, and other athletes with large muscle size are typical examples. Some of these athletes who appear to be 20 or 30 pounds overweight really have little body fat.

The inaccuracy of height/weight charts was illustrated clearly when a young man who weighed about 225 pounds applied to join a city police force but was turned down without having been granted an interview. The reason? He was "too fat," according to the height/weight charts. When this young man's body composition later was assessed at a preventive medicine clinic, he was shocked to find out that only 5% of his total body weight was in the form of fat — considerably lower than the recommended standard. In the words of the technical director of the clinic, "The only way this fellow could come down to the chart's target weight would have been through surgical removal of a large amount of his muscle tissue."

At the other end of the spectrum, some people who weigh very little and are viewed by many as skinny or underweight actually can be classified as obese because of their high body fat content. People who weigh as little as 100 pounds but are more than 30% fat (about one-third of their total body weight) are not uncommon. These cases are found more readily in sedentary people and those who are always dieting. Physical inactivity and constant negative caloric balance both lead to a loss in lean body mass (see Chapter 4). From these examples, body weight alone clearly does not always tell the true story.

ESSENTIAL AND STORAGE FAT

Total fat in the human body is classified into two types: essential fat and storage fat. Essential fat is needed for normal physiological functions, and without it, human health deteriorates. This essential fat constitutes about 3% of the total fat in men and 12% in women. The percentage is higher in women because it includes sex-specific fat, such as that found in the breast tissue, the uterus, and other sex-related fat deposits.

Storage fat is the fat stored in adipose tissue, mostly beneath the skin (subcutaneous fat) and around major organs in the body. This fat serves three basic functions:

1. As an insulator to retain body heat.

2. As energy substrate for metabolism.
3. As padding against physical trauma to the body.

The amount of storage fat does not differ between men and women, except that men tend to store fat around the waist and women more so around the hips and thighs.

TECHNIQUES FOR ASSESSING BODY COMPOSITION

Body composition can be determined through several different procedures. The most common techniques are: (a) hydrostatic or underwater weighing, (b) skinfold thickness, (c) girth measurements, and (d) bioelectrical impedance.

When using the different techniques, slightly different values are obtained. Therefore, when assessing body composition, the same technique should be used for pre- and post-test comparisons.

HYDROSTATIC WEIGHING

Hydrostatic weighing (Figure 3.1) has been called the "gold standard" of body composition. Almost all other techniques to determine body composition are validated against hydrostatic weighing. It is the most accurate technique available if it is administered properly and if the individual is able to perform the test adequately.

The procedure for hydrostatic weighing, as outlined in Figure 3.2, requires a considerable amount

FIGURE 3.1
Hydrostatic weighing technique for body composition assessment.

HYDROSTATIC WEIGHING

A small tank or pool, an autopsy scale, and a submergible chair are needed. The scale should measure up to about 10 kilograms (kg) and should be readable to the nearest 100th of a kilogram. The chair is suspended from the scale and submerged in a tank of water or pool measuring at least 5 × 5 × 5 feet (see Figure 3.1). A swimming pool can also be used in place of the tank.

The procedure for the technician is:

1. Ask the person to be weighed to fast for approximately six to eight hours and to have a bladder and bowel movement prior to underwater weighing.

2. Measure the individual's residual lung volume (RV or amount of air left in the lungs following complete exhalation). If no equipment (spirometer) is available to measure the residual volume, estimate it using the following predicting equations* (to convert inches to centimeters, multiply inches by 2.54):

   Men: RV = [(0.027 × height in
   centimeters) + (0.017 × age)] – 3.447

   Women: RV = [(0.032 × height in
   centimeters) + (0.009 × age)] – 3.9

3. Have the person remove all jewelry prior to weighing or testing. Weigh the person on land in a swimsuit, and subtract the weight of the suit. Convert the weight from pounds to kilograms (divide pounds by 2.2046).

4. Record the water temperature in the tank in degrees Centigrade. Use that temperature to obtain the water density factor provided below, which is required in the formula to compute body density.

Temp (°C)	Water Density (gr/ml)	Temp (°C)	Water Density (gr/ml)
28	0.99626	35	0.99406
29	0.99595	36	0.99371
30	0.99567	37	0.99336
31	0.99537	38	0.99299
32	0.99505	39	0.99262
33	0.99473	40	0.99224
34	0.99440		

5. Ask the person, dressed in the swimsuit, to enter the tank and completely wipe off all air clinging to the skin and hair. Have the person sit in the chair with the water at chin level (raise or lower the chair as needed). Make sure the water and scale remain as still as possible during the entire procedure, as this allows for a better underwater reading. (During underwater weighing, you can decrease scale movement by holding and slowly releasing the neck of the scale until the subject is floating freely in the water).

6. Place a clip on the person's nose and have him or her forcefully exhale all of the air out of the lungs. The individual then totally submerges underwater. (Make sure that all the air is exhaled from the lungs prior to submerging. Record the reading on the scale. Repeat this procedure 8 to 10 times, as practice and experience increases the accuracy of the underwater weight. Use the average of the three heaviest underwater weights as the gross underwater weight.

7. Because tare weight (the weight of the chair and chain or rope used to suspend the chair) accounts for part of the gross underwater weight, subtract this weight to obtain the person's net underwater weight. To determine tare weight, place a clothespin on the chain or rope at the water level when the person is submerged completely. After the person comes out of the water, lower the chair into the water to the pin level. Now record tare weight. Determine the net underwater weight by subtracting the tare weight from the gross underwater weight.

8. Compute body density and percent fat using the following equations:

$$\text{Body density} = \frac{BW}{\dfrac{BW - UW}{WD} - RV - .1}$$

$$\text{Percent fat**} = \frac{495}{BD} - 450$$

Where:

BW = body weight in kg
UW = net underwater weight
WD = water density (determined by water temperature)
RV = residual volume
BD = body density

A sample computation for body fat assessment according to hydrostatic weighing is provided in Lab 3A.

---

*From: "Respiratory Function Tests: Normal Values at Medium Altitudes and the Prediction of Normal Results," by H. L. Goldman and M. R. Becklake, in *American Review of Tuberculosis* 79 (1959):457–467.

**From *Body Composition from Fluid Spaces and Density*, by W. E. Siri. Berkeley, CA: University of California, Donner Laboratory of Medical Physics, March 19, 1956.

FIGURE 3.2
Hydrostatic weighing procedure for body composition assessment.

of time, skill, space, and equipment. An experienced instructor must train all technicians who will administer this test.

Because each individual assessment can take as long as 30 minutes, hydrostatic weighing is not feasible when testing large numbers of people. Furthermore, the person's residual lung volume (amount of air left in the lungs following complete forceful exhalation) has to be measured prior to testing. If residual volume cannot be measured, as is the case in many laboratories or health/fitness centers, it can be estimated using the predicting equations in Figure 3.2. Estimating residual volume, however, may decrease the accuracy of hydrostatic weighing.

A major concern during hydrostatic weighing is the person's ability to follow the test procedures. Also, the psychological variables in being weighed while submerged underwater makes hydrostatic weighing difficult to administer to aquaphobic people (those with a fear of water). For each underwater weighing trial, the person has to: (a) force out all of the air in the lungs, (b) lean forward and completely submerge underwater in a sitting position for about 5 to 10 seconds (long enough to take a reading on the scale), and (c) remain as calm as possible (chair movement makes reading the scale difficult). This procedure has to be repeated 8 to 10 times.

Forcing all of the air out of the lungs is not easy for everyone. Leaving additional air (beyond residual volume) in the lungs makes a person more buoyant. Because fat is less dense than water, overweight individuals weigh less in water. Additional air in the lungs makes a person lighter in water, yielding a false higher body fat percentage.

Because of the cost, time, and complexity of hydrostatic weighing, most health and fitness programs prefer anthropometric measurement techniques, which correlate quite well with hydrostatic weighing. These techniques, primarily skinfold thickness and girth measurements, allow a quick, simple, and inexpensive estimate of body composition.

SKINFOLD THICKNESS

Assessing body composition using skinfold thickness is based on the principle that approximately half of the body's fatty tissue is directly beneath the skin. Valid and reliable estimates of this tissue give a good indication of percent body fat.

The skinfold test is done with the aid of pressure calipers (see Figures 3.3 and 3.4). Several sites must

be measured to reflect the total percentage of fat: triceps, suprailium, and thigh skinfolds for women; and chest, abdomen, and thigh for men (Figure 3.5). All measurements should be taken on the right side of the body.

Even with the skinfold technique, some training is necessary to obtain accurate measurements. Also, different technicians may produce slightly different measurements from the same person. Therefore, the same technician should take pre- and post-measurements.

Measurements should be done at the same time of the day, preferably in the morning, as changes in water hydration from activity and exercise can increase skinfold girth. The procedures for assessing

FIGURE 3.3
Skinfold thickness technique for body composition assessment.

FIGURE 3.4
Various types of skinfold calipers used to assess skinfold thickness.

Chest (men)

Abdominal (men)

Thigh (men and women)

FIGURE 3.5
Anatomical landmarks for
skinfold measurements.

Triceps (women)

Suprailium (women)

percent body fat using skinfold thickness is given in Figure 3.6. If skinfold calipers* are available to you, you may proceed to assess your percent body fat with the help of your instructor or an experienced technician.

---

*This instrument is available at most colleges and universities. If unavailable, you can purchase an inexpensive, yet reliable skinfold caliper from: Fat Control Inc., P. O. Box 10117, Towson, MD 21204, Phone 301/296–1993.

BODY FAT ASSESSMENT ACCORDING TO SKINFOLD THICKNESS TECHNIQUE

1. Select the proper anatomical sites. For men, chest, abdomen, and thigh skinfolds are used. For women, use triceps, suprailium, and thigh skinfolds (*see* Figure 3.5). All measurements should be taken on the right side of the body with the person standing. The correct anatomical landmarks for skinfolds are:

   Chest: a diagonal fold halfway between the shoulder crease and the nipple.

   Abdomen: a vertical fold taken about one inch to the right of the umbilicus.

   Triceps: a vertical fold on the back of the upper arm, halfway between the shoulder and the elbow.

   Thigh: a vertical fold on the front of the thigh, midway between the knee and hip.

   Suprailium: a diagonal fold above the crest of the ilium (on the side of the hip).

2. Measure each site by grasping a double thickness of skin firmly with the thumb and forefinger, pulling the fold slightly away from the muscular tissue. The calipers are held perpendicular to the fold, and the measure-ment is taken one-half inch below the finger hold. Each site is measured three times and the values are read to the nearest .1 to .5 mm. The average of the two closest readings is recorded as the final value. The readings should be taken without delay to avoid excessive com-pression of the skinfold. Releasing and refolding the skinfold is required between readings.

3. When doing pre- and post-assessments, the measure-ment should be conducted at the same time of day. The best time is early in the morning to avoid water hydra-tion changes resulting from activity or exercise.

4. Percent fat is obtained by adding the three skinfold measurements and looking up the respective values on Tables 3.1 for women, 3.2 for men under age forty, and 3.3 for men over forty.

5. For example, if the skinfold measurements for an eigh-teen-year-old female are: (a) triceps = 16, (b) suprailium = 4, and (c) thigh = 30 (total = 50), the percent body fat would be 20.6%

FIGURE 3.6
Procedure for body fat assessment according to skinfold thickness technique.

TABLE 3.1
Percent Fat Estimates for Women Calculated From Triceps, Suprailium, and Thigh Skinfold Thickness

Sum of 3 Skinfolds	Under 22	23 to 27	28 to 32	33 to 37	38 to 42	43 to 47	48 to 52	53 to 57	Over 58
23- 25	9.7	9.9	10.2	10.4	10.7	10.9	11.2	11.4	11.7
26- 28	11.0	11.2	11.5	11.7	12.0	12.3	12.5	12.7	13.0
29- 31	12.3	12.5	12.8	13.0	13.3	13.5	13.8	14.0	14.3
32- 34	13.6	13.8	14.0	14.3	14.5	14.8	15.0	15.3	15.5
35- 37	14.8	15.0	15.3	15.5	15.8	16.0	16.3	16.5	16.8
38- 40	16.0	16.3	16.5	16.7	17.0	17.2	17.5	17.7	18.0
41- 43	17.2	17.4	17.7	17.9	18.2	18.4	18.7	18.9	19.2
44- 46	18.3	18.6	18.8	19.1	19.3	19.6	19.8	20.1	20.3
47- 49	19.5	19.7	20.0	20.2	20.5	20.7	21.0	21.2	21.5
50- 52	20.6	20.8	21.1	21.3	21.6	21.8	22.1	22.3	22.6
53- 55	21.7	21.9	22.1	22.4	22.6	22.9	23.1	23.4	23.6
56- 58	22.7	23.0	23.2	23.4	23.7	23.9	24.2	24.4	24.7
59- 61	23.7	24.0	24.2	24.5	24.7	25.0	25.2	25.5	25.7
62- 64	24.7	25.0	25.2	25.5	25.7	26.0	26.2	26.4	26.7
65- 67	25.7	25.9	26.2	26.4	26.7	26.9	27.2	27.4	27.7
68- 70	26.6	26.9	27.1	27.4	27.6	27.9	28.1	28.4	28.6
71- 73	27.5	27.8	28.0	28.3	28.5	28.8	29.0	29.3	29.5
74- 76	28.4	28.7	28.9	29.2	29.4	29.7	29.9	30.2	30.4
77- 79	29.3	29.5	29.8	30.0	30.3	30.5	30.8	31.0	31.3
80- 82	30.1	30.4	30.6	30.9	31.1	31.4	31.6	31.9	32.1
83- 85	30.9	31.2	31.4	31.7	31.9	32.2	32.4	32.7	32.9
86- 88	31.7	32.0	32.2	32.5	32.7	32.9	33.2	33.4	33.7
89- 91	32.5	32.7	33.0	33.2	33.5	33.7	33.9	34.2	34.4
92- 94	33.2	33.4	33.7	33.9	34.2	34.4	34.7	34.9	35.2
95- 97	33.9	34.1	34.4	34.6	34.9	35.1	35.4	35.6	35.9
98-100	34.6	34.8	35.1	35.3	35.5	35.8	36.0	36.3	36.5
101-103	35.2	35.4	35.7	35.9	36.2	36.4	36.7	36.9	37.2
104-106	35.8	36.1	36.3	36.6	36.8	37.1	37.3	37.5	37.8
107-109	36.4	36.7	36.9	37.1	37.4	37.6	37.9	38.1	38.4
110-112	37.0	37.2	37.5	37.7	38.0	38.2	38.5	38.7	38.9
113-115	37.5	37.8	38.0	38.2	38.5	38.7	39.0	39.2	39.5
116-118	38.0	38.3	38.5	38.8	39.0	39.3	39.5	39.7	40.0
119-121	38.5	38.7	39.0	39.2	39.5	39.7	40.0	40.2	40.5
122-124	39.0	39.2	39.4	39.7	39.9	40.2	40.4	40.7	40.9
125-127	39.4	39.6	39.9	40.1	40.4	40.6	40.9	41.1	41.4
128-130	39.8	40.0	40.3	40.5	40.8	41.0	41.3	41.5	41.8

Body density calculated based on the generalized equation for predicting body density of women developed by A. S. Jackson, M. L. Pollock, and A. Ward. *Medicine and Science in Sports and Exercise* 12:175–182, 1980. Percent body fat determined from the calculated body density using the Siri formula.

TABLE 3.2
Percent Fat Estimates for Men 40 and Under Calculated From Chest, Abdomen, and Thigh Skinfold Thickness

Sum of 3 Skinfolds	Under 19	20 to 22	23 to 25	26 to 28	29 to 31	32 to 34	35 to 37	38 to 40
8- 10	.9	1.3	1.6	2.0	2.3	2.7	3.0	3.3
11- 13	1.9	2.3	2.6	3.0	3.3	3.7	4.0	4.3
14- 16	2.9	3.3	3.6	3.9	4.3	4.6	5.0	5.3
17- 19	3.9	4.2	4.6	4.9	5.3	5.6	6.0	6.3
20- 22	4.8	5.2	5.5	5.9	6.2	6.6	6.9	7.3
23- 25	5.8	6.2	6.5	6.8	7.2	7.5	7.9	8.2
26- 28	6.8	7.1	7.5	7.8	8.1	8.5	8.8	9.2
29- 31	7.7	8.0	8.4	8.7	9.1	9.4	9.8	10.1
32- 34	8.6	9.0	9.3	9.7	10.0	10.4	10.7	11.1
35- 37	9.5	9.9	10.2	10.6	10.9	11.3	11.6	12.0
38- 40	10.5	10.8	11.2	11.5	11.8	12.2	12.5	12.9
41- 43	11.4	11.7	12.1	12.4	12.7	13.1	13.4	13.8
44- 46	12.2	12.6	12.9	13.3	13.6	14.0	14.3	14.7
47- 49	13.1	13.5	13.8	14.2	14.5	14.9	15.2	15.5
50- 52	14.0	14.3	14.7	15.0	15.4	15.7	16.1	16.4
53- 55	14.8	15.2	15.5	15.9	16.2	16.6	16.9	17.3
56- 58	15.7	16.0	16.4	16.7	17.1	17.4	17.8	18.1
59- 61	16.5	16.9	17.2	17.6	17.9	18.3	18.6	19.0
62- 64	17.4	17.7	18.1	18.4	18.8	19.1	19.4	19.8
65- 67	18.2	18.5	18.9	19.2	19.6	19.9	20.3	20.6
68- 70	19.0	19.3	19.7	20.0	20.4	20.7	21.1	21.4
71- 73	19.8	20.1	20.5	20.8	21.2	21.5	21.9	22.2
74- 76	20.6	20.9	21.3	21.6	22.0	22.2	22.7	23.0
77- 79	21.4	21.7	22.1	22.4	22.8	23.1	23.4	23.8
80- 82	22.1	22.5	22.8	23.2	23.5	23.9	24.2	24.6
83- 85	22.9	23.2	23.6	23.9	24.3	24.6	25.0	25.3
86- 88	23.6	24.0	24.3	24.7	25.0	25.4	25.7	26.1
89- 91	24.4	24.7	25.1	25.4	25.8	26.1	26.5	26.8
92- 94	25.1	25.5	25.8	26.2	26.5	26.9	27.2	27.5
95- 97	25.8	26.2	26.5	26.9	27.2	27.6	27.9	28.3
98-100	26.6	26.9	27.3	27.6	27.9	28.3	28.6	29.0
101-103	27.3	27.6	28.0	28.3	28.6	29.0	29.3	29.7
104-106	27.9	28.3	28.6	29.0	29.3	29.7	30.0	30.4
107-109	28.6	29.0	29.3	29.7	30.0	30.4	30.7	31.1
110-112	29.3	29.6	30.0	30.3	30.7	31.0	31.4	31.7
113-115	30.0	30.3	30.7	31.0	31.3	31.7	32.0	32.4
116-118	30.6	31.0	31.3	31.6	32.0	32.3	32.7	33.0
119-121	31.3	31.6	32.0	32.3	32.6	33.0	33.3	33.7
122-124	31.9	32.2	32.6	32.9	33.3	33.6	34.0	34.3
125-127	32.5	32.9	33.2	33.5	33.9	34.2	34.6	34.9
128-130	33.1	33.5	33.8	34.2	34.5	34.9	35.2	35.5

Body density calculated based on the generalized equation for predicting body density of men developed by A. S. Jackson, and M. L. Pollock. *British Journal of Nutrition* 40:497-504, 1978. Percent body fat determined from the calculated body density using the Siri formula.

TABLE 3.3
Percent Fat Estimates for Men Over 40 Calculated From Chest, Abdomen, and Thigh Skinfold Thickness

				Age to the Last Year				
Sum of 3 Skinfolds	41 to 43	44 to 46	47 to 49	50 to 52	53 to 55	56 to 58	59 to 61	Over 62
8- 10	3.7	4.0	4.4	4.7	5.1	5.4	5.8	6.1
11- 13	4.7	5.0	5.4	5.7	6.1	6.4	6.8	7.1
14- 16	5.7	6.0	6.4	6.7	7.1	7.4	7.8	8.1
17- 19	6.7	7.0	7.4	7.7	8.1	8.4	8.7	9.1
20- 22	7.6	8.0	8.3	8.7	9.0	9.4	9.7	10.1
23- 25	8.6	8.9	9.3	9.6	10.0	10.3	10.7	11.0
26- 28	9.5	9.9	10.2	10.6	10.9	11.3	11.6	12.0
29- 31	10.5	10.8	11.2	11.5	11.9	12.2	12.6	12.9
32- 34	11.4	11.8	12.1	12.4	12.8	13.1	13.5	13.8
35- 37	12.3	12.7	13.0	13.4	13.7	14.1	14.4	14.8
38- 40	13.2	13.6	13.9	14.3	14.6	15.0	15.3	15.7
41- 43	14.1	14.5	14.8	15.2	15.5	15.9	16.2	16.6
44- 46	15.0	15.4	15.7	16.1	16.4	16.8	17.1	17.5
47- 49	15.9	16.2	16.6	16.9	17.3	17.6	18.0	18.3
50- 52	16.8	17.1	17.5	17.8	18.2	18.5	18.8	19.2
53- 55	17.6	18.0	18.3	18.7	19.0	19.4	19.7	20.1
56- 58	18.5	18.8	19.2	19.5	19.9	20.2	20.6	20.9
59- 61	19.3	19.7	20.0	20.4	20.7	21.0	21.4	21.7
62- 64	20.1	20.5	20.8	21.2	21.5	21.9	22.2	22.6
65- 67	21.0	21.3	21.7	22.0	22.4	22.7	23.0	23.4
68- 70	21.8	22.1	22.5	22.8	23.2	23.5	23.9	24.2
71- 73	22.6	22.9	23.3	23.6	24.0	24.3	24.7	25.0
74- 76	23.4	23.7	24.1	24.4	24.8	25.1	25.4	25.8
77- 79	24.1	24.5	24.8	25.2	25.5	25.9	26.2	26.6
80- 82	24.9	25.3	25.6	26.0	26.3	26.6	27.0	27.3
83- 85	25.7	26.0	26.4	26.7	27.1	27.4	27.8	28.1
86- 88	26.4	26.8	27.1	27.5	27.8	28.2	28.5	28.9
89- 91	27.2	27.5	27.9	28.2	28.6	28.9	29.2	29.6
92- 94	27.9	28.2	28.6	28.9	29.3	29.6	30.0	30.3
95- 97	28.6	29.0	29.3	29.7	30.0	30.4	30.7	31.1
98-100	29.3	29.7	30.0	30.4	30.7	31.1	31.4	31.8
101-103	30.0	30.4	30.7	31.1	31.4	31.8	32.1	32.5
104-106	30.7	31.1	31.4	31.8	32.1	32.5	32.8	33.2
107-109	31.4	31.8	32.1	32.4	32.8	33.1	33.5	33.8
110-112	32.1	32.4	32.8	33.1	33.5	33.8	34.2	34.5
113-115	32.7	33.1	33.4	33.8	34.1	34.5	34.8	35.2
116-118	33.4	33.7	34.1	34.4	34.8	35.1	35.5	35.8
119-121	34.0	34.4	34.7	35.1	35.4	35.8	36.1	36.5
122-124	34.7	35.0	35.4	35.7	36.1	36.4	36.7	37.1
125-127	35.3	35.6	36.0	36.3	36.7	37.0	37.4	37.7
128-130	35.9	36.2	36.6	36.9	37.3	37.6	38.0	38.5

Body density calculated based on the generalized equation for predicting body density of men developed by A. S. Jackson and M. L. Pollock. *British Journal of Nutrition* 40:497-504, 1978. Percent body fat determined from the calculated body density using the Siri formula.

GIRTH MEASUREMENTS

A simpler method to determine body fat is by measuring circumferences at various body sites. All this technique requires is a standard measuring tape, and good accuracy can be achieved with little practice. The limitation is that it may not be valid for athletic individuals (men or women) who actively participate in strenuous physical activity or people who can be classified visually as thin or obese.

The required procedure for girth measurements is given in Figure 3.7. Measurements for women include the upper arm, hip, and wrist; for men, the waist and wrist.

GIRTH MEASUREMENTS

Girth Measurements for Women*

1. Using a regular tape measure, determine the following girth measurements in centimeters (cm):

   Upper Arm: the measure is taken halfway between the shoulder and the elbow.

   Hip: measure at the point of largest circumference.

   Wrist: take the girth in front of the bones where the wrist bends.

2. Obtain the age of the subject.

3. Using Table 3.4, find the girth measurement for each site and age in the lefthand columns. Look up the constant values in the righthand columns. These values will allow you to derive body density (BD) by substituting the constants in the following formula:

   $BD = A - B - C + D$

4. Using the derived body density, calculate percent body fat (%F) according to the following equation:

   $\%F = (495 \div BD) - 450$**

5. Example: Jane is twenty years old, and the following girth measurements were taken: biceps = 27 cm, hip = 99.5 cm, wrist = 15.4 cm.

Data	Constant
Upper Arm = 27 cm	A = 1.0813
Age = 20	B = .0102
Hip = 99.5 cm	C = .1206
Wrist = 15.4 cm	D = .0971

   $BD = A - B - C + D$
   $BD = 1.0813 - .0102 - .1206 + .0971 = 1.0476$

   $\%F = (495 \div BD) - 450$
   $\%F = (495 \div 1.0476) - 450 = 22.5$

Girth Measurements for Men***

1. Using a regular tape measure, determine the following girth measurements in inches (the men's measurements are taken in inches as opposed to centimeters for women):

   Waist: measure at the umbilicus (belly button)
   Wrist: measure in front of the bones where the wrist bends.

2. Subtract the wrist from the waist measurement.

3. Obtain the weight of the subject in pounds.

4. Look up the percent body fat (%F) in Table 3.5 by using the difference obtained in number 2 above and the subjects' body weight.

5. Example: John weighs 160 pounds, and his waist and wrist girth measurements are 36.5 and 7.5 inches, respectively.

   Waist girth = 36.5 inches
   Wrist girth = 7.5 inches
   Difference = 29.0 inches
   Body weight = 160.0 lbs.
   %F = 22

---

* Reproduced with permission from Lambson, R. B. "Generalized Body Density Prediction Equations for Women Using Simple Anthropometric Measurements." Unpublished doctoral dissertation, Brigham Young University, August 1987.

** From Siri, W. E. *Body Composition From Fluid Spaces and Density*. Berkeley, CA: University of California, Donner Laboratory of Medical Physics, 1956.

*** Table 3.5 reproduced by permission from Fisher, A. G., and P. E. Allsen. *Jogging*. Dubuque, IA: Wm. C. Brown, 1987. This table was developed according to the generalized body composition equation for men using simple measurement techniques by K. W. Penrouse, A. G Nelson, and A G. Fisher. Medicine and Science in Sports and Exercise 17(2):189, 1985. © American College of Sports Medicine 1985..

FIGURE 3.7
Procedure for body fat assessment according to girth measurements.

TABLE 3.4
Conversion Constants from Girth Measurements (Centimeters) to Calculate Body Density for Women

Upper Arm (cm)	Constant A	Age	Constant B	Hip (cm)	Constant C	Hip (cm)	Constant C	Wrist (cm)	Constant D
20.5	1.0966	17	.0086	79	.0957	114.5	.1388	13.0	.0819
21	1.0954	18	.0091	79.5	.0963	115	.1394	13.2	.0832
21.5	1.0942	19	.0096	80	.0970	115.5	.1400	13.4	.0845
22	1.0930	20	.0102	80.5	.0976	116	.1406	13.6	.0857
22.5	1.0919	21	.0107	81	.0982	116.5	.1412	13.8	.0807
23	1.0907	22	.0112	81.5	.0988	117	.1418	14.0	.0882
23.5	1.0895	23	.0117	82	.0994	117.5	.1424	14.2	.0895
24	1.0883	24	.0122	82.5	.1000	118	.1430	14.4	.0908
24.5	1.0871	25	.0127	83	.1006	118.5	.1436	14.6	.0920
25	1.0860	26	.0132	83.5	.1012	119	.1442	14.8	.0933
25.5	1.0848	27	.0137	84	.1018	119.5	.1448	15.0	.0946
26	1.0836	28	.0142	84.5	.1024	120	.1454	15.2	.0958
26.5	1.0824	29	.0147	85	.1030	120.5	.1460	15.4	.0971
27	1.0813	30	.0152	85.5	.1036	121	.1466	15.6	.0983
27.5	1.0801	31	.0157	86	.1042	121.5	.1472	15.8	.0996
28	1.0789	32	.0162	86.5	.1048	122	.1479	16.0	.1009
28.5	1.0777	33	.0168	87	.1054	122.5	.1485	16.2	.1021
29	1.0775	34	.0173	87.5	.1060	123	.1491	16.4	.1034
29.5	1.0754	35	.0178	88	.1066	123.5	.1497	16.6	.1046
30	1.0742	36	.0183	88.5	.1072	124	.1503	16.8	.1059
30.5	1.0730	37	.0188	89	.1079	124.5	.1509	17.0	.1072
31	1.0718	38	.0193	89.5	.1085	125	.1515	17.2	.1084
31.5	1.0707	39	.0198	90	.1091	125.5	.1521	17.4	.1097
32	1.0695	40	,0203	90.5	.1097	126	.1527	17.6	.1109
32.5	1.0683	41	.0208	91	.1103	126.5	.1533	17.8	.1122
33	1.0671	42	.0213	91.5	.1109	127	.1539	18.0	.1135
33.5	1.0666	43	.0218	92	.1115	127.5	.1545	18.2	.1147
34	1.0648	44	.0223	92.5	.1121	128	.1551	18.4	.1160
34.5	1.0636	45	.0228	93	.1127	128.5	.1558	18.6	.1172
35	1.0624	46	.0234	93.5	.1133	129	.1563		
35.5	1.0612	47	.0239	94	.1139	129.5	.1569		
36	1.0601	48	,0244	94.5	.1145	130	.1575		
36.5	1.0589	49	.0249	95	.1151	130.5	.1581		
37	1.0577	50	.0254	95.5	.1157	131	.1587		
37.5	1.0565	51	.0259	96	.1163	131.5	.1593		
38	1.0554	52	.0264	96.5	.1169	132	.1600		
38.5	1.0542	53	.0269	97	.1176	132.5	.1606		
39	1.0530	54	.0274	97.5	.1182	133	.1612		
39.5	1.0518	55	.0279	98	.1188	133.5	.1618		
40	1.0506	56	.0284	98.5	.1194	134	.1624		
40.5	1.0495	57	.0289	99	.1200	134.5	.1630		
41	1.0483	58	.0294	99.5	.1206	135	.1636		
41.5	1.0471	59	.0300	100	.1212	135.5	.1642		
42	1.0459	60	.0305	100.5	.1218	136	.1648		
42.5	1.0448	61	.0310	101	.1224	136.5	.1654		
43	1.0434	62	.0315	101.5	.1230	137	.1660		

(Continued)

TABLE 3.4 *(Continued)*
Conversion Constants from Girth Measurements (Centimeters) to Calculate Body Density for Women

Upper Arm (cm)	Constant A	Age	Constant B	Hip (cm)	Constant C	Hip (cm)	Constant C	Wrist (cm)	Constant D
43.5	1.0424	63	.0320	102	.1236	137.5	.1666		
44	1.0412	64	.0325	102.5	.1242	138	.1672		
		65	.0330	103	.1248	138.5	.1678		
		66	.0335	103.5	.1254	139	.1685		
		67	.0340	104	.1260	139.5	.1691		
		68	.0345	104.5	.1266	140	.1697		
		69	.0350	105	.1272	140.5	.1703		
		70	.0355	105.5	.1278	141	.1709		
		71	.0360	106	.1285	141.5	.1715		
		72	.0366	106.5	.1291	142	.1721		
		73	.0371	107	.1297	142.5	.1728		
		74	.0376	107.5	.1303	143	.1733		
		75	.0381	108	.1309	143.5	.1739		
				108.5	.1315	144	.1745		
				109	.1321	144.5	.1751		
				109.5	.1327	145	.1757		
				110	.1333	145.5	.1763		
				110.5	.1339	146	.1769		
				111	.1345	146.5	.1775		
				111.5	.1351	147	.1781		
				112	.1357	147.5	.1787		
				112.5	.1363	148	.1794		
				113	.1369	148.5	.1800		
				113.5	.1375	149	.1806		
				114	.1382	149.5	.1812		
						150	.1818		

TABLE 3.5
Estimated Percent Body Fat for Men Obtained from Waist Minus Wrist Girth Measurements (Inches) and Body Weight

Weight	22	22.5	23	23.5	24	24.5	25	25.5	26	26.5	27	27.5	28	28.5	29	29.5	30	30.5	31	31.5	32	32.5	33	33.5	34	34.5	35	35.5	36	36.5	37	37.5	38	38.5	39	39.5	40	40.5	41	41.5	42	42.5	43	43.5	44	44.5	45	45.5	46	46.5	47	47.5	48	48.5	49	49.5	50
120	4	6	8	10	12	14	16	18	20	21	23	25	27	29	31	33	35	37	39	41	43	45	47	49	50	52	54	56	58																												
125	4	6	7	9	11	13	15	17	19	20	22	24	26	28	30	32	33	35	37	39	41	43	45	46	48	50	52	54	56	58																									
130	3	5	7	9	11	13	15	16	18	20	21	23	25	27	28	30	32	34	35	37	39	41	43	44	46	48	50	52	53	55	57																							
135	3	5	7	8	10	12	14	15	17	19	20	22	24	26	27	29	31	32	34	36	38	39	41	43	44	46	48	49	51	53	54	56																						
140	3	5	6	8	10	11	13	15	16	18	20	21	23	25	26	28	30	31	33	34	36	38	39	41	43	44	46	48	49	51	53	54	56																				
145	3	4	6	7	9	11	12	14	16	17	19	20	22	24	25	27	29	30	32	33	35	36	38	40	41	43	44	46	47	49	51	52	54	55																		
150	2	4	6	7	9	10	12	14	15	17	18	20	21	23	24	26	28	29	31	32	34	35	37	38	40	41	43	44	46	47	49	50	52	53	55																
155	2	4	5	7	8	10	12	13	15	16	18	19	21	22	24	25	27	28	30	31	33	34	36	37	39	40	42	44	45	47	48	50	52	53	55	55														
160	2	4	5	6	8	9	11	13	14	16	17	19	20	22	23	25	26	28	29	31	32	34	35	37	38	40	41	43	44	46	47	49	50	52	53	54													
165	2	3	5	6	8	9	11	12	14	15	17	18	20	21	23	24	26	27	29	30	32	33	35	36	38	39	41	42	44	45	47	48	50	51	53	54	54											
170	2	3	5	6	7	9	10	12	13	15	16	18	19	21	22	24	25	27	28	30	31	33	34	36	37	39	40	42	43	45	46	48	49	51	52	54	54										
175	2	3	4	6	7	9	10	12	13	14	16	17	19	20	22	23	25	26	28	29	31	32	34	35	37	38	40	41	43	44	46	47	49	50	52	53										
180		3	4	6	7	8	10	11	13	14	16	17	18	20	21	23	24	26	27	29	30	32	33	35	36	38	39	40	42	43	45	46	48	49	51	52	53								
185		2	4	5	7	8	10	11	12	14	15	17	18	19	21	22	24	25	27	28	30	31	32	34	35	37	38	40	41	43	44	45	47	48	50	51	53							
190		2	4	5	6	8	9	11	12	14	15	16	18	19	20	22	23	25	26	28	29	30	32	33	35	36	37	39	40	42	43	44	46	47	49	50	51	52					
195		2	3	5	6	7	9	10	12	13	14	16	17	19	20	21	23	24	25	27	28	30	31	32	34	35	36	38	39	41	42	43	45	46	47	49	50	51	52				
200		2	3	4	6	7	9	10	11	13	14	15	17	18	19	21	22	23	25	26	28	29	30	32	33	34	36	37	38	40	41	42	44	45	46	48	49	50	51	52			
205		2	3	4	6	7	8	10	11	12	14	15	16	18	19	20	22	23	24	26	27	28	30	31	32	34	35	36	38	39	40	42	43	44	45	47	48	49	51	51	52		
210		2	3	4	5	7	8	9	11	12	13	15	16	17	19	20	21	23	24	25	26	28	29	30	32	33	34	36	37	38	39	41	42	43	45	46	47	48	50	51			
215		2	3	4	5	6	8	9	10	11	13	14	15	16	18	19	20	22	23	24	26	27	28	29	31	32	33	34	36	37	38	39	41	42	43	44	46	47	48	49	50	51	
220			2	3	4	6	7	8	9	11	12	13	14	16	17	18	19	21	22	23	24	26	27	28	29	31	32	33	34	35	37	38	39	40	41	43	44	45	46	47	49	50	51
225			2	3	4	6	7	8	9	10	11	13	14	15	16	18	19	20	21	22	24	25	26	27	28	30	31	32	33	34	36	37	38	39	40	42	43	44	45	46	47	49	50	51
230			2	3	4	5	6	8	9	10	11	12	13	15	16	17	18	19	21	22	23	24	25	27	28	29	30	31	32	34	35	36	37	38	40	41	42	43	44	45	46	48	49	50	51
235			2	3	4	5	6	7	9	10	11	12	13	14	15	17	18	19	20	21	22	24	25	26	27	28	29	30	32	33	34	35	36	37	38	40	41	42	43	44	45	46	48	49	50
240			2	3	4	5	6	7	8	9	10	12	13	14	15	16	17	18	19	21	22	23	24	25	26	27	28	30	31	32	33	34	35	36	37	39	40	41	42	43	44	45	46	48	49	50
245			2	3	4	5	6	7	8	9	10	11	12	13	15	16	17	18	19	20	21	22	23	24	25	26	27	28	30	31	32	33	34	35	36	37	38	39	40	41	42	43	44	45	46	47	48	49	50
250				2	3	4	5	6	7	8	9	10	11	12	13	15	16	16	17	18	19	20	21	22	23	24	25	26	27	28	29	30	31	32	33	34	35	36	37	38	39	40	41	42	43	44	45	46	47	48	49	50
255				2	3	4	5	6	7	8	9	10	11	12	13	14	15	16	17	18	19	20	21	22	23	24	25	26	27	28	29	30	31	32	33	34	35	36	37	38	39	40	41	42	43	44	45	46	47	48	49	50
260					2	3	4	5	6	7	8	8	9	10	11	12	13	14	15	16	17	18	19	20	21	22	23	24	25	26	26	27	28	29	30	31	32	33	34	35	36	37	38	39	40	41	42	43	44	45	46	47	48	49
265					2	3	4	5	6	7	8	8	9	10	11	12	13	14	15	16	17	18	19	20	20	21	22	23	24	25	26	27	28	29	30	31	32	33	34	35	36	37	38	39	40	41	42	43	44	45	46	47	48	49
270					2	3	4	5	6	6	7	8	9	10	11	12	12	13	14	15	16	17	18	19	20	21	22	23	24	25	26	27	28	29	30	31	32	33	34	35	36	37	37	38	39	40	41	42	43	44	45	46	47	48
275						2	3	4	5	6	7	7	8	9	10	11	12	13	14	15	16	16	17	18	19	20	21	22	23	24	25	26	27	28	29	30	31	32	33	33	34	35	36	37	38	39	40	41	42	43	44	45	46	47
280						2	3	4	5	6	6	7	8	9	10	11	12	12	13	14	15	16	17	18	19	20	21	22	23	24	24	25	26	27	28	29	30	31	32	33	34	35	36	37	38	38	39	40	41	42	43	44	45	46
285						2	3	4	5	5	6	7	8	9	10	11	11	12	13	14	15	16	17	17	18	19	20	21	22	23	24	24	25	26	27	28	29	30	31	32	33	34	34	35	36	37	38	39	40	41	42	43	44	45
290						2	3	4	5	5	6	7	8	9	10	10	11	12	13	14	15	16	16	17	18	19	20	21	22	23	24	24	25	26	27	28	29	30	30	31	32	33	34	35	36	37	38	39	40	40	41	42	43	44
295						2	3	4	4	5	6	7	8	9	9	10	11	12	13	14	14	15	16	17	18	19	20	21	21	22	23	24	25	26	27	28	29	29	30	31	32	33	34	35	36	37	38	39	40	41	42	43	43	44
300						2	2	3	4	5	6	7	8	8	9	10	11	12	13	14	15	15	16	17	18	19	20	21	22	22	23	24	25	26	27	28	29	30	31	32	33	34	35	36	36	37	38	39	40	41	42	43		

BIOELECTRICAL IMPEDANCE

The bioelectrical impedance technique is much simpler to administer, but it does require costly equipment. In this technique, the individual is hooked up to a machine and a weak electrical current (totally painless) is run through the body to analyze body composition (body fat, lean body mass, and body water). The technique is based on the principle that fat tissue is not as good a conductor of an electrical current as lean tissue is. The easier the conductance, the leaner the individual.

The accuracy of current equations used in estimating percent body fat with this technique is still questionable. More research is required before the equations approach the accuracy of hydrostatic weighing, skinfolds, or girth measurements.

An advantage of bioelectrical impedance is that results are highly reproducible. Unlike other techniques, in which experienced technicians are necessary to obtain valid results, almost anyone can administer bioelectrical impedance. And, although the test results may not be completely accurate, this instrument is valuable in assessing body composition changes over time.

If this instrument or some other type of equipment for body composition assessment is available to you, you can use it to determine your percent body fat. You may want to compare the results with other techniques. Following all manufacturer's instructions will ensure the best possible result

WAIST-TO-HIP RATIO

Scientific evidence suggests that the way people store fat affects the risk for disease. Some individuals tend to store fat in the abdominal area (called the "apple" shape). Others store it primarily around the hips and thighs (gluteal femoral fat or "pear" shape).

Obese individuals with a lot of abdominal fat clearly are at higher risk for coronary heart disease, congestive heart failure, hypertension, adult-onset diabetes (Type II), and strokes than are obese people with similar amounts of total body fat that is stored primarily in the hips and thighs. Relatively new evidence also indicates that, among individuals with high abdominal fat, those whose fat deposits are around internal organs (visceral fat) are at even greater risk for disease than those whose abdominal fat is primarily beneath the skin (subcutaneous fat).

Because of the higher risk for disease in individuals who tend to store a lot of fat in the abdominal area, as contrasted with the hips and thighs, a waist-to-hip ratio test recently was designed by a panel of scientists appointed by the National Academy of Sciences and the Dietary Guidelines Advisory Council for the U.S. Departments of Agriculture and Health and Human Services. The waist measurement is taken at the point of smallest circumference, and the hip measurement is taken at the point of greatest circumference.

The waist-to-hip ratio differentiates the "apples" from the "pears." Most men are apples, and most women are pears. The panel recommends that men need to lose weight if the waist-to-hip ratio is 1.0 or higher. Women need to lose weight if the ratio is .85 or higher. More conservative estimates indicate that the risk starts to increase when the ratio exceeds .95 and .80 for men and women, respectively. For example, the waist-to-hip ratio for a man with a 40-inch waist and a 38-inch hip would be 1.05 (40 ÷ 38). This ratio may indicate higher risk for disease.

BODY MASS INDEX

Another technique scientists use to determine thinness and excessive fatness is the Body Mass Index (BMI). This index incorporates height and weight to estimate critical fat values at which the risk for disease increases.

BMI is calculated by multiplying your weight in pounds by 705, dividing this figure by your height in inches, and then dividing by the same height again (or weight in kilograms divided by the square of the height in meters). For example, the BMI for an individual who weighs 172 pounds and is 67 inches tall would be 27 (172 × 705 ÷ 67 ÷ 67).

According to BMI, the lowest risk for chronic disease is in the 22 to 25 range (see Table 3.6). Individuals are classified as overweight between 25 and 30. BMIs above 30 are defined as obesity and below 20 as underweight.

BMI is a useful tool to screen the general population, but, similar to height/weight charts, it fails to differentiate fat from lean body mass or where most of the fat is located (see waist-to-hip ratio). Using BMI, athletes with a large amount of muscle mass

TABLE 3.6
Disease Risk According to Body Mass Index (BMI)

BMI	Disease Risk
<20.00	Moderate to Very High
20.00 to 21.99	Low
22.00 to 24.99	Very Low
25.00 to 29.99	Low
30.00 to 34.99	Moderate
35.00 to 39.99	High
≥40.00	Very High

(body builders, football players) easily can fall in the moderate or even high-risk categories. Therefore, body composition and waist-to-hip ratios are better procedures to determine health risk and recommended body weight.

DETERMINING RECOMMENDED BODY WEIGHT

After finding out your percent body fat, you can determine your current body composition classification according to Table 3.7. In this table you will find the health fitness and the high physical fitness percent fat standards.

For example, the recommended health fitness fat percentage for a 20-year-old female is 28% or less. The health fitness standard is established at the point at which there seems to be no harm to health in terms of percent body fat. A high physical fitness range for this same woman would be between 18% and 23%.

The high physical fitness standard does not mean you cannot be somewhat below this number. Many highly trained male athletes are as low as 3%, and some female distance runners have been measured at 6% body fat (which may not be healthy).

Although people generally agree that the mortality rate is greater for obese people, some evidence indicates that the same is true for underweight people. "Underweight" and "thin" do not necessarily mean the same thing. A healthy thin person has total body fat around the high fitness percentage, whereas an underweight person has extremely low body fat, even to the point of compromising the essential fat.

The 3% essential fat for men and 12% for women seem to be the lower limits for people to maintain good health. Below these percentages normal physiologic functions can be seriously impaired. Some experts point out that a little storage fat (over the essential fat) is better than none at all.

TABLE 3.7
Body Composition Classification According to Percent Body Fat

			MEN		
Age	Excellent	Good	Moderate	Overweight	Obese
≤19	12.0	12.1-17.0	17.1-22.0	22.1-27.0	≥ 27.1
20-29	13.0	13.1-18.0	18.1-23.0	23.1-28.0	≥ 28.1
30-39	14.0	14.1-19.0	19.1-24.0	24.1-29.0	≥ 29.1
40-49	15.0	15.1-20.0	20.1-25.0	25.1-30.0	≥ 30.1
≥ 50	16.0	16.1-21.5	21.1-26.0	26.1-31.0	≥ 31.1
			WOMEN		
Age	Excellent	Good	Moderate	Overweight	Obese
≤19	17.0	17.1-22.0	22.1-27.0	27.1-32.0	≥ 32.1
20-29	18.0	18.1-23.0	23.1-28.0	28.1-33.0	≥ 33.1
30-39	19.0	19.1-24.0	24.1-29.0	29.1-34.0	≥ 34.1
40-49	20.0	20.1-25.0	25.1-30.0	30.1-35.0	≥ 35.1
≥ 50	21.0	21.1-26.5	26.1-31.0	31.1-36.0	≥ 36.1

☐ High physical fitness standard
☐ Health fitness standard

See Chapter 1, Fitness Standards: Health vs Physical Fitness, p. 6.

As a result, the health and high fitness standards for percent fat in Table 3.7 are set higher than the minimum essential fat requirements, at a point beneficial to optimal health and well-being. Finally, because lean tissue decreases with age, one extra percentage point is allowed for every additional decade of life.

Your recommended body weight is computed based on the selected health or high fitness fat percentage for your age and gender. Your decision to select a "desired" fat percentage should be based on your current percent body fat and your personal health/fitness objectives. To compute your own recommended body weight:

1. Determine the pounds of body weight in fat (FW). Multiply body weight (BW) by the current percent fat (%F) expressed in decimal form (FW = BW × %F).
2. Determine lean body mass (LBM) by subtracting the weight in fat from the total body weight (LBM = BW − FW). (Anything that is not fat must be part of the lean component.)
3. Select a desired body fat percentage (DFP) based on the health or high fitness standards given in Table 3.7.
4. Compute recommended body weight (RBW) according to the formula: RBW = LBM ÷ (1.0 − DFP).

As an example of these computations, a 19-year-old female who weighs 160 pounds and is 30% fat would like to know what her recommended body weight would be at 22%:

Gender: female
Age: 19
BW: 160 lbs.
%F: 30% (.30 in decimal form)

1. FW = BW × %F
   FW = 160 × .30 = 48 lbs.

2. LBM = BW − FW
   LBM = 160 − 48 = 112 lbs.

3. DFP: 22% (.22 in decimal form)

4. RBW = LBM ÷ (1.0 − DFP)
   RBW = 112 ÷ (1.0 − .22)
   RBW = 112 ÷ (.78) = 143.6 lbs.

In Labs 3A and 3B you will have the opportunity to determine your own body composition and recommended body weight using the procedures outlined in this chapter. In Lab 3C you can determine your disease risk according to waist-to-hip ratio and BMI.

Other than hydrostatic weighing, skinfold thickness seems to be the most practical and valid technique to estimate body fat. If skinfold calipers are available, use this technique to assess percent body fat. If calipers are unavailable, you can estimate your percent fat according to the girth measurements technique or another technique available to you. (You may wish to use several techniques and compare the results.)

If you are on a diet/exercise program, you should repeat the computations about once a month to monitor changes in body composition. This is important because lean body mass is affected by weight reduction programs and amount of physical activity. As lean body mass changes, so will your recommended body weight. To make valid comparisons, the same technique should be used between pre- and post-assessments.

Changes in body composition resulting from a weight control/exercise program were illustrated in a co-ed aerobic dance course taught during a six-week summer term. Students participated in aerobic dance routines four times a week, 60 minutes each time. On the first and last days of class, several physiological parameters, including body composition, were assessed. Students also were given information on diet and nutrition, and they basically followed their own weight control program.

At the end of the six weeks, the average weight loss for the entire class was 3 pounds (see Figure 3.8). But since body composition was assessed, class members were surprised to find that the average fat loss was actually 6 pounds, accompanied by a 3-pound increase in lean body mass.

When dieting, body composition should be reassessed periodically because of the effects of negative caloric balance on lean body mass. As is discussed in Chapter 4, dieting does decrease lean body mass. This lean body mass loss can be reduced or eliminated by combining a sensible diet with physical exercise.

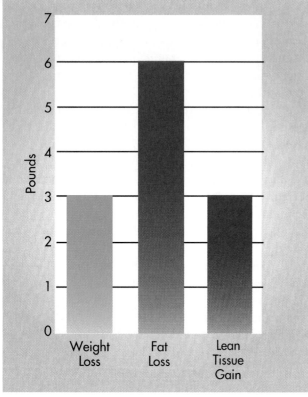

FIGURE 3.8
Effects of a six-week aerobics program on body composition.

LABORATORY EXPERIENCE

LAB 3A
Hydrostatic Weighing

Lab Preparation
Bring a swimsuit and towel to this lab. A six- to eight-hour fast and bladder and bowel movements are recommended prior to underwater weighing. If pulmonary function equipment is available, measure residual lung volume before going into the water.

LAB 3B
Anthropometric Measurements for Body Comparison Assessment and Recommended Body Weight Determination

Lab Preparation
Wear shorts and a loose fitting t-shirt (no leotards). Do not use lotion on your skin the day of this lab.

LAB 3C
Weight and Health: Disease Risk Assessment

Lab Preparation
None required.

REFERENCES

1. Bouchard, C., and F. E. Johnson, Editors. *Fat Distribution During Growth and Later Health Outcomes.* New York: Alan R. Liss, 1988.
2. Bouchard, C., G. A. Bray, and V. S. Hubbard. "Basic and Clinical Aspects of Regional Fat Distribution." *American Journal of Clinical Nutrition* 52 (1990):946–950.
3. Bray, G. A. "Pathophysiology of Obesity." *American Journal of Clinical Nutrition,* 55 (1992): 488S–494S.
4. Fisher, A. G., and P. E. Allsen. *Jogging.* Dubuque, IA: Wm. C. Brown, 1987.
5. Goldman, H. L., and M. R. Becklake. "Respiratory Function Tests: Normal Values at Medium Altitudes and the Prediction of Normal Results." *American Review of Tuberculosis* 79 (1959): 457–467.

6. Hoeger, W. W. K., and S. A. Hoeger. *Lifetime Physical Fitness & Wellness: A Personalized Program.* Englewood, CO: Morton Publishing, 1992.
7. Jackson, A. S., and M. L. Pollock. "Generalized Equations for Predicting Body Density of Men." *British Journal of Nutrition* 40 (1978):497–504.
8. Jackson, A. S., M. L. Pollock, and A. Ward. "Generalized Equations for Predicting Body Density of Women." *Medicine and Science in Sports and Exercise* 3 (1980):175–182.
9. Lambson, R. B. "Generalized Body Density Prediction Equations for Women Using Simple Anthropometric Measurements." Unpublished doctoral dissertation, Brigham Young University, Provo, Utah, August 1987.

10. Penrouse, K. W., A. G. Nelson, and A. G. Fisher. "Generalized Body Composition Equation for Men Using Simple Measurement Techniques." *Medicine and Science in Sports and Exercise* 17(2), 1985:189.
11. Siri, W. E. *Body Composition from Fluid Spaces and Density.* Berkeley, CA: Donner Laboratory of Medical Physics, University of California, 1956.
12. Stensland, S. H., and S. Margolis. "Simplifying the Calculation of Body Mass Index for Quick Reference." *Journal of the American Dietetic Association,* 90 (1990):856.

PRINCIPLES OF WEIGHT CONTROL

4

Two terms commonly are used in reference to people who weigh more than recommended: overweight and obesity. **Overweight** indicates *an excess amount of weight against a given standard* such as height or recommended percent body fat. **Obesity** is defined as *a chronic disease characterized by an excessively high amount of body fat in relation to lean body mass.* Obesity levels are established at a point at which the excess body fat can lead to serious health problems.

Scientific evidence also recognizes problems with being underweight. The social pressure to be thin has decreased slightly in recent years, but the pressure to attain model-like thinness is still with us and contributes to the gradual increase in the number of people who develop eating disorders (anorexia nervosa and bulimia, discussed later in this chapter).

Extreme weight loss can lead to medical conditions such as heart damage, gastrointestinal problems, shrinkage of internal organs, immune system abnormalities, disorders of the reproductive system, loss of muscle tissue, damage to the nervous system, and even death. About 14% of the American people are underweight.

OBESITY AND OVERWEIGHT

Obesity is a health hazard of epidemic proportions in most developed countries around the world. An estimated 35% of the adult population in industrialized nations is obese.

Children in the United States do not start with a weight problem. Although a small group struggles with weight throughout life, most are not overweight when they reach age 20. *According to 1993 estimates, 65% of adults in the United States was over recommended body weight.* The prevalence continues to increase.

When Yankee Stadium in New York was renovated several years ago, total seating capacity had to be reduced to accommodate the wider bodies of the spectators. During the last decade, the average weight of American adults increased by about 15 pounds. In 1991, 33% of adults were at least 10% above recommended body weight. In 1993, this figure grew to 40%.

Obesity by itself has been associated with several serious health problems and accounts for 15% to 20% of the annual mortality rate in the United States. Obesity is a major risk factor for diseases of the cardiovascular system, including coronary heart disease, hypertension, congestive heart failure, high levels of blood lipids, atherosclerosis, strokes, thromboembolitic disease, osteoarthritis, varicose veins, and intermittent claudication.

> *The health consequences of obesity apply primarily to the severely overweight individual.*

Other research points toward a possible link between obesity and cancer of the colon, rectum, prostate, gallbladder, breast, uterus, and ovaries. In addition, obesity has been associated with diabetes, ruptured intervertebral discs, gallstones, gout, respiratory insufficiency, and complications during pregnancy and delivery. Furthermore, it is implicated in psychological maladjustment and increased accidental death rate.

Achieving and maintaining recommended body weight is a major objective of a good physical fitness and wellness program (Figure 4.1). The assessment of recommended body weight was discussed in detail in Chapter 3. Next to poor cardiovascular fitness, obesity is the problem encountered most commonly in fitness and wellness assessments.

Approximately 65 million Americans are either overweight or consider themselves to be overweight. Of these, 30 million are obese. About 50% of all women and 25% of all men are on diets at any given moment. People spend about $40 billion yearly attempting to lose weight. More than $10 billion goes to memberships in weight reduction centers and another $30 billion to diet food sales.

Overweight and obesity are not the same thing. Most overweight people are not obese. The health consequences of obesity apply primarily to the severely overweight individual.

Granted, genetic differences exist. Some moderately overweight people have health problems, but, such is not the case for most. Moderately overweight

FIGURE 4.1
Recommended body weight is best determined through the assessment of body composition.

people with diabetes and other cardiovascular risk factors benefit from weight loss.

Many people want to lose weight so they will look better. That's a noteworthy goal. The problem, however, is that they have a distorted image of what they would really look like if they were to reduce to what they think is their ideal weight. Hereditary factors play a big role and only a small fraction of the population have the genes for a "perfect body."

As people set their own target weight, they should be realistic. Attaining the excellent percent body fat figure in Table 3.7, Chapter 3, is extremely difficult for some. It is even more difficult to maintain, unless they are willing to make a commitment to a vigorous lifetime exercise program and permanent dietary changes. Few people are willing to do that. The moderate percent body fat category may be more realistic for many people.

A question you should ask yourself is: Are you happy with your weight? Part of enjoying a higher quality of life is being happy with yourself. If you are not, you either need to do something about it or learn to live with it!

If you are above the moderate percent body fat category, you should try to come down and stay in this category, for health reasons. This is the category in which there appears to be no detriment to health.

If you are in the moderate category but would like to be lower, you need to ask yourself a second question: How bad do I want it? Do you want it bad enough to implement lifetime exercise and dietary changes? *If you are not willing to change, you should stop worrying about your weight and deem the moderate category as "tolerable" for you.*

THE WEIGHT LOSS DILEMMA

Constantly gaining and losing weight — *yo-yo dieting* — carries as great a health risk as being overweight and remaining overweight in the first place. Epidemiological data are beginning to show that frequent fluctuations in weight (up or down) markedly increase the risk of dying from cardiovascular disease.

Based on the findings that constant losses and regains can be hazardous to health, quick fix diets should be replaced by a slow but permanent weight loss program, as described in this chapter. The benefits of recommended body weight are reaped when people get to their recommended body weight and stay there throughout life.

Unfortunately, only about 10% of all people who begin a traditional weight loss program, without exercise, are able to lose the desired weight. Worse, only one in 200 is able to keep the weight off. The body is highly resistant to permanent weight changes through caloric restrictions alone.

Traditional diets have failed because few of them incorporate lifetime changes in food selection and exercise as fundamental to successful weight loss. When the diet stops, weight gain begins. The $40 billion diet industry tries to capitalize on the idea that weight can be lost quickly without taking into consideration the consequences of fast weight loss or the importance of lifetime behavioral changes to ensure proper weight loss and maintenance.

In addition, various studies indicate that most people tend to underestimate their energy intake, especially obese people. Those who try to lose weight, but apparently fail to do so, are often referred to as "diet-resistant" individuals. A study published in 1992 by Dr. Steven Lichtman and colleagues in the *New England Journal of Medicine* found that, while on a "diet," a group of obese individuals with a self-reported history of diet resistance

underreported their average daily caloric intake by almost 50% (1,028 self-reported versus 2,081 actual, see Figure 4.2). These individuals also overestimated their amount of daily physical activity by about 25% (1022 calories self-reported versus 771 actual calories). These differences represent an additional 1304 calories of energy unaccounted for by the subjects in the study. These findings indicate that failing to lose weight often is related to misreports of actual food intake and level of physical activity.

Fad diets continue to appeal to people. These diets deceive people and claim the person indeed will lose weight by following all instructions. Most fad diets are very low in calories and deprive the body of certain nutrients, generating a metabolic imbalance. Under these conditions, a lot of the weight lost is in the form of water and protein, and not fat.

On a crash diet close to half the weight loss is in lean (protein) tissue. When the body uses protein instead of a combination of fats and carbohydrates as a source of energy, weight is lost as much as 10 times faster.[12] A gram of protein produces half the amount of energy that fat does. In the case of muscle protein, one-fifth of protein is mixed with four-fifths

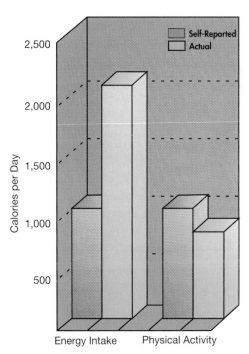

Source: "Discrepancy Between Self-Reported and Actual Caloric Intake and Exercise in Obese Subjects" by S. W. Lichtman et al., in *New England Journal of Medicine* 327 (1992): 1893-1898.

FIGURE 4.2
Differences between self-reported and actual daily caloric intake and exercise in obese individuals attempting to lose weight.

water. Each pound of muscle yields only one-tenth the amount of energy of a pound of fat. As a result, most of the weight loss is in the form of water, which on the scale, of course, looks good.

Some diets allow only certain specialized foods. If people would realize that no magic foods will provide all of the necessary nutrients, and that a person has to eat a variety of foods to be well-nourished, the diet industry would not be as successful. Most of these diets create a nutritional deficiency, which at times can be fatal.

The reason some of these diets succeed is that people eventually get tired of eating the same thing day in and day out and start eating less. If they happen to achieve the lower weight but do not make permanent dietary changes they quickly regain the weight once they go back to their old eating habits.

A few diets recommend exercise along with caloric restrictions — the best method for weight reduction, of course. A lot of the weight lost is because of the exercise, so the diet has achieved its purpose. Unfortunately, if the people do not change their food selection and activity level, permanently, they quickly gain back the weight once they discontinue dieting and exercise.

EATING DISORDERS

Anorexia nervosa and bulimia are physical and emotional problems, thought to develop from individual, family, or social pressures, characterized by an intense fear of becoming fat, which does not disappear even when losing extreme amounts of weight. These medical disorders are steadily increasing in most industrialized nations where society encourages low-calorie diets and thinness.

ANOREXIA NERVOSA

Anorexia nervosa is a condition of self-imposed starvation to lose and then maintain very low body weight. Approximately 19 of every 20 anorexics are young women. An estimated 1% of the female population in the United States is anorexic. Anorexic individuals seem to fear weight gain more than death from starvation. Furthermore, they have a distorted image of their body and think of themselves as being fat even when they are emaciated.

Although a genetic predisposition may contribute, the anorexic person often comes from a mother-dominated home, with other possible drug addictions in the family. The syndrome may emerge following a stressful life event and the uncertainty about the ability to cope efficiently.

Because the female role in society is changing more rapidly, women seem to be especially susceptible. Life experiences such as gaining weight, starting menstrual periods, beginning college, losing a boyfriend, having poor self-esteem, being socially rejected, starting a professional career, or becoming a wife or mother may trigger the syndrome.

These individuals typically begin a diet and at first feel in control and happy about the weight loss, even if they are not overweight. To speed up the weight loss, they frequently combine extreme dieting with exhaustive exercise and overuse of laxatives and diuretics.

Anorexic individuals seem to fear weight gain more than death from starvation.

Anorexics commonly develop obsessive and compulsive behaviors and emphatically deny their condition. They are preoccupied with food, meal planning, grocery shopping, and unusual eating habits. As they lose weight and their health begins to deteriorate, anorexics feel weak and tired and may realize they have a problem but will not stop the starvation and refuse to consider the behavior as abnormal.

Once they have lost a lot of weight and malnutrition sets in, physical changes become more visible. Some typical changes are amenorrhea (stopping menstruation), digestive problems, extreme sensitivity to cold, hair and skin problems, fluid and electrolyte abnormalities (which may lead to an irregular heartbeat and sudden stopping of the heart), injuries to nerves and tendons, abnormalities of immune function, anemia, growth of fine body hair, mental confusion, inability to concentrate, lethargy, depression, skin dryness, and lower skin and body temperature.

Many of the changes of anorexia nervosa can be reversed. Treatment almost always requires professional help, and the sooner it is started, the better the chances for reversibility and cure. Therapy consists of a combination of medical and psychological techniques to restore proper nutrition, prevent medical complications, and modify the environment or events that triggered the syndrome.

Seldom are anorexics able to overcome the problem by themselves. Unfortunately, they strongly deny their condition. They are able to hide it and deceive friends and relatives quite effectively. Based on their behavior, many of them meet all of the characteristics of anorexia nervosa, but it goes undetected because both thinness and dieting are socially acceptable. Only a well-trained clinician is able to make a positive diagnosis. The criteria recommended by the American Psychiatric Association for clinicians to diagnose anorexia nervosa are described in Figure 4.3.

BULIMIA

A pattern of binge eating and purging, bulimia is more prevalent than anorexia nervosa. For many years it was thought to be a variant of anorexia nervosa, but now it is identified as a separate condition. It afflicts mainly young people, and as many as one in every five women on college campuses may be bulimic, according to some estimates. Bulimia also is more prevalent than anorexia nervosa in males.

- Refusal to maintain body weight over a minimal normal weight for age and height, e.g., weight loss leading to maintenance of body weight 15% below that expected; or failure to make expected weight gain during period of growth, leading to body weight 15% below that expected.
- Intense fear of gaining weight or becoming fat, even though underweight.
- Disturbance in the way in which one's body weight, size, or shape is experienced; e.g., the person claims to "feel fat" even when emaciated or believes that one area of the body is "too fat" even when obviously underweight.
- In females, absence of at least three consecutive menstrual cycles when otherwise expected to occur (primary or secondary amenorrhea). (A woman is considered to have amenorrhea if her periods occur only following hormone, e.g., estrogen, administration.)

Source: American Psychiatric Association, *Diagnostic and Statistical Manual of Mental Disorders* (Washington, DC, Association, 1987), p. 67.

FIGURE 4.3
Diagnostic criteria for anorexia nervosa.

Bulimics usually are healthy-looking people, well-educated, near recommended body weight, who enjoy food and often socialize around it. In actuality, they are emotionally insecure, rely on others, and lack self-confidence and esteem. Recommended weight and food are important to them.

The binge-purge cycle usually occurs in stages. As a result of stressful life events or the simple compulsion to eat, bulimics periodically engage in binge eating that may last an hour or longer.

The sooner treatment for eating disorders is initiated, the better the chances for recovery.

With some apprehension, bulimics anticipate and plan the cycle. Next they feel an urgency to begin, followed by a large and uncontrollable food consumption during which they may eat several thousand calories (up to 10,000 calories in extreme cases). After a short period of relief and satisfaction, feelings of deep guilt, shame, and intense fear of gaining weight ensue. Purging seems to be an easy answer, as the binging cycle can continue without the fear of gaining weight.

The most common form of purging is self-induced vomiting, although bulimics frequently ingest strong laxatives and emetics. Near-fasting diets and strenuous bouts of exercise are seen commonly in bulimics. Medical problems associated with bulimia include cardiac arrhythmias, amenorrhea, kidney and bladder damage, ulcers, colitis, tearing of the esophagus or stomach, tooth erosion, gum damage, and general muscular weakness.

Unlike anorexics, bulimics realize their behavior is abnormal and feel great shame about it. Fearing social rejection, they pursue the binge-purge cycle in secrecy and at unusual hours of the day.

Bulimia can be treated successfully when the person realizes this destructive behavior is not the solution to life's problems. A change in attitude can prevent permanent damage or death. The guidelines by the American Psychiatric Association for the diagnosis of bulimia are given in Figure 4.4.

Treatment for anorexia nervosa and bulimia are available on most school campuses through the school's counseling center or the health center. Local hospitals also offer treatment for these conditions. Many communities have support groups, frequently

■ Recurrent episodes of binge eating (rapid consumption of a large amount of food in a discrete period of time).

■ A feeling of lack of control over eating behavior during the eating binges.

■ Regular practice of either self-induced vomiting, use of laxatives or diuretics, strict dieting or fasting, or vigorous exercise to prevent weight gain.

■ A minimum average of two binge eating episodes a week for at least three months.

■ Persistent overconcern with body shape and weight.

Source: American Psychiatric Association, *Diagnostic and Statistical Manual of Mental Disorders* (Washington, DC, Association), p. 68-69, 1987.

FIGURE 4.4
Diagnostic criteria for bulimia.

led by professional personnel and usually free of charge.

PHYSIOLOGY OF WEIGHT LOSS

Only a few years ago the principles governing a weight loss and maintenance program seemed to be fairly clear, but we now know the final answers are not yet in. Traditional concepts related to weight control have centered on three assumptions: (a) that balancing food intake against output allows a person to achieve recommended weight, (b) that all fat people just eat too much, and (c) that the human body doesn't care how much (or little) fat it stores. Although these statements have some truth, they are still open to much debate and research.

THE ENERGY-BALANCING EQUATION

The energy-balancing equation basically states that as long as caloric input equals caloric output, the person will not gain or lose weight. If caloric intake exceeds output, the individual gains weight. When output exceeds input, the person loses weight.

This principle is simple. If daily energy requirements could be determined, accurately, it seems reasonable that caloric intake could be balanced against output. This is not always the case, though, because genetic and lifestyle-related individual differences determine the number of calories required to maintain or lose body weight.

Table 4.1, on page 77, offers some general guidelines for estimating daily caloric intake according to lifestyle patterns. This is only an estimated figure and, as discussed later in the chapter, it serves only as a starting point from which individual adjustments have to be made.

One pound of fat equals 3,500 calories. Assuming that a person's basic daily caloric expenditure is 2,500 calories, if this person were to decrease the daily intake by 500 calories per day, it should result in a loss of one pound of fat in 7 days (500 × 7 = 3,500). But research has shown, and many dieters probably have experienced, that even when they carefully balance caloric input against caloric output, weight loss does not always happen as predicted. Furthermore, two people with similar measured caloric intake and output seldom lose weight at the same rate.

The most common explanation regarding individual differences in weight loss and weight gain has been the variation in human metabolism from one person to another. We are all familiar with people who can eat "all day long" and not gain an ounce of weight, while others cannot even "dream" about food without gaining weight. Because experts did not believe that human metabolism alone could account for such extreme differences, they developed several theories that may better explain these individual variations.

SETPOINT THEORY

Results of several research studies point toward a weight-regulating mechanism (WRM) in the hypothalamus of the brain that regulates how much the body should weigh. This mechanism has a setpoint that controls both appetite and the amount of fat stored.

Setpoint is hypothesized to work like a thermostat for body fat, maintaining fairly constant body weight because it knows at all times the exact amount of adipose tissue stored in the fat cells. Some people have high settings; others have low settings.

If body weight decreases (as in dieting), the setpoint senses this change and triggers the WRM to increase the person's appetite or make the body conserve energy to maintain the "set" weight. The opposite also may be true. Some people have a hard time gaining weight. In this case the WRM decreases appetite or causes the body to waste energy to maintain the lower weight.

Dieting Makes People Fat!

Every person has his or her own certain body fat percentage (as established by the setpoint) that the body attempts to maintain. The genetic instinct to survive tells the body that fat storage is vital, and therefore it sets an acceptable fat level. This level remains somewhat constant or may gradually climb because of poor lifestyle habits.

For instance, under strict calorie reduction the body may make extreme metabolic adjustments in an effort to maintain its setpoint for fat. The basal metabolic rate (amount of energy the body needs to maintain life at complete rest) may drop dramatically against a consistent negative caloric balance, and a person may be on a plateau for days or even weeks without losing much weight. A low metabolic rate compounds a person's problems in maintaining recommended body weight.

Dietary restriction alone will not lower the setpoint, even though the person may lose weight and fat. When the dieter goes back to the normal or even below-normal caloric intake, at which the weight may have been stable for a long time, he or she quickly regains the fat loss as the body strives to regain a comfortable fat store.

Let's use a practical illustration. A person would like to lose some body fat and assumes that a stable body weight has been reached at an average daily caloric intake of 1,800 calories (no weight gain or loss occurs at this daily intake). In an attempt to lose weight rapidly, this person now goes on a strict low-calorie diet, or even worse, a near-fasting diet. Immediately the body activates its survival mechanism and readjusts its metabolism to a lower caloric balance. After a few weeks of dieting at fewer than 400 to 600 calories per day, the body now can maintain its normal functions at 1,000 calories per day.

Having lost the desired weight, the person terminates the diet but realizes the original intake of 1,800 calories per day will have to be lower to maintain the new lower weight. To adjust to the new lower body weight, the intake is restricted to about 1,500 calories per day. The individual is surprised to find that, even at this lower daily intake (300 fewer calories), weight comes back at a rate of one pound every one to two weeks. After ending the diet, this new lowered metabolic rate may take several months to kick back up to its normal level.

From this explanation, individuals clearly should never go on very low-calorie diets. Not only will this slow down resting metabolic rate, but it also will deprive the body of basic daily nutrients required for normal function.

Under no circumstances should a person go on a diet that calls for below 1,200 and 1,500 calories for women and men, respectively. Weight (fat) is gained over months and years, not overnight. Likewise, weight loss should be gradual, not abrupt.

Daily caloric intakes of 1,200 to 1,500 calories provide the necessary nutrients if they are distributed properly over the five basic food groups (meeting the daily required servings from each group). Of course, the individual will have to learn which foods meet the requirements and yet are low in fat and sugar.

Setpoint and Nutrition

A second way in which the setpoint may work is by keeping track of the nutrients and calories consumed daily. It is thought that the body, like a cash register, records the daily food intake and the brain will not feel satisfied until the calories and nutrients have been "registered."

This setpoint for calories and nutrients seems to work for some people, even when they participate in moderately intense exercise. Some studies have shown that people do not become hungrier with moderate physical activity. Therefore, people can choose to lose weight either by going hungry or by stepping up their daily physical activity. The greater number of calories burned through exercise will help lower body fat.

The most common question regarding the setpoint is how it can be lowered so the body will feel comfortable at a lesser fat percentage. Several factors seem to affect the setpoint directly by lowering the fat thermostat:

1. Aerobic exercise.
2. A diet high in complex carbohydrates.
3. Nicotine.
4. Amphetamines.

The last two, however, are more destructive than the overfatness, so they are not reasonable alternatives (as far as the extra strain on the heart is concerned, smoking one pack of cigarettes per day is said to be the equivalent of carrying 50 to 75 pounds of excess body fat).

On the other hand, a diet high in fats and refined carbohydrates, near-fasting diets, and perhaps even artificial sweeteners seem to raise the setpoint. Therefore, the only practical and sensible way to lower the setpoint and lose fat weight seems to be a combination of aerobic exercise and a diet high in complex carbohydrates and low in fat.

Because of the effects of proper food management on the body's setpoint, many nutritionists believe the total number of calories should not be the main concern in a weight control program. Rather, it should be the source of those calories. In this regard, most of the effort is spent in retraining eating habits, increasing the intake of complex carbohydrates and high-fiber foods, and decreasing the consumption of refined carbohydrates (sugars) and fats. In most cases, this change in eating habits will bring about a decrease in total daily caloric intake.

A "diet" is no longer viewed as a temporary tool to aid in weight loss but, instead, as a permanent change in eating behaviors to ensure weight management and better health. The role of increased physical activity also must be considered, because successful weight loss, maintenance, and recommended body composition seldom are attained without a moderate reduction in caloric intake combined with a regular exercise program.

Diet and Metabolism

Fat can be lost by selecting the proper foods, with exercise, or restricting calories. When a person tries to lose weight by dietary restrictions alone, lean body mass (muscle protein, along with vital organ protein) always decreases. The amount of lean body mass lost depends entirely on caloric limitation.

When obese people go on a near-fasting diet, up to half of the weight loss is lean body mass and the other half is actual fat loss (see Figure 4.5). When the diet is combined with exercise, close to 100% of the weight loss is in the form of fat, and lean tissue actually may increase.

Loss of lean body mass is never good, because it weakens the organs and muscles and slows down metabolism. Large losses in lean tissue can cause disturbances in heart function and damage to other organs. Equally important is not to overindulge (binge) following very-low-calorie diets. This may

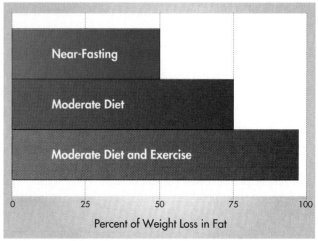

Adapted from Shephard, R. J. *Alive Man: The Physiology of Physical Activity.* Springfield, IL: Charles C. Thomas, 484–488, 1975.

FIGURE 4.5
Effects of three forms of diet on fat loss.

cause changes in metabolic rate and electrolyte balance, which could trigger fatal cardiac arrhythmias.

Contrary to some beliefs, aging is not the main reason for the lower metabolic rate. It is not so much that metabolism slows down as that people slow down. As people age they tend to rely more on the amenities of life (remote controls, cellular telephones, intercoms, single-level homes, riding lawn mowers) that lull a person into sedentary living.

Basal metabolism is related directly to lean body weight. The more the lean tissue, the higher the metabolic rate. As a consequence of sedentary living and less physical activity, the lean component decreases and fat tissue increases. The human body, though, requires a certain amount of oxygen per pound of lean body mass. As fat is considered metabolically inert from the point of view of caloric use, the lean tissue uses most of the oxygen, even at rest. As muscle and organ mass decreases (lean body mass), so do the energy requirements at rest.

Reductions in lean body mass are common in aging people (because of physical inactivity) and those on severely restricted diets. The loss of lean body mass also may account for a lower metabolic rate (described earlier) and the longer time it takes to kick back up.

Diets with caloric intakes below 1,200 to 1,500 calories cannot guarantee the retention of lean body mass. Even at this intake level, some loss is inevitable unless the diet is combined with exercise. Despite the claims of many diets that they do not alter the lean component, the simple truth is that, regardless of what nutrients may be added to the diet, severe caloric restrictions always prompt a loss of lean tissue. Too many people constantly go on low-calorie diets. Every time they do, the metabolic rate slows down as more lean tissue is lost.

You may run across people in their 40s or older who weigh the same as they did when they were 20 and think they are at recommended body weight. During this span of 20 years or more, these people may have dieted many times without participating in an exercise program. They regain the weight shortly after they terminate each diet, but most of that gain is in fat. Maybe at age 20 they weighed 150 pounds and had only 15% fat. Now at age 40, even though they still weigh 150 pounds, they might be 30% fat. At recommended body weight, they wonder why they are eating very little and still having trouble staying at that weight.

EXERCISE: THE KEY TO WEIGHT LOSS AND WEIGHT MAINTENANCE

Based on the preceding discussion, exercise is vital to weight loss and weight maintenance (Figure 4.6). Not only will exercise maintain lean tissue, but advocates of the setpoint theory say that exercise resets the fat thermostat to a new, lower level. This change may be rapid, or it may take time. A few overweight individuals have exercised faithfully almost daily, 60 minutes at a time, for a whole year before weight change is significant. People with a "sticky" setpoint have to be patient and persistent.

If a person is trying to lose weight, a combination of aerobic and strength-training exercises works best. Aerobic exercise is the best to offset the setpoint, and the continuity and duration of these types of activities cause many calories to be burned in the process. The role of aerobic exercise in successful lifetime weight management cannot be over-estimated. As illustrated in Figure 4.7, greater weight loss is achieved by combining a diet with an aerobic exercise program.

Of even greater significance, only the individuals who participated in an 18-month post-diet aerobic exercise program were able to keep the weight off. Those who discontinued exercise gained weight. Furthermore, all those who initiated or resumed exercise during the 18-month follow-up were able to lose weight again. Individuals who only dieted and never exercised regained 60% and 92% of their weight loss at the 6 and 18-month follow-up, respectively.

Weight loss comes more rapidly when aerobic exercise is combined with a strength-training program. Two exercise groups — a 30-minute aerobic group and a 15-minute aerobic plus 15-minute strength-training (30 minutes total) group — participated in an eight-week, three-days-per-week study. Both groups followed a dietary plan that consisted of approximately 60% carbohydrates, 20% fats, and 20% proteins.

The aerobic group lost an average of 3½ pounds, 3 of which were fat and the remaining half pound lean tissue. The combined aerobic and strength-training group lost an average of 8 pounds. Changes in body composition, however, indicated that the latter group actually lost 10 pounds of fat and gained 2 pounds of lean tissue (see Figure 4.8). These findings indicate that a sensible strength-training program is better to lose weight and maintain or increase muscle mass and metabolic rate.

Based on estimates, each additional pound of muscle tissue can raise the basal metabolic rate

FIGURE 4.6
Regular participation in a lifetime exercise program is the key to successful weight management.

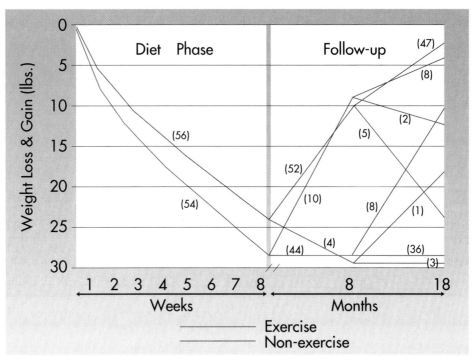

Source: Pavlou, K. N., S. Krey, and W. P. Steffe. "Exercise as an Adjunct to Weight Loss and Maintenance in Moderately Obese Subjects." *American Journal of Clinical Nutrition,* 49:1115-1123, 1989.

FIGURE 4.7
Value of aerobic exercise and weight loss and maintenance in moderately obese individuals (numbers in parenthesis indicate number of participants).

between 30 and 50 calories per day. Using the conservative estimate of 30 calories per day, an individual who adds 5 pounds of muscle tissue as a result of strength training increases the basal metabolic rate by 150 calories per day, which equals 54,750

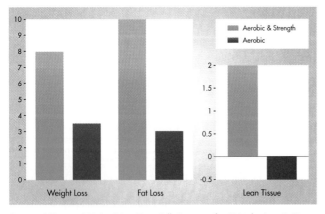

Source: Wescott, W. L. "You Can Sell Exercise for Weight Loss." *Fitness Management,* 7(12):33–34, 1991.

FIGURE 4.8
Changes in body composition through an aerobic exercise program and a combined aerobic/strength-training exercise program.

calories per year, or the equivalent of 15.6 pounds of fat.

Strength training is recommended especially for people who think they are at their ideal body weight, yet their body fat percentage is higher than recommended. The number of calories burned during a typical hour-long strength-training session is much less than during an hour of aerobic exercise. Because of the high intensity of strength training, the person needs frequent rest intervals to recover from each set of exercise. The average person actually lifts weights only 10 to 12 minutes in each hour of exercise.

Weight can be lost through a regular strength-training program, but much more slowly than through aerobics. In the long run, however, the person enjoys the benefits of gains in lean tissue. Guidelines for developing aerobic and strength-training programs are given in Chapters 6 and 8.

Because exercise results in more lean body mass, body weight often remains the same or even increases after beginning an exercise program, while inches and percent body fat decrease. More lean tissue means more functional capacity of the human body. With exercise, most of the weight loss becomes apparent after a few weeks of training, after the lean component has stabilized.

Although we now know that a negative caloric balance of 3,500 calories does not always result in a loss of exactly one pound of fat, the role of exercise in achieving a negative balance by burning additional calories is significant in weight reduction and maintenance programs. Sadly, some individuals claim that the amount of calories burned during exercise is hardly worth the effort. They think that cutting their daily intake by some 300 calories is easier than participating in some sort of exercise that would burn the same amount of calories. The problem is that the willpower to cut those 300 calories lasts only a few weeks, and then the person goes right back to the old eating patterns.

The lack of exercise, not the weight problem itself, possibly is the cause of many of the health risks associated with obesity.

If a person gets into the habit of exercising regularly, say three times a week, running 3 miles per exercise session (about 300 calories burned), this represents 900 calories in one week, about 3,600 in one month, or 46,800 calories per year. This minimal amount of exercise could mean as many as 13.5 extra pounds of fat in one year, 27 in two, and so on.

We tend to forget that our weight creeps up gradually over the years, not just overnight. Hardly worth the effort? And we have not even taken into consideration the increase in lean tissue, the possible resetting of the setpoint, the benefits to the cardiovascular system, and most important, the improved quality of life. The fundamental reasons for overfatness and obesity, few could argue, are lack of physical activity and sedentary living.

In terms of preventing disease, many of the health benefits people try to achieve by losing weight are reaped through exercise alone, even without weight loss. Exercise offers protection against premature morbidity and mortality for everyone, including people who already have risk factors for disease (see Chapter 12). *The lack of exercise, not the weight problem itself, possibly is the cause of many of the health risks associated with obesity.*

HEALTHY WEIGHT GAIN

"Skinny" people, too, should realize that the only healthy way to gain weight is through exercise (mainly strength-training exercises) and a slight increase in caloric intake. Attempting to gain weight just by overeating will raise the fat component and not the lean component — which is not the path to better health. Exercise is the best solution to weight (fat) reduction and weight (lean) gain.

A strength-training program such as the one outlined in Chapter 8 is the best approach to add body weight. To produce the most muscle hypertrophy, the training program should include at least two exercises of three to five sets for each major body part (see Principles Involved in Strength Training, Chapter 8). Each set should consist of about 10 repetitions maximum.

Even though the metabolic cost of synthesizing a pound of muscle tissue is still unclear, an estimated 500 additional calories daily, including 15 grams of protein above the RDA, are recommended to gain an average of 1 pound of muscle tissue per week. Based on the typical American diet, the extra 15 grams of protein are not necessary. Each day, the average American already consumes 30 to 60 grams of protein above the RDA. The extra 500 calories should be in the form of complex carbohydrates, because most diets already are too high in fat. If the higher caloric intake is not accompanied by a strength-training program, the increase in body weight will be in the form of fat and not muscle tissue.

WEIGHT LOSS MYTHS

Spot reducing and losing "cellulite" (as some people refer to the fat deposits that bulge out on certain body parts) are mythical concepts. These deposits are nothing but enlarged fat cells, from accumulated body fat. Doing several sets of daily sit-ups will not get rid of fat in the midsection of the body.

When fat comes off, it does so throughout the entire body, not just the exercised area. The greatest proportion of fat may come off the biggest fat deposits, but the caloric output of a few sets of sit-ups has practically no effect on reducing total body fat. A person has to exercise much longer to really see results.

Other touted means toward quick weight loss — rubberized sweatsuits, steam baths, mechanical vibrators — are misleading. When a person wears a sweatsuit or steps into a sauna, the weight lost is not fat but merely a significant amount of water. Sure, it looks nice when you step on the scale immediately afterward, but this represents a false loss of weight. As soon as you replace body fluids, you gain back the weight quickly.

Wearing rubberized sweatsuits not only hastens the rate of body fluid loss — fluid that is vital during prolonged exercise — but at the same time it raises core temperature. This combination puts a person in danger of dehydration, which impairs cellular function and in extreme cases can even cause death.

Similarly, mechanical vibrators are worthless in a weight control program. Vibrating belts and turning rollers may feel good, but they require no effort whatsoever. Fat cannot be shaken off; it is primarily lost by burning it in muscle tissue.

LOSING WEIGHT THE SOUND AND SENSIBLE WAY

Dieting never has been fun and never will be. People who are overweight and are serious about losing weight, however, have to include regular exercise in their life along with proper food management and a sensible reduction in caloric intake.

Some precautions are in order, as excessive body fat is a risk factor for cardiovascular disease. Depending on the extent of the weight problem, a medical examination and possibly a stress ECG (see Figure 1.13, Chapter 1) may be a good idea before undertaking the exercise program. A physician should be consulted in this regard.

Significantly overweight individuals also may have to choose activities in which they will not have to support their own body weight but that still will be effective in burning calories. Joint and muscle injuries are common in overweight individuals who participate in weight-bearing exercises such as walking, jogging, and aerobics.

Swimming may not be a good exercise either. More body fat makes a person more buoyant, and most people are not at the skill level to swim fast

enough to get the best training effect. They tend to just float along, limiting the amount of calories burned as well as the benefits to the cardiovascular system.

Some better alternatives are riding a bicycle (either road or stationary), walking in a shallow pool, doing water aerobics (Figure 4.9), or running in place in deep water (treading water). These forms of water exercise are gaining popularity and have proven to be effective in weight reduction without the "pain" and fear of injuries. Through the caloric expenditure of selected physical activities given in Table 4.2, you will be able to determine your own daily caloric requirement in Lab 4A.

How long should each exercise session last? To develop and maintain cardiovascular fitness, 20 to 30 minutes of exercise at the ideal target rate, three to five times per week, is suggested (see Chapter 6). For weight loss purposes, many experts recommend exercising at least 45 minutes at a time, five to six times a week.

A person should not try to do too much too fast. Unconditioned beginners should start with about 15 minutes of aerobic exercise three times a week, gradually increasing the duration by approximately 5 minutes each week and the frequency by one day per week during the next three to four weeks.

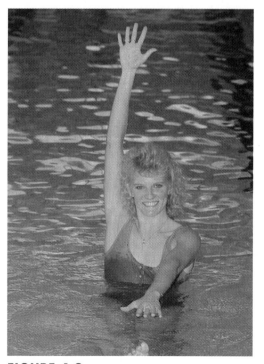

FIGURE 4.9
Water aerobics is a relatively new form of aerobic exercise.

One final benefit of exercise for weight control is that it allows fat to be burned more efficiently. As both carbohydrates and fats are sources of energy, when the glucose levels begin to drop during prolonged exercise, more fat is used as energy substrate.

Equally important is that fat-burning enzymes increase with aerobic training. Essentially, fat is lost by burning it in muscle. Therefore, as the concentration of the enzymes increases, so does the ability to burn fat.[12]

In addition to exercise and adequate food management, sensible adjustments in caloric intake are recommended. Most research finds that a negative caloric balance is required to lose weight. Perhaps the only exception is in people who are eating too few calories. A nutrient analysis (see Chapter 2) often reveals that faithful dieters are not consuming enough calories. These people actually need to increase their daily caloric intake (combined with an exercise program) to get metabolism to kick back up to a normal level.

The reasons for prescribing a lower caloric figure to lose weight are:

1. Most people underestimate their caloric intake and are eating more than they should be eating.

2. Developing new behaviors takes time, and some people have trouble changing and adjusting to new eating habits.

3. Many individuals are in such poor physical condition that it takes them a long time to increase their activity level enough to offset the setpoint and burn enough calories to aid in body fat loss.

4. Some dieters have difficulty succeeding unless they can count calories.

5. A few people simply will not alter their food selection. For those who will not change their food selection (which will still increase the risk for chronic diseases), a large increase in physical activity, a negative caloric balance, or a combination of the two is the only solution to successfully lose weight.

An estimated daily caloric requirement can be determined by consulting Tables 4.1 and 4.2. This activity is conducted in Lab 4A. As this is only an estimated value, individual adjustments related to many of the factors discussed in this chapter may be necessary to establish a more precise value. Nevertheless, the estimated value does offer a beginning guideline for weight control or reduction.

The average daily caloric requirement without exercise is based on typical lifestyle patterns, total body weight, and gender. Individuals who hold jobs that require heavy manual labor burn more calories during the day than those who have sedentary jobs such as working behind a desk.

To find your activity level:

1. Refer to Table 4.1 and rate yourself accordingly. The number given in Table 4.1 is per pound of body weight, so you should multiply your current weight by that number. For example, the typical caloric requirement to maintain body weight for a moderately active male who weighs 160 pounds is 2,400 calories (160 lbs × 15 cal/lb).

2. Determine the average number of calories burned on a daily basis as a result of exercise. To get this number, figure out the total number of minutes you exercise weekly, and then figure the daily average exercise time. For instance, a person cycling at 13 miles per hour, five times a week, 30 minutes each time, exercises 150 minutes per week (5 × 30). The average daily exercise time is 21 minutes (150 ÷ 7). Round off to the lowest unit.

3. Referring to Table 4.2, find the energy requirement for the activity (or activities) chosen for the exercise program. In the case of cycling (13 miles per hour), the requirement is .071 calories per pound of body weight per minute of activity (cal/lb/min). With a body weight of 160 pounds, this man burns 11.4 calories each minute (body weight × .071, or 160 × .071). In 21 minutes, he burns approximately 240 calories (21 × 11.4).

4. Obtain the estimated total caloric requirement, with exercise, needed to maintain body weight. To do this, add the typical daily requirement (without exercise) and the average calories

TABLE 4.1
Average Caloric Requirement Per Pound of Body Weight Based on Lifestyle Patterns and Gender

	Calories Per Pound	
	Men	Women*
Sedentary — Limited physical activity	13.0	12.0
Moderate physical activity	15.0	13.5
Hard Labor — Strenuous physical effort	17.0	15.0

*Pregnant or lactating women add three calories to these values.

TABLE 4.2
Caloric Expenditure of Selected Physical Activities (expressed in calories per pound of body weight per minute of activity)

Activity*	Cal/lb/min	Activity*	Cal/lb/min	Activity*	Cal/lb/min
Aerobelt Exercise		Dance		StairMaster	
Aero-belt Jogging/6 mph	0.098	Moderate	0.030	Moderate	0.070
Aero-belt Step-Aerobics/8"	0.105	Vigorous	0.055	Vigorous	0.090
Aero-belt Walking/4 mph	0.073	Golf	0.030	Stationary Cycling	
Aerobics		Gymnastics		Moderate	0.055
Moderate	0.065	Light	0.030	Vigorous	0.070
Vigorous	0.095	Heavy	0.056	Strength Training	0.050
Step-Aerobics	0.070	Handball	0.064	Swimming (crawl)	
Archery	0.030	Hiking	0.040	20 yds/min	0.031
Badminton		Judo/Karate	0.086	25 yds/min	0.040
Recreation	0.038	Racquetball	0.065	45 yds/min	0.057
Competition	0.065	Rope Jumping	0.060	50 yds/min	0.070
Baseball	0.031	Rowing (vigorous)	0.090	Table Tennis	0.030
Basketball		Running		Tennis	
Moderate	0.046	11.0 min/mile	0.070	Moderate	0.045
Competition	0.063	8.5 min/mile	0.090	Competition	0.064
Bowling	0.030	7.0 min/mile	0.102	Volleyball	0.030
Calisthenics	0.033	6.0 min/mile	0.114	Walking	
Cycling (level)		Deep water**	0.100	4.5 mph	0.045
5.5 mph	0.033	Skating (moderate)	0.038	Shallow pool	0.090
10.0 mph	0.050	Skiing		Water Aerobics	
13.0 mph	0.071	Downhill	0.060	Moderate	0.050
		Level (5 mph)	0.078	Vigorous	0.070
		Soccer	0.059	Wrestling	0.085

*Values are only for actual time engaged in the activity.   **Treading water

Adapted from:
Allsen, P. E., J. M. Harrison, and B. Vance. *Fitness for Life: An Individualized Approach.* Dubuque, IA: Wm. C. Brown, 1989.
Bucher, C. A., and W. E. Prentice, *Fitness for College and Life.* St. Louis: Times Mirror/Mosby College Publishing, 1989.
Consolazio, C. F., R. E. Johnson, and L. J. Pecora. *Physiological Measurements of Metabolic Functions in Man.* New York: McGraw-Hill, 1963.
Hockey, R. V. *Physical Fitness: The Pathway to Healthful Living.* St. Louis: Times Mirror/Mosby College Publishing, 1989.
Hoeger, W. W. K., et al. Research conducted at Boise State Univesrity, 1986-1993.

burned through exercise. In our example, it is 2,640 calories (2,400 + 240). If a negative caloric balance is recommended to lose weight, this person has to consume fewer than 2,640 daily calories to achieve the objective. Because of the many factors that play a role in weight control, the previous value is only an estimated daily requirement.

Furthermore, to lose weight, a person can't predict that exactly one pound of fat will be lost in one week by reducing daily intake by 500 calories (500 × 7 = 3,500 calories, or the equivalent of one pound of fat). The estimated daily caloric figure provides only a target guideline for weight control. Periodic readjustments are necessary because individuals differ, and the estimated daily cost changes as you lose weight and modify your exercise habits.

The recommended number of calories to be subtracted from the daily intake to obtain a negative caloric balance depends on the typical daily requirement. At this point, the best recommendation is to moderately decrease the daily intake, never below 1,200 calories for women and 1,500 for men.

A good rule to follow is to restrict the intake by no more than 500 calories if the daily requirement is below 3,000 calories. For caloric requirements in excess of 3,000, as many as 1,000 calories per day may be subtracted from the total intake. The daily distribution should be approximately 60% carbohydrates (mostly complex carbohydrates), less than 30% fat, and about 12% protein.

Many experts believe that a person may take off weight more efficiently by reducing the amount of daily fat intake to 10% to 20% of the total daily caloric intake. Because 1 gram of fat supplies more than twice the amount of calories that carbohydrates and protein do, the general tendency is not to overeat.

Further, it takes only 3% to 5% of ingested calories to store fat as fat, whereas it takes approximately 25% of ingested calories to convert carbohydrates to fat. Other research points to the fact that if people eat the same amount of calories as carbohydrate or fat, those on the fat diet will store more fat. Successful weight-loss programs only allow small amounts of fat in the diet.

Many people have trouble adhering to a 10% to 20% fat-calorie diet. During weight loss periods, however, you are strongly encouraged to do so. Start with a 20% fat-calorie diet. Refer to Table 4.3 to aid you in determining the grams of fat at 10%, 20%, and 30% of the total calories for selected energy intakes. Also use the form provided in Lab 2B to monitor your daily fat intake.

The time of day when food is consumed also may play a part in weight reduction. A study conducted at the Aerobics Research Center in Dallas, Texas, indicated that, when a person is on a diet, weight is lost most effectively if most of the calories are consumed before 1:00 p.m. and not during the evening meal. This center recommends that, when a person is attempting to lose weight, intake should consist of a minimum of 25% of the total daily calories for breakfast, 50% for lunch, and 25% or less at dinner.

Other experts have reported that if most of the daily calories are consumed during one meal, the body may perceive that something is wrong and will slow down the metabolism so it can store a greater amount of calories in the form of fat. Eating most of the calories in one meal also causes a person to go hungry the rest of the day, making it harder to adhere to the diet.

The principle of consuming most of the calories earlier in the day not only seems helpful in losing weight but also in managing atherosclerosis. According to research, the time of day when most of the fats and cholesterol are consumed can influence blood lipids and coronary heart disease. Peak digestion time following a heavy meal is about seven hours after that meal. If most lipids are consumed during the evening meal, digestion peaks while the person is sound asleep, when the metabolism is at its lowest rate. Consequently, the body may not metabolize fats and cholesterol as well, leading to a higher blood lipid count and increasing the risk for atherosclerosis and coronary heart disease.

To monitor daily progress, you may use a form such as given in Figure 2B.1 (Lab 2B). Meeting the basic requirements from each food group should get top priority. The caloric content for each food is given in the Nutritive Value of Selected Foods list, Appendix A, Table A.1. For a more precise record, the information should be recorded immediately after each meal. According to the person's progress, adjustments can be made in the typical daily requirement or the exercise program, or both.

TABLE 4.3
Grams of Fat as a Percentage of Total Calories for Selected Energy Intakes

Caloric Intake	Grams of Fat		
	10%	20%	30%
1,200	13	27	40
1,300	14	29	43
1,400	16	31	47
1,500	17	33	50
1,600	18	36	53
1,700	19	38	57
1,800	20	40	60
1,900	21	42	63
2,000	22	44	67
2,100	23	47	70
2,200	24	49	73
2,300	26	51	77
2,400	27	53	80
2,500	28	56	83
2,600	29	58	87
2,700	30	60	90
2,800	31	62	93
2,900	32	64	97
3,000	33	67	100

TIPS FOR BEHAVIOR MODIFICATION AND ADHERENCE TO A WEIGHT MANAGEMENT PROGRAM

Achieving and maintaining recommended body composition is by no means impossible, but it does require desire and commitment. If weight management is to become a priority in life, people must realize they have to retrain behavior to some extent.

Modifying old habits and developing new positive behaviors take time. Individuals have applied the following management techniques to successfully change detrimental behavior and adhere to a positive lifetime weight control program. In developing a retraining program, people are not expected to incorporate all of the strategies listed but should note the ones that apply to them. The form provided in Lab 4C will allow you to evaluate and monitor your own weight management behaviors.

1. **Make a commitment to change.** The first ingredient to modify behavior is the desire to do so. The reasons for change must be more compelling than those for continuing present lifestyle patterns. People must accept the fact that they have a problem and decide by themselves whether they really want to change. If a sincere commitment is there, the chances for success are enhanced already.

2. **Set realistic goals.** Most people with a weight problem would like to lose weight in a relatively short time but fail to realize that the weight problem developed over a span of several years. A sound weight reduction and maintenance program can be accomplished only by establishing new lifetime eating and exercise habits, both of which take time to develop. In setting a realistic long-term goal, short-term objectives also should be planned. The long-term goal may be to decrease body fat to 20% of total body weight. The short-term objective may be to decrease body fat 1% each month. Objectives like these allow for regular evaluation and help maintain motivation and renewed commitment to attain the long-term goal.

3. **Incorporate exercise into the program.** Choosing enjoyable activities, places, times, equipment, and people to exercise with helps a person adhere to an exercise program. Details on developing a complete exercise program are found in Chapters 6 (cardiovascular), 8 (strength), and 10 (flexibility).

4. **Develop healthy eating patterns.** Plan to eat three regular meals per day consistent with the body's nutritional requirements. Learn to differentiate hunger from appetite. Hunger is the actual physical need for food. Appetite is a desire for food, usually triggered by factors such as stress, habit, boredom, depression, food availability, or just the thought of food itself. Eat only when you have a physical need. In this

regard, developing and sticking to a regular meal pattern helps control hunger.

5. **Avoid automatic eating.** Many people associate certain daily activities with eating. For example, people eat while cooking, watching television, reading, talking on the telephone, or visiting with neighbors. Most of the time, the foods consumed in these situations lack nutritional value or are high in sugar and fat.

6. **Stay busy.** People tend to eat more when they sit around and do nothing. Occupying the mind and body with activities not associated with eating helps take away the desire to eat. Try walking, cycling, playing sports, gardening, sewing, or visiting a library, a museum, a park. Develop other skills and interests, or try something new and exciting to break the routine of life.

7. **Plan your meals ahead of time.** Sensible shopping is required to accomplish this objective (by the way, shop on a full stomach, because hungry shoppers tend to buy unhealthy foods impulsively, and then snack on the way home). Include whole-grain breads and cereals, fruits and vegetables, low-fat milk and dairy products, lean meats, fish, and poultry.

8. **Cook wisely.** Use less fat and refined foods in food preparation. Trim all visible fat off meats, and remove skin from poultry before cooking. Skim the fat off gravies and soups. Bake, broil, and boil instead of frying. Sparingly use butter, cream, mayonnaise, and salad dressings. Avoid coconut oil, palm oil, and cocoa butter. Prepare plenty of bulky foods. Add whole-grain breads and cereals, vegetables, and legumes to most meals. Try fruits for dessert. Beware of soda pop, fruit juices, and fruit-flavored drinks. In addition to sugar, cut down on other refined carbohydrates such as corn syrup, malt sugar, dextrose, and fructose. Drink plenty of water — at least eight glasses a day.

9. **Do not serve more food than you should eat.** Measure the food portions and keep serving dishes away from the table. This means you will eat less, have a harder time getting seconds, and have less appetite because food is not visible. People should not be forced to eat when they are satisfied (including children after they have already had a healthy, nutritious serving).

10. **Learn to eat slowly and at the table only.** Eating is one of the pleasures of life, and we need to take time to enjoy it. Eating on the run is not good because the body doesn't have enough time to "register" nutritive and caloric consumption and people overeat before the body perceives the signal of fullness. Always eating at the table also forces people to take time out to eat, and it deters snacking between meals, primarily because of the extra time and effort required to sit down and eat. When done eating, do not sit around the table. Clean up and put away the food to keep from unnecessary snacking.

11. **Avoid social binges.** Social gatherings commonly entice self-defeating behavior. Plan ahead and visualize yourself in that gathering. Do not feel pressured to eat or drink, and don't rationalize in these situations. Choose low-calorie foods, and entertain yourself with other activities such as dancing and talking.

Successful weight management is accomplished by making a lifetime commitment to physical activity and proper food selection.

12. **Beware of raids on the refrigerator and the cookie jar.** When you find yourself in these tempting situations, take control. Stop and think what is happening. If you have the propensity for raids, try environmental management. Do not bring high-calorie, high-sugar, or high-fat foods into the house. If they are already in the house, store them where they are hard to get to or see. If they are out of sight or not readily available, the temptation is less. Keeping food in places such as the garage and the basement tends to discourage people from taking the time and effort to get them. By no means should you have to completely eliminate treats, but all things should be done in moderation.

13. **Avoid eating out.** Most meals served at restaurants (especially fast food restaurants) are high in calories and fat. People who regularly eat out often have a difficult time managing weight. When eating out, plan your choices ahead of time by selecting low-fat and low-calorie meals.

14. **Practice stress management techniques.** Many people snack and increase food consumption in stressful situations. Eating is not a stress-releasing activity and actually can aggravate the problem if weight control is an issue. Several stress management techniques are set forth in Chapter 14.

15. **Monitor changes and reward accomplishments.** Feedback on fat loss, lean tissue gain, and weight loss is a reward in itself. Awareness of changes in body composition also helps reinforce new behaviors. Being able to exercise without interruption for 15, 20, 30, 60 minutes, cycling a certain distance, running a mile — all these accomplishments deserve recognition. Meeting objectives calls for rewards, but not related to eating. Buy new clothing, a tennis racquet, a bicycle, exercise shoes, or something else that is special and you would not have acquired otherwise.

16. **Think positive.** Avoid negative thoughts on how difficult changing your past behaviors might be. Instead, think of the benefits you will reap, such as feeling, looking, and functioning better, plus enjoying better health and improving your quality of life. Attempt to stay away from negative environments and people who will not be supportive. Avoid those who do not have the same desires and who encourage self-defeating behaviors.

IN CONCLUSION

There is no simple and quick way to take off excessive body fat and keep it off for good. Weight management is accomplished by making a lifetime commitment to physical activity and proper food selection. When taking part in a weight (fat) reduction program, people also have to moderately decrease their caloric intake and implement strategies to modify unhealthy eating behaviors.

During the process of behavior modification, relapses into past negative behaviors are almost inevitable. The three most common reasons for relapse are:

1. Stress-related factors (major life changes, depression, job changes, illness).

2. Social reasons (entertaining, eating out, business travel).

3. Self-enticing behaviors (placing yourself in a situation to see how much you can get away with: "One small taste won't hurt," leading to "I'll eat just one slice," and finally, "I haven't done so well so I might as well eat some more").

Making mistakes is human and does not necessarily mean failure. Failure comes to those who give up and do not use previous experiences to build upon and, in turn, develop skills that will prevent self-defeating behaviors in the future. Where there's a will, there's a way, and those who persist will reap the rewards.

LABORATORY EXPERIENCE

LAB 4A
Estimation of Daily Caloric Requirement

Lab Preparation
None required.

LAB 4B
Behavioral Objectives for Weight Management

Lab Preparation
Read Chapters 2, 3, and 4 of this textbook.

LAB 4C
Weight Management: Behavior Modification Progress Form

Lab Preparation
Read the section on tips for behavior modification and adherence to a lifetime weight management program.

REFERENCES

1. Anderson, A. J., et.al. "Body Fat Distribution, Plasma Lipids and Lipoproteins." *Arteriosclerosis* 8:88-94, 1988.

2. Bennett, W., and J. Gurin. "Do Diets Really Work?" *Science* 42-50, March 1982.

3. "Brown Fat is Good Fat." The *Health Letter.* December 11, 1981.

4. Committee on Diet and health, Food and Nutrition Board. "*Diet and health: Implications for Reducing Chronic Disease Risk.*" Washington, D.C.: National Academy Press, 1989.

5. Hafen, B. Q., A. L. Thygerson, K. J. Frandsen. *Behavioral Guidelines for Health & Wellness.* Englewood, CO: Morton Publishing Company, 1988.

6. Health Implications of Obesity: National Institutes of Health Consensus Development Conference. *Annals of Internal medicine,* 103:977-1077, 1985.

7. Morgan, B. L. G. *The Lifelong Nutrition Guide.* Englewood Cliffs, NJ: Prentice-Hall, 1983.

8. National Academy of Sciences. "*Diet and Health: Implications for Reducing Chronic Disease Risk.*" Washington, D.C.National Academy Press, 1989.

9. Jenkins, D. J. A., et.al. "Nibbling versus Gorging: Metabolic Advantages of Increased Meal Frequency." The *New England Journal of Medicine* 321 (14): 929-934, 1989.

10. Lichtman, S. W., et al. "Discrepancy Between Self-Reported and Actual Caloric Intake and Exercise in Obese Subjects." The *New England Journal of Medicine,* 327(27):1893-1898, 1992.

11. Perkins, K. A., L. H. Epstein, B. L. Marks, R. L. Stiller, and R. G. Jacob. "The Effect of Nicotine on Energy Expenditure During Light Physical Activity." The *New England Journal of Medicine* 320(14):898-903, 1989.

12. Remington, D., A. G. Fisher, and E. A. Parent. *How to Lower Your Fat Thermostat.* Provo, UT: Vitality House International, Inc., 1983.

13. Sims, E. A. H. "Obesity is Hazardous to Your Health: Affirmative." *Debates in Medicine* 2:103-137, 1989.

14. Steen, S. N., R. A. Oppliger, and K. D. Brownell. "Metabolic Effects of Repeated Weight Loss and Regain in Adolescent Wrestlers." *Journal of the American Medical Association* 260:47-50, 1988.

15. Stunkard, A. J., T. I. A. Sorensen, C. Hanis, T. W. Teasdale, R. Chakraborty, W. J. Schull, and F. Schulsinger. "An Adoption Study of Human Obesity." The *New England Journal of Medicine* 314(4):193-198, 1986.

16. Wadden, T. A., T. B. Van Itallie, and G. L. Blackburn. "Responsible and Irresponsible Use of Very-Low-Calorie Diets in the Treatment of Obesity." *Journal of the American Medical Association* 263:83-85, 1990.

17. Whitney, E. N., and E. V. N. Hamilton. *Understanding Nutrition.* St. Paul, MN: West Publishing Co., 1994.

18. Wolf, M. D. "The Battle Against Body Fat." *Fitness Management* 3(3):48-49, 1987.

CARDIOVASCULAR ENDURANCE ASSESSMENT

5

The most important component of physical fitness and best indicator of overall health is cardiovascular endurance. Physical activity is no longer a natural part of our existence. We live in an automated world, one in which most of the activities that used to require strenuous physical exertion can be done by machines with the simple pull of a handle or push of a button. For instance, if there is a need to go to a store only a couple of blocks away, most people drive their automobiles and then spend a couple of minutes driving around the parking lot to find a spot ten yards closer to the store's entrance. They do not even have to carry out the groceries any more. A youngster working at the store usually takes them out in a cart and places them in the vehicle.

> ***Modern-day commodities have reduced the amount of daily physical activity, thus enhancing the deterioration rate of the human body.***

Similarly, during a visit to a multi-level shopping mall, almost everyone chooses to ride the escalators instead of taking the stairs (see Figure 5.1). Automobiles, elevators, escalators, telephones, intercoms, remote controls, electric garage door openers — all are modern-day commodities that minimize the amount of movement and effort required of the human body.

One of the most harmful effects of modern-day technology is an increase in chronic conditions related to a lack of physical activity. These include hypertension, heart disease, chronic low back pain, and obesity. They are referred to as *hypokinetic diseases*. The term "hypo" means low or little, and "kinetic" implies motion. Lack of adequate physical activity is a fact of modern life that most people can no longer avoid. To enjoy modern-day commodities and still expect to live life to its fullest, however, a personalized lifetime exercise program must become a part of daily living.

FIGURE 5.1
Advances in modern technology have almost completely eliminated the need for physical activity, significantly enhancing the deterioration rate of the human body.

For most people around the world, modern-day technology has led to a decrement in the level of cardiovascular endurance, *the ability of the lungs, heart, and blood vessels to deliver adequate amounts of oxygen to the cells to meet the demands of prolonged physical activity* (Figure 5.2).

FIGURE 5.2
Cardiovascular endurance is the ability of the lungs, heart, and blood vessels to deliver adequate amounts of oxygen to the cells to meet the demands of prolonged physical activity.

As a person breathes, part of the oxygen in the air is taken up in the lungs and transported in the blood to the heart. The heart then is responsible for pumping the oxygenated blood through the circulatory system to all organs and tissues of the body. At the cellular level, oxygen is used to convert food substrates, primarily carbohydrates and fats, into energy necessary to conduct body functions and maintain constant internal equilibrium. During physical exertion, more energy is needed to perform the activity. As a result, the heart, lungs, and blood vessels have to deliver more oxygen to the cells to supply the required energy.

> *Good aerobic or cardiovascular fitness implies an efficient system to deliver and utilize oxygen.*

During prolonged exercise, an individual with a high level of cardiovascular endurance is able to deliver the required amount of oxygen to the tissues with relative ease. The cardiovascular system of a person with a low level of endurance has to work much harder, as the heart has to pump more often to supply the same amount of oxygen to the tissues and, consequently, fatigues faster. Hence, a higher capacity to deliver and utilize oxygen (oxygen uptake) indicates a more efficient cardiovascular system.

AEROBIC AND ANAEROBIC EXERCISE

Cardiovascular endurance activities often are called aerobic exercises. The word "aerobic" means "with oxygen." Whenever an activity requires oxygen to produce energy, it is considered an aerobic exercise. Examples of cardiovascular or aerobic exercises are walking, jogging, swimming, cycling, cross-country skiing, water aerobics, rope skipping, and aerobics.

Anaerobic activities, on the other hand, are carried out "without oxygen." The intensity of anaerobic exercise is so high that oxygen is not utilized to produce energy. Because energy production is limited in the absence of oxygen, these activities can be carried out for only short periods (two to three minutes). The higher the intensity of the activity, the shorter the duration.

Activities such as the 100, 200, and 400 meters in track and field, the 100 meters in swimming, gymnastics routines, and strength training are good examples of anaerobic activities. Anaerobic activities do not contribute much to development of the cardiovascular system. Only aerobic activities will help increase cardiovascular endurance. The basic guidelines for cardiovascular exercise prescription are set forth in Chapter 6.

BENEFITS OF CARDIOVASCULAR ENDURANCE TRAINING

Everyone who participates in a cardiovascular or aerobic exercise program can expect a number of physiological adaptations from training. Among these benefits are:

1. *An increase in the oxygen-carrying capacity of the blood.* As a result of training, the red blood cell count goes up. Red blood cells contain hemoglobin, which transports oxygen in the blood.

2. *A higher maximal oxygen uptake (Max VO$_2$).* The amount of oxygen the body is able to use during physical activity increases significantly. This allows the individual to exercise longer and at a higher rate before becoming fatigued. Depending on the initial fitness level, maximal oxygen uptake may increase as much as 30%, although higher increases have been reported in people with very low initial levels of fitness.

3. *A decrease in resting heart rate and an increase in cardiac muscle strength.* During resting conditions, the heart ejects between five and six liters of blood per minute (a liter is slightly larger than a quart). This amount of blood, also referred to as cardiac output, meets the energy demands in the resting state. Like any other muscle, the heart responds to training by increasing in strength and size. As the heart gets stronger, the muscle can produce a more forceful contraction, which causes a greater ejection of blood with each beat (stroke volume), yielding a lower heart rate. This lower heart rate also allows the heart to rest longer between beats. Average resting and maximal cardiac outputs, stroke volumes and heart rates for sedentary, trained, and highly trained (elite) individuals are shown in Table 5.1.

TABLE 5.1
Average Resting and Maximal Cardiac Outputs (Q̇), Stroke Volumes (SV), and Heart Rates (HR), for Sedentary, Trained, and Highly Trained (elite athletes) Male Individuals

	RESTING			MAXIMAL		
	Q̇ (l/min)	SV (ml)	HR (bpm)	Q̇ (L/min)	SV (ml)	HR (bpm)
Sedentary	5	68	74	20	100	200
Trained	5	90	56	30	150	200
Highly Trained	5	110	45	35	175	200

Resting heart rates frequently are decreased by 10 to 20 beats per minute (bpm) after only six to eight weeks of training. A reduction of 20 bpm saves the heart about 10,483,200 beats per year. The average heart beats between 70 and 80 bpm. As seen in Table 5.1, resting heart rates in highly trained athletes are often around 45 bpm.

4. *A lower heart rate at given workloads.* When compared with untrained individuals, a trained person has a lower heart rate response to a given task. This is because of the greater efficiency of the cardiovascular system. Individuals also are surprised to find that, following several weeks of training, a given workload (let's say a 10-minute mile) elicits a much lower heart rate response as compared to the response when training first started.

5. *An increase in the number and size of the mitochondria.* All energy necessary for cell function is produced in the mitochondria. As the size and number increase, so does the potential to produce energy for muscular work.

6. *An increase in the number of functional capillaries.* These smaller vessels allow for the exchange of oxygen and carbon dioxide between the blood and the cells. As more vessels open up, more gas exchange can take place, delaying the onset of fatigue during prolonged exercise. This increase in capillaries also speeds up the rate at which waste products of cell metabolism can be removed. Increased capillarization also is seen in the heart, which enhances the oxygen delivery capacity to the heart muscle itself.

7. *A decrease in recovery time.* Trained individuals recover more rapidly after exercising. A fit system is able to restore more quickly any internal equilibrium disrupted during exercise.

8. *A decrease in blood pressure and blood lipids.* A regular aerobic exercise program leads to lower blood pressure and fats such as cholesterol and triglycerides, all of which have been linked to the formation of atherosclerotic plaque, which obstructs the arteries. This decreases the risk of coronary heart disease (see Chapter 12). High blood pressure also is a leading risk factor for strokes.

9. *An increase in fat-burning enzymes.* The role of fat-burning enzymes is significant because fat is primarily lost by burning it in muscle. As the concentration of the enzymes increases, so does the ability to burn fat.

ASSESSMENT OF CARDIOVASCULAR ENDURANCE

The level of cardiovascular endurance, cardiovascular fitness, or aerobic capacity is determined by the maximal amount of oxygen (Max VO$_2$) the human body is able to utilize per minute of physical activity. This value can be expressed in liters per minute (l/min) or milliliters per kilogram per minute (ml/kg/min). The relative value in ml/kg/min is used most often because it considers total body mass (weight). When comparing two individuals with the same absolute value, the one with the lesser body mass will have a higher relative value, indicating that more oxygen is available to each kilogram (2.2 pounds) of body weight. Because all tissues and organs of the body need oxygen to function, a higher oxygen consumption indicates a more efficient cardiovascular system.

The most precise way to determine maximal oxygen uptake is through direct gas analysis. This is done by using a metabolic cart through which the amount of oxygen consumption can be measured directly (see Figure 5.3). This type of equipment is not available in most health/fitness centers. Therefore several alternative methods of estimating maximal oxygen uptake have been developed using limited equipment.

Even though most cardiovascular endurance tests probably are safe to administer to apparently healthy individuals (those with no major coronary

FIGURE 5.3
Determining maximal oxygen uptake (cardiovascular fitness) through gas analysis.
Photo Courtesy of Quinton Instrument Co., 2121 Terry Ave., Seattle, WA 98121-2791.

risk factors or symptoms), the American College of Sports Medicine recommends that a physician be present for all maximal exercise tests on apparently healthy men over age 40 and women over age 50. A maximal test is any test that requires the participant's all-out or nearly all-out effort. For submaximal exercise tests a physician should be present when testing higher risk/symptomatic individuals or diseased people, regardless of the participant's current age.

Five exercise tests used to assess cardiovascular fitness are introduced in this chapter: the 1.5-Mile Run Test, 1.0-Mile Walk Test, Step Test, Astrand-Ryhming Test, and 12-Minute Swim Test. The tests procedures are explained in detail in Figures 5.4, 5.7, 5.8, 5.10, and 5.12, respectively.

Depending on time, equipment, and individual physical limitations, you may perform one or more of these tests. For example, people who can't jog or walk could take the bike or swim test. Because these are different tests, they will not necessarily yield the exact same results. Therefore, to make valid comparisons, you should take the same test when doing pre- and post-assessments.

A sixth test, the University of Houston Non-Exercise Test, also is presented at the end of this chapter (Figure 5.13). This non-exercise test is a valuable tool for making initial estimates of maximal oxygen uptake, hopefully to motivate people to exercise. The test is also valuable for mass screening, because the required information is collected through a self-reported method.

THE 1.5-MILE RUN TEST

This test is used most frequently to predict cardiovascular fitness according to the time the person takes to run or walk a 1.5-mile course (see Figure 5.4). Maximal oxygen uptake is estimated based on the time the person takes to cover the distance (see Table 5.2).

The only equipment necessary to conduct this test is a stopwatch and a track or premeasured 1.5-mile course. This perhaps is the easiest test to administer, but a note of caution is in order when conducting the test. As the objective is to cover the distance in the shortest time, it is considered a maximal exercise test. The 1.5-Mile Run Test should be limited to conditioned individuals who have been cleared for exercise. The test is not recommended for unconditioned beginners, men over age 40 and women over age 50 without proper medical

clearance, symptomatic individuals, and those with known disease or coronary heart disease risk factors. A program of at least six weeks of aerobic training is recommended before unconditioned individuals take this test.

**TABLE 5.2
Estimated Maximal Oxygen Uptake (Max VO$_2$)
in ml/kg/min for the 1.5-Mile Run Test**

Time	Max VO$_2$	Time	Max VO$_2$
6:10	80.0	12:40	39.8
6:20	79.0	12:50	39.2
6:30	77.9	13:00	38.6
6:40	76.7	13:10	38.1
6:50	75.5	13:20	37.8
7:00	74.0	13:30	37.2
7:10	72.6	13:40	36.8
7:20	71.3	13:50	36.3
7:30	69.9	14:00	35.9
7:40	68.3	14:10	35.5
7:50	66.8	14:20	35.1
8:00	65.2	14:30	34.7
8:10	63.9	14:40	34.3
8:20	62.5	14:50	34.0
8:30	61.2	15:00	33.6
8:40	60.2	15:10	33.1
8:50	59.1	15:20	32.7
9:00	58.1	15:30	32.2
9:10	56.9	15:40	31.8
9:20	55.9	15:50	31.4
9:30	54.7	16:00	30.9
9:40	53.5	16:10	30.5
9:50	52.3	16:20	30.2
10:00	51.1	16:30	29.8
10:10	50.4	16:40	29.5
10:20	49.5	16:50	29.1
10:30	48.6	17:00	28.9
10:40	48.0	17:10	28.5
10:50	47.4	17:20	28.3
11:00	46.6	17:30	28.0
11:10	45.8	17:40	27.7
11:20	45.1	17:50	27.4
11:30	44.4	18:00	27.1
11:40	43.7	18:10	26.8
11:50	43.2	18:20	26.6
12:00	42.3	18:30	26.3
12:10	41.7	18:40	26.0
12:20	41.0	18:50	25.7
12:30	40.4	19:00	25.4

Source: Adapted from "A Means of Assessing Maximal Oxygen Intake," by K. H. Cooper, in *Journal of the American Medical Association* 203(1968):201-204; *Health and Fitness Through Physical Activity*, by M. L. Pollock, J. H. Wilmore, and S. M. Fox III (New York: John Wiley & Sons, 1978); and *Training for Sport and Activity*, by J. H. Wilmore and D. L. Costill (Dubuque, IA: Wm. C. Brown Publishers, 1988).

1.5 MILE RUN TEST

1. Make sure that you qualify for this test. This test is contraindicated for unconditioned beginners, individuals with symptoms of heart disease, and those with known heart disease or risk factors.

2. Select the testing site. Find a school track (each lap is one-fourth of a mile) or a premeasured 1.5-mile course.

3. Have a stopwatch available to determine your time.

4. Conduct a few warm-up exercises prior to the test. Do some stretching exercises, some walking, and slow jogging.

5. Initiate the test and try to cover the distance in the fastest time possible (walking or jogging). Time yourself during the run to see how fast you have covered the distance. If any unusual symptoms arise during the test, do not continue. Stop immediately and retake the test after another six weeks of aerobic training.

6. At the end of the test, cool down by walking or jogging slowly for another three to five minutes. Do not sit or lie down after the test.

7. According to your performance time, look up your estimated maximal oxygen uptake in Table 5.2.

8. Example: A twenty-year-old female runs the 1.5-mile course in 12 minutes and 40 seconds. Table 5.2 shows a maximal oxygen uptake of 39.8 ml/kg/min for a time of 12:40. According to Table 5.8, this maximal oxygen uptake would place her in the good cardiovascular fitness category.

FIGURE 5.4
Procedure for the 1.5-Mile Run Test.

THE 1.0-MILE WALK TEST

This test can be used by individuals who are unable to run because of low fitness levels or injuries. All that is required is a brisk 1.0-mile walk that will elicit an exercise heart rate of at least 120 beats per minute at the end of the test.

You will need to know how to take your heart rate by counting your pulse. This can be done on the wrist by placing two fingers over the radial artery (inside the wrist on the side of the thumb) or over the carotid artery in the neck just below the jaw, next to the voice box (see Figures 5.5 and 5.6).

FIGURE 5.5
Pulse taken at the radial artery.

FIGURE 5.6
Pulse taken at the carotid artery.

Maximal oxygen uptake is estimated according to a prediction equation that requires the following data: 1.0-mile walk time, exercise heart rate at the end of the walk, age, gender, and body weight in pounds. The procedure for this test and the equation are given in Figure 5.7.

THE STEP TEST

The Step Test requires little time and equipment and can be administered to almost anyone, as a submaximal workload is used to estimate maximal oxygen uptake. Symptomatic and diseased individuals should not take this test. Significantly overweight individuals and those with joint problems in the lower extremities may have difficulty performing the test.

The actual test takes only three minutes. A 15-second recovery heart rate is taken between 5 and 20 seconds following the test (see Figure 5.8 and Table 5.3). The equipment required is a bench or gymnasium bleacher 16¼ inches high, a stopwatch, and a metronome.

You also will need to know how to take your heart rate by counting your pulse (explained under the 1.0-Mile Walk Test). By teaching people to take their own heart rate, a large group of people can be tested at once, using gymnasium bleachers.

1.0 MILE WALK TEST*

1. Select the testing site. Use a 440-yard track (4 laps to a mile) or a premeasured 1.0-mile course.

2. Determine your body weight in pounds prior to the test.

3. Have a stopwatch available to determine total walking time and exercise heart rate.

4. Walk the 1.0-mile course at a brisk pace (the exercise heart rate at the end of the test should be above 120 beats per minute).

5. At the end of the 1.0-mile walk, check your walking time and immediately count your pulse for 10 seconds. Multiply the 10-second pulse count by 6 to obtain the exercise heart rate in beats per minute.

6. Convert the walking time from minutes and seconds to minute units. Because there are 60 seconds in one minute, divide the seconds by 60 to obtain the fraction of a minute. For instance, a walking time of 12 minutes and 15 seconds would equal 12 + (15 ÷ 60), or 12.25 minutes.

7. To obtain the estimated maximal oxygen uptake (Max VO_2) in ml/kg/min, plug your values in the following equation:

   Max VO_2 = 132.853 − (.0769 × W) − (.3877 × A) + (6.315 × G) − (3.2649 × T) − (.1565 × HR)

   Where:
   W = Weight in pounds
   A = Age in years
   G = Gender (use 0 for women and 1 for men)
   T = Total time for the one-mile walk in minutes (see item 6 above)
   HR = Exercise heart rate in beats per minute at the end of the one-mile walk

8. Example: A nineteen-year-old female subject who weighs 140 pounds completed the one-mile walk in 14 minutes 39 seconds and with an exercise heart rate of 148 beats per minute. The estimated maximal oxygen uptake would be:

   W = 140 lbs
   A = 19
   G = 0 (female gender = 0)
   T = 14:39 = 14 + (39 ÷ 60) = 14.65 min
   HR = 148 bpm

   Max VO_2 = 132.853 − (.0769 × 140) − (.3877 × 19) + (6.315 × 0) − (3.2649 × 14.65) − (.1565 × 148)

   Max VO_2 = 43.7 ml/kg/min

*Source: Kline, G. et al. "Estimation of VO_2max from a one-mile track walk, gender, age, and body weight." *Medicine and Science in Sports and Exercise* 19(3):253259, 1987. © American College of Sports Medicine.

FIGURE 5.7
Procedure for the 1.0-Mile Walk Test.

STEP TEST

1. The test is conducted with a bench or gymnasium bleacher 16¼ inches high.

2. The stepping cycle is performed to a four-step cadence (up-up-down-down). Men should perform twenty-four complete step-ups per minute, regulated with a metronome set at 96 beats per minute. Women perform twenty-two step-ups per minute, or 88 beats per minute on the metronome.

3. Allow a brief practice period of five to ten seconds to familiarize yourself with the stepping cadence.

4. Begin the test and perform the step-ups for exactly three minutes.

5. Upon completion of the three minutes, remain standing and take your heart rate for a fifteen-second interval from five to twenty seconds into recovery. Convert recovery heart rate to beats per minute (multiply 15-second heart rate by 4).

6. Maximal oxygen uptake in ml/kg/min is estimated according to the following equations:
   Men:
   maximal oxygen uptake =
   111.33 − (0.42 × recovery heart rate in bpm)
   Women:
   maximal oxygen uptake =
   65.81 − (0.1847 × recovery heart rate in bpm)

7. Example: The recovery fifteen-second heart rate for a male subject following the three-minute step test is found to be 39 beats. Maximal oxygen uptake is estimated as follows:
   Fifteen-second heart rate = 39 beats
   Minute heart rate = 39 × 4 = 156 bpm
   Maximal oxygen uptake =
   111.33 − (0.42 × 156) = 45.81 ml/kg/min

8. Maximal oxygen uptake also can be obtained according to recovery heart rates in Table 5.3.

From McArdle, W. D., et al. *Exercise Physiology: Energy, Nutrition, and Human Performance.* Philadelphia: Lea & Febiger, 1991.

FIGURE 5.8
Procedure for the Step Test.

TABLE 5.3
Predicted Maximal Oxygen Uptake (Max VO$_2$)
for the Step Test in ml/kg/min

15-Sec HR	HR-bpm	Max VO$_2$ Men	Max VO$_2$ Women
30	120	60.9	43.6
31	124	59.3	42.9
32	128	57.6	42.2
33	132	55.9	41.4
34	136	54.2	40.7
35	140	52.5	40.0
36	144	50.9	39.2
37	148	49.2	38.5
38	152	47.5	37.7
39	156	45.8	37.0
40	160	44.1	36.3
41	164	42.5	35.5
42	168	40.8	34.8
43	172	39.1	34.0
44	176	37.4	33.3
45	180	35.7	32.6
46	184	34.1	31.8
47	188	32.4	31.1
48	192	30.7	30.3
49	196	29.0	29.6
50	200	27.3	28.9

ASTRAND-RYHMING TEST

Because of its simplicity and practicality, the Astrand-Ryhming has become one of the most popular tests used to estimate maximal oxygen uptake in the laboratory setting. The test is conducted on a bicycle ergometer (see Figure 5.9), and, similar to the Step Test, it requires only submaximal workloads and little time to administer.

The cautions given for the Step Test also apply to the Astrand-Ryhming Test. Nevertheless, because the participant does not have to support his or her own body weight while riding the bicycle, overweight individuals and those with limited joint problems in the lower extremities can take this test.

The bicycle ergometer to be used for this test should allow for the regulation of workloads (see the test procedure in Figure 5.10 and Tables 5.4, 5.5, and 5.6). Besides the bicycle ergometer, a stopwatch and an additional technician to monitor the heart rate are needed to conduct the test.

The heart rate is taken every minute for six minutes. At the end of the test, the heart rate should be in the range given for each workload in Table 5.5 (generally between 120 and 170 beats per minute).

When administering the test to older people, good judgment is essential. Low workloads should be used, because if the higher heart rates are reached (around 150 to 170 bpm), these individuals could be working near or at their maximal capacity, making it an unsafe test without adequate medical supervision. When choosing workloads for older people, final exercise heart rates should not exceed 130 to 140 bpm.

FIGURE 5.9
Monitoring heart rate on carotid artery during Astrand-Ryhming Test.

ASTRAND-RYHMING TEST

1. Adjust the bike seat so that the knees are almost completely extended as the foot goes through the bottom of the pedaling cycle.

2. During the test, keep the speed constant at fifty revolutions per minute. Test duration is six minutes.

3. Select the appropriate work load for the bike based on age, weight, health, and estimated fitness level. For unconditioned individuals: women, use 300 kpm (kilopounds per meter) or 450 kpm; men, 300 kpm or 600 kpm. Conditioned adults: women, 450 kpm or 600 kpm; men, 600 kpm or 900 kpm.ª

4. Ride the bike for six minutes and check the heart rate every minute, during the last ten seconds of each minute. Determine heart rate by recording the time it takes to count thirty pulse beats, and then converting to beats per minute using Table 5.4.

5. Average the final two heart rates (fifth and sixth minutes). If these two heart rates are not within five beats per minute of each other, continue the test for another few minutes until this is accomplished. If the heart rate continues to climb significantly after the sixth minute, stop the test and rest for fifteen to twenty minutes. You may then retest, preferably at a lower work load. The final average heart rate should also fall between the ranges given for each work load in Table 5.5 (e.g., men: 300 kpm = 120 to 140 beats per minute; 600 kpm = 120 to 170 beats per minute).

6. Based on the average heart rate of the final two minutes and your work load, look up the maximal oxygen uptake in Table 5.5 (e.g., men: 600 kpm and average heart rate = 145, maximal oxygen uptake = 2.4 liters/minute).

7. Correct maximal oxygen uptake using the correction factors found in Table 5.6 (e.g., maximal oxygen uptake = 2.4 and age thirty-five, correction factor = .870. Multiply 2.4 × .870 and final corrected maximal oxygen uptake = 2.09 liters/minute).

8. To obtain maximal oxygen uptake in ml/kg/min, multiply the maximal oxygen uptake by 1,000 (to convert liters to milliliters) and divide by body weight in kilograms (to obtain kilograms, divide your body weight in pounds by 2.2046).

9. Example: Corrected maximal oxygen uptake = 2.09 liters/minute
Body weight = 132 pounds or 60 kilograms (132 ÷ 2.2046 = 60)

Maximal oxygen uptake in ml/kg/min =
2.09 × 1,000 = 2,090
2,090 divided by 60 = 34.8 ml/kg/min

ª On the Monarch bicycle ergometer when riding at a speed of fifty revolutions per minute, a load of 1 kp = 300 kpm, 1.5 kp = 450, 2 kp = 600 kpm, and so forth, with increases of 150 kpm to each half kp.

FIGURE 5.10
Procedure for the Astrand-Ryhming Test.

TABLE 5.4
Conversion of the Time for 30 Pulse Beats to Pulse Rate Per Minute

Sec.	bpm	Sec.	bpm	Sec.	bpm	Sec.	bpm	Sec.	bpm	Sec.	bpm	Sec.	bpm
22.0	82	19.9	90	17.8	101	15.7	115	13.6	132	11.5	157	9.4	191
21.9	82	19.8	91	17.7	102	15.6	115	13.5	133	11.4	158	9.3	194
21.8	83	19.7	91	17.6	102	15.5	116	13.4	134	11.3	159	9.2	196
21.7	83	19.6	92	17.5	103	15.4	117	13.3	135	11.2	161	9.1	198
21.6	83	19.5	92	17.4	103	15.3	118	13.2	136	11.1	162	9.0	200
21.5	84	19.4	93	17.3	104	15.2	118	13.1	137	11.0	164	8.9	202
21.4	84	19.3	93	17.2	105	15.1	119	13.0	138	10.9	165	8.8	205
21.3	85	19.2	94	17.1	105	15.0	120	12.9	140	10.8	167	8.7	207
21.2	85	19.1	94	17.0	106	14.9	121	12.8	141	10.7	168	8.6	209
21.1	85	19.0	95	16.9	107	14.8	122	12.7	142	10.6	170	8.5	212
21.0	86	18.9	95	16.8	107	14.7	122	12.6	143	10.5	171	8.4	214
20.9	86	18.8	96	16.7	108	14.6	123	12.5	144	10.4	173	8.3	217
20.8	87	18.7	96	16.6	108	14.5	124	12.4	145	10.3	175	8.2	220
20.7	87	18.6	97	16.5	109	14.4	125	12.3	146	10.2	176	8.1	222
20.6	87	18.5	97	16.4	110	14.3	126	12.2	148	10.1	178	8.0	225
20.5	88	18.4	98	16.3	110	14.2	127	12.1	149	10.0	180		
20.4	88	18.3	98	16.2	111	14.1	128	12.0	150	9.9	182		
20.3	89	18.2	99	16.1	112	14.0	129	11.9	151	9.8	184		
20.2	89	18.1	99	16.0	113	13.9	129	11.8	153	9.7	186		
20.1	90	18.0	100	15.9	113	13.8	130	11.7	154	9.6	188		
20.0	90	17.9	101	15.8	114	13.7	131	11.6	155	9.5	189		

TABLE 5.5
Maximal Oxygen Uptake (Max VO₂) Estimates for the Astrand-Ryhming Test in Liters per Minute (L/min)

Heart Rate	MEN					WOMEN				
	300	600	900	1200	1500	300	450	600	750	900
120	2.2	3.4	4.8			2.6	3.4	4.1	4.8	
121	2.2	3.4	4.7			2.5	3.3	4.0	4.8	
122	2.2	3.4	4.6			2.5	3.2	3.9	4.7	
123	2.1	3.4	4.6			2.4	3.1	3.9	4.6	
124	2.1	3.3	4.5	6.0		2.4	3.1	3.8	4.5	
125	2.0	3.2	4.4	5.9		2.3	3.0	3.7	4.4	
126	2.0	3.2	4.4	5.8		2.3	3.0	3.6	4.3	
127	2.0	3.1	4.3	5.7		2.2	2.9	3.5	4.2	
128	2.0	3.1	4.2	5.6		2.2	2.8	3.5	4.2	4.8
129	1.9	3.0	4.2	5.6		2.2	2.8	3.4	4.1	4.8
130	1.9	3.0	4.1	5.5		2.1	2.7	3.4	4.0	4.7
131	1.9	2.9	4.0	5.4		2.1	2.7	3.4	4.0	4.6
132	1.8	2.9	4.0	5.3		2.0	2.7	3.3	3.9	4.5
133	1.8	2.8	3.9	5.3		2.0	2.6	3.2	3.8	4.4
134	1.8	2.8	3.9	5.2		2.0	2.6	3.2	3.8	4.4
135	1.7	2.8	3.8	5.1		2.0	2.6	3.1	3.7	4.3
136	1.7	2.7	3.8	5.0		1.9	2.5	3.1	3.6	4.2
137	1.7	2.7	3.7	5.0		1.9	2.5	3.0	3.6	4.2
138	1.6	2.7	3.7	4.9		1.8	2.4	3.0	3.5	4.1
139	1.6	2.6	3.6	4.8		1.8	2.4	2.9	3.5	4.0
140	1.6	2.6	3.6	4.8	6.0	1.8	2.4	2.8	3.4	4.0
141		2.6	3.5	4.7	5.9	1.8	2.3	2.8	3.4	3.9
142		2.5	3.5	4.6	5.8	1.7	2.3	2.8	3.3	3.9
143		2.5	3.4	4.6	5.7	1.7	2.2	2.7	3.3	3.8
144		2.5	3.4	4.5	5.7	1.7	2.2	2.7	3.2	3.8
145		2.4	3.4	4.5	5.6	1.6	2.2	2.7	3.2	3.7
146		2.4	3.3	4.4	5.6	1.6	2.2	2.6	3.2	3.7
147		2.4	3.3	4.4	5.5	1.6	2.1	2.6	3.1	3.6
148		2.4	3.2	4.3	5.4	1.6	2.1	2.6	3.1	3.6
149		2.3	3.2	4.3	5.4		2.1	2.6	3.0	3.5
150		2.3	3.2	4.2	5.3		2.0	2.5	3.0	3.5
151		2.3	3.1	4.2	5.2		2.0	2.5	3.0	3.4
152		2.3	3.1	4.1	5.2		2.0	2.5	2.9	3.4
153		2.2	3.0	4.1	5.1		2.0	2.4	2.9	3.3
154		2.2	3.0	4.0	5.1		2.0	2.4	2.8	3.3
155		2.2	3.0	4.0	5.0		1.9	2.4	2.8	3.2
156		2.2	2.9	4.0	5.0		1.9	2.3	2.8	3.2
157		2.1	2.9	3.9	4.9		1.9	2.3	2.7	3.2
158		2.1	2.9	3.9	4.9		1.8	2.3	2.7	3.1
159		2.1	2.8	3.8	4.8		1.8	2.2	2.7	3.1
160		2.1	2.8	3.8	4.8		1.8	2.2	2.6	3.0
161		2.0	2.8	3.7	4.7		1.8	2.2	2.6	3.0
162		2.0	2.8	3.7	4.6		1.8	2.2	2.6	3.0
163		2.0	2.8	3.7	4.6		1.7	2.2	2.6	2.9
164		2.0	2.7	3.6	4.5		1.7	2.1	2.5	2.9
165		2.0	2.7	3.6	4.5		1.7	2.1	2.5	2.9
166		1.9	2.7	3.6	4.5		1.7	2.1	2.5	2.8
167		1.9	2.6	3.5	4.4		1.6	2.1	2.4	2.8
168		1.9	2.6	3.5	4.4		1.6	2.0	2.4	2.8
169		1.9	2.6	3.5	4.3		1.6	2.0	2.4	2.8
170		1.8	2.6	3.4	4.3		1.6	2.0	2.4	2.7

From Astrand, I. *Acta Physiologica Scandinavica* 49(1960). Supplementum 169:45-60.

TABLE 5.6
Age-Based Correction Factors for Maximal Oxygen Uptake

Age	Correction Factor	Age	Correction Factor	Age	Correction Factor	Age	Correction Factor
14	1.11	27	.974	40	.830	53	.726
15	1.10	28	.961	41	.820	54	.718
16	1.09	29	.948	42	.810	55	.710
17	1.08	30	.935	43	.800	56	.704
18	1.07	31	.922	44	.790	57	.698
19	1.06	32	.909	45	.780	58	.692
20	1.05	33	.896	46	.774	59	.686
21	1.04	34	.883	47	.768	60	.680
22	1.03	35	.870	48	.762	61	.674
23	1.02	36	.862	49	.756	62	.668
24	1.01	37	.854	50	.750	63	.662
25	1.00	38	.846	51	.742	64	.656
26	.987	39	.838	52	.734	65	.650

Adapted from Astrand, I. *Acta Physiologica Scandinavica* 49(1960). Supplementum 169:45-60.

THE 12-MINUTE SWIM TEST

Similar to the 1.5-Mile Run test, the 12-Minute Swim Test is considered a maximal exercise test, and the same precautions apply. The objective is to swim as far as possible during the 12-minute test.

A swimming test (Figures 5.11 and 5.12) is practical only for those who are planning to take part in a swimming program. Unlike land-based tests, predicting maximal oxygen uptake through a swimming test is difficult. Differences in skill level, swimming conditioning, and body composition greatly affect the energy requirements (oxygen uptake) of swimming.

A skilled swimmer is able to swim more efficiently and expend much less energy than an unskilled swimmer. Improper breathing patterns cause premature fatigue. Overweight individuals are more buoyant in the water, and the larger surface area (body size) produces greater friction against movement in the water medium.

Lack of conditioning affects swimming test results as well. An unconditioned skilled swimmer who is in good cardiovascular shape because of a regular jogging program will not perform as effectively in a swimming test. Swimming conditioning is important for adequate performance on this test.

Because of these limitations, maximal oxygen uptake cannot be estimated for a swimming test and the fitness categories given in Table 5.7 are only estimated ratings. This test should be limited to people who cannot perform any of the other tests and whose primary aerobic exercise will be a swimming program. Unskilled and unconditioned swimmers can expect lower cardiovascular fitness ratings than those obtained with a land-based test.

FIGURE 5.11
Swimming efficiency requires skill and proper conditioning.

12-MINUTE SWIM TEST

1. Enlist a friend to time the test. The only other requisites are a stopwatch and a swimming pool. Do not attempt to do this test in an unsupervised pool.

2. Warm up by swimming slowly and doing a few stretching exercises before taking the test.

3. Start the test and swim as many laps as possible in 12 minutes. Pace yourself throughout the test, and do not swim to the point of complete exhaustion.

4. After completing the test, cool down by swimming another two or three minutes at a slower pace.

5. Determine the total distance you swam during the test, and look up your fitness category in Table 5.7.

FIGURE 5.12
Procedure for the 12-Minute Swim Test.

TABLE 5.7
12-Minute Swim Test Fitness Categories

Distance (yards)	Fitness Categories
≥700	Excellent
500–700	Good
400–500	Average
200–400	Fair
≤200	Poor

Source: Adapted from *The Aerobics Program for Total Well-Being,* by K. H. Cooper (New York: Bantam Books, 1982).

UNIVERSITY OF HOUSTON NON-EXERCISE TEST

The University of Houston Non-Exercise Test (N-Ex) is a method used to estimate maximal oxygen uptake that does not involve any form of exercise testing. As indicated earlier, this protocol can be used as an initial estimate of maximal oxygen uptake and for mass screening purposes. The information for this test is collected through self-reports.

This N-Ex test is especially useful when testing individuals who are taking high blood pressure medication. Hypertensive medication lowers the heart rate. Therefore, tests based on heart rate (walk test, step test, and Astrand-Ryhming) cannot be used with these people. Maximal exercise tests (1.5-Mile Run) also are not to be administered to hypertensive people. The N-Ex equations to predict maximal oxygen uptake have a high degree of accuracy with men on anti-hypertensive medication.

The non-exercise test is based on research findings in exercise physiology indicating that maximal oxygen uptake is negatively related to age and body composition but positively related to exercise habits. Based on these variables, multiple regression equations were developed to estimate maximal oxygen uptake in ml/kg/min. The procedure for the Houston Non-Exercise Test is outlined in Figures 5.13 and 5.14. The test is suitable for men and women alike.

UNIVERSITY OF HOUSTON NON-EXERCISE TEST

Use the appropriate number (0-7) which best describes your general physical activity rating (PAR) for the previous month:

I. Do not participate regularly in programmed recreation sport or physical activity.

0   Avoid walking or exertion, e.g., always use elevator, drive whenever possible instead of walking.

1   Walk for pleasure, routinely use stairs, occasionally exercise sufficiently to cause heavy breathing or perspiration.

II. Participate regularly in recreation or work requiring modest physical activity, such as golf, horseback riding, calisthenics, gymnastics, table tennis, bowling, weight lifting, yard work.

2   10 to 60 minutes per week.

3   Over one hour per week.

III. Participate regularly in heavy physical exercise such as running or jogging, swimming, cycling, rowing, skipping rope, running in place or engaging in vigorous aerobic activity type exercise such as tennis, basketball or handball.

4   Run less than one mile per week or spend less than 30 minutes per week in comparable physical activity.

5   Run 1 to 5 miles per week or spend 30 to 60 minutes per week in comparable physical activity.

6   Run 5 to 10 miles per week or spend 1 to 3 hours per week in comparable physical activity.

7   Run over 10 miles per week or spend over 3 hours per week in comparable physical activity.

FIGURE 5.13
Physical activity code for the University of Houston Non-Exercise Test.

UNIVERSITY OF HOUSTON NON-EXERCISE TEST*

Multiple regression equations have been developed to estimate maximal oxygen uptake in ml/kg/min according to physical activity rating (PAR), age (A), and percent body fat (%Fat) or body mass index (BMI). The first equation uses percent body fat determined through skinfolds (N-EX %Fat). The procedures to determine percent body fat through skinfolds are outlined in Figure 3.6 in Chapter 3. The second equation uses body mass index (N-Ex BMI). The N-Ex %Fat equation is slightly more accurate than the N-Ex BMI equation. The physical activity rating code provided in Figure 5.13 is used for a global, self-rating of physical activity. The subject uses the code to rate his or her physical activity during the past month. The selected number is a global rating of the subject's exercise habits. This value is used in the equation. The regression equations are as follows:

N-Ex %Fat Model

Men $\text{Max VO}_2 = 56.370 - (.289 \times A) - (.552 \times \%\text{Fat}) + (1.589 \times \text{PAR})$

Women $\text{Max VO}_2 = 50.513 - (.289 \times A) - (.552 \times \%\text{Fat}) + (1.589 \times \text{PAR})$

N-Ex BMI Model (BMI = Weight in pounds × 705 ÷ Height in inches ÷ Height in inches

Men $\text{Max VO}_2 = 67.350 - (.381 \times A) - (.754 \times \text{BMI}) + (1.951 \times \text{PAR})$

Women $\text{Max VO}_2 = 56.363 - (.381 \times A) - (.754 \times \text{BMI}) + (1.951 \times \text{PAR})$

Examples

The N-Ex %fat model is illustrated with a 40-year-old man with 17 percent body fat and an activity rating of 6. Estimated Max VO$_2$ for the man would be:

$$\text{Max VO}_2 = 56.37 - (.289 \times 40) - (.552 \times 17) + (1.589 \times 6)$$

$$\text{Max VO}_2 = 45.0 \text{ ml/kg/min}$$

The N-Ex BMI for a 30-year-old woman who weighs 130 pounds, with a height of 64 inches, and a physical activity rating of 5 would be:

BMI = Weight in pounds × 705 ÷ Height in inches ÷ Height in inches

BMI = 130 × 705 ÷ 64 ÷ 64

$$\text{Max VO}_2 = 56.363 - (.381 \times 30) - (.754 \times 22.38) + (1.951 \times 5)$$

$$\text{Max VO}_2 = 37.8 \text{ ml/kg/min}$$

*University of Houston Non-Exercise Test reproduced with permission from *Exercise Concepts, Calculations, & Computer Applications* by R. M. Ross and A. S. Jackson; Benchmark Press, Inc., pp. 108–110, 1990.

FIGURE 5.14
Procedure for the University of Houston Non-Exercise Test.

INTERPRETING YOUR MAXIMAL OXYGEN UPTAKE RESULTS

After obtaining your maximal oxygen uptake, you can determine your current level of cardiovascular fitness by consulting Table 5.8. Locate the maximal oxygen uptake in your age category, and on the top row you will find your present level of cardiovascular fitness. For example, a 19-year-old male with a maximal oxygen uptake of 35 ml/kg/min would be classified in the average cardiovascular fitness category. After you initiate your personal cardiovascular exercise program (see Chapter 6), you may wish to retest yourself periodically to evaluate your progress.

Good cardiovascular fitness has been linked to better health and increased longevity.

TABLE 5.8
Cardiovascular Fitness Classification According to Maximal Oxygen Uptake (Max VO₂) in ml/kg/min

Gender	Age	FITNESS CLASSIFICATION				
		Poor	Fair	Average	Good	Excellent
Men	≤29	≤24.9	25-33.9	34-43.9	44-52.9	≥53
	30-39	≤22.9	23-30.9	31-41.9	42-49.9	≥50
	40-49	≤19.9	20-26.9	27-38.9	39-44.9	≥45
	50-59	≤17.9	18-24.9	25-37.9	38-42.9	≥43
	60-69	≤15.9	16-22.9	23-35.9	36-40.9	≥41
Women	≤29	≤23.9	24-30.9	31-38.9	39-48.9	≥49
	30-39	≤19.9	20-27.9	28-36.9	37-44.9	≥45
	40-49	≤16.9	17-24.9	25-34.9	35-41.9	≥42
	50-59	≤14.9	15-21.9	22-33.9	34-39.9	≥40
	60-69	≤12.9	13-20.9	21-32.9	33-36.9	≥37

■ High physical fitness standard
■ Health fitness standard

See Chapter 1, Fitness Standards: Health vs. Physical Fitness, p. 6.

LABORATORY EXPERIENCE

LAB 5A
Cardiovascular Endurance Assessment Protocols

Lab Preparation
Wear appropriate exercise clothing and jogging or walking shoes as required. Be prepared to take the 1.5-Mile Run Test, 1.0-Mile Walk Test, Step Test, Astrand-Ryhming Test, or 12-Minute Swim Test. Avoid vigorous physical activity 24 hours prior to this lab.

REFERENCES

1. American College of Sports Medicine. *Guidelines for Graded Exercise Testing and Exercise Prescription.* Philadelphia: Lea & Febiger, 1991.
2. Astrand, I. *Acta Physiologica Scandinavica* 49 (1960) (Supplement) 169(1960):45-60.
3. Astrand, P. O., and K. Rodahl. *Textbook of Work Physiology.* New York: McGraw-Hill, 1986.
4. Cooper, K. H. "A Means of Assessing Maximal Oxygen Intake." *Journal of the American Medical Association* 203(1968):201-204.
5. Cooper, K. H. *The Aerobics Program for Total Well-Being.* New York: Mount Evans and Co., 1982.
6. Jackson, A. S., et al. "Prediction of VO₂max Without Exercise Testing." *Medicine and Science in Sports and Exercise* 21(2), 1898:S115.
7. Kline, G., et al. "Estimation of VO₂max from a one-mile track walk, gender, age, and body weight." *Medicine and Science in Sports and Exercise* 19(3),1987:253-259.
8. McArdle, W. D., F. I. Katch, and V. L. Katch. *Exercise Physiology: Energy, Nutrition and Human Performance.* Philadelphia: Lea & Febiger, 1991.
9. Pollock, M. L., J. H. Wilmore, and S. M. Fox III. *Health and Fitness Through Physical Activity.* New York: John Wiley & Sons, 1978.
10. Ross, R. M. and A. S. Jackson. *Exercise Concepts, Calculations, & Computer Applications.* Carmel, IN: Benchmark Press, 1990.
11. Wilmore, J. H. and D. L. Costill. *Training for Sport and Activity.* Dubuque, IA: Wm. C. Brown Publishers, 1988.

PRINCIPLES OF CARDIOVASCULAR EXERCISE PRESCRIPTION

6

A sound cardiovascular endurance program greatly contributes to the enhancement and maintenance of good health. Of the four components of physical fitness (see Chapter 1), cardiovascular endurance is the single most important. A person needs a certain amount of muscular strength and flexibility to engage in normal daily activities. Nevertheless, a person can get by without a lot of strength and flexibility but cannot do without a good cardiovascular system.

Cardiovascular endurance is the most important component of health-related physical fitness.

Aerobic exercise is especially important in preventing coronary heart disease. A poorly conditioned heart, which has to pump more often just to keep a person alive, is subject to more wear-and-tear than a well-conditioned heart. In situations that place strenuous demands on the heart, such as doing yard work, lifting heavy objects or weights, or running to catch a bus, the unconditioned heart may not be able to sustain the strain. Regular participation in cardiovascular endurance activities also helps a person achieve and maintain recommended body weight, the fourth component of health-related physical fitness.

READINESS FOR EXERCISE

Surveys indicate that more than half of the people who start exercising drop out during the first six months of the program. Sports psychologists are trying to find out why some people exercise habitually and many do not. All of the benefits of exercise cannot help unless people commit to a lifetime program of physical activity.

If you are not exercising now, are you willing to give exercise a try? The first step is to decide positively that you will try. Lab 6A will help you make this decision.

Make list of the advantages and disadvantages of incorporating exercise into your lifestyle. Your list may include things such as: It will make me feel better. I will lose weight. I will have more energy. It will lower risk for chronic diseases. Your list of disadvantages might include: I don't want to take the time. I'm too out of shape. There's no good place to exercise. I don't have the willpower to do it. When the reasons for exercise outweigh the reasons for not exercising, it will become easier to try.

Lab 6B may answer the question: Am I ready to start an exercise program? You are evaluated in four categories: mastery (self-control), attitude, health, and commitment. The higher you score in any category — mastery, for example — the more important that reason is for you to exercise.

Scores can vary from 4 to 16. A score of 12 and above is a strong indicator that that factor is important to you, whereas 8 and below is low. If you score 12 or more points in each category, your chances of initiating and sticking to an exercise program are good. If you do not score at least 12 points in three categories, your chances of succeeding at exercise may be slim. You need to be better informed about the benefits of exercise, and a retraining process may be helpful. More tips on how you can become committed to exercise are provided later in the chapter.

GUIDELINES FOR CARDIOVASCULAR EXERCISE PRESCRIPTION

All too often individuals who exercise regularly and then take a cardiovascular endurance test are surprised to find their maximal oxygen uptake is not as good as they think it is. Although these individuals may be exercising regularly, they most likely are not following the basic principles for cardiovascular exercise prescription. Therefore, they do not reap significant improvements in cardiovascular endurance.

To develop the cardiovascular system, the heart muscle has to be overloaded like any other muscle in the human body. Just as the biceps muscle in the upper arm is developed through strength-training exercises, the heart muscle has to be exercised to increase in size, strength, and efficiency. To better understand how the cardiovascular system can be developed, we have to be familiar with four basic principles: intensity, mode, duration, and frequency of exercise (also see Appendix B).

Before discussing cardiovascular prescription principles, you should be aware that the American College of Sports Medicine recommends that a medical exam and a diagnostic exercise stress test (see Figure 1.13, Chapter 1) be administered prior to vigorous exercise by apparently healthy men over age 40 and women over age 50.[1]

The four basic principles for improving the cardiovascular system are intensity, mode, duration, and frequency of exercise.

The American College of Sports Medicine has defined *vigorous exercise* as an exercise intensity above 60% of maximal oxygen uptake. This intensity is the equivalent of exercise that provides a "substantial challenge" to the participant or one that cannot be maintained for 20 continuous minutes.

INTENSITY OF EXERCISE

When trying to develop the cardiovascular system, intensity of exercise perhaps is the factor that is ignored most often. This principle refers to how hard a person has to exercise to improve cardiovascular endurance.

For muscles to develop they have to be overloaded to a given point. The training stimulus to develop the biceps muscle can be accomplished with curl-up exercises, but the stimulus for the cardiovascular system is provided by making the heart pump faster for a certain period of time.

Cardiovascular development occurs when working between 50% and 85% of heart rate reserve.[2] Working closer to 85% of heart rate reserve yields quicker results. For this reason, many experts prescribe exercise between 70% and 85% for young people. Exercise intensity can be calculated easily, and training can be monitored by checking your pulse.

Determining Training Intensity

To determine the intensity of exercise or cardio-vascular training zone:

1. Estimate your maximal heart rate (MHR). The maximal heart rate depends on the person's age and can be estimated according to the formula: MHR = 220 minus age (220 – age)
2. Check your resting heart rate (RHR) sometime after you have been sitting quietly for 15 to 20 minutes. You may take your pulse for 30 seconds and multiply by 2, or take it for a full minute.
3. Determine the heart rate reserve (HRR). This is done by subtracting the resting heart rate from the maximal heart rate (HRR = MHR – RHR). The heart rate reserve indicates the number of beats available to go from resting conditions to an all-out maximal effort.
4. Calculate the training intensities (TI) at 50%, 70%, and 85%. Multiply the heart rate reserve by the respective 50, 70, and 85 percentages, and then add the resting heart rate to these three figures (for example, 85% TI = HRR × .85 + RHR).

5. *Example:* The 50%, 70%, and 85% training intensities for a 20-year-old person with a resting heart rate of 68 bpm is:

    MHR: 220 – 20 = 200 beats per minute (bpm)

    RHR = 68 bpm

    HRR: 200 – 68 = 132 beats

    50% TI = (132 × .50) + 68 = 134 bpm

    70% TI = (132 × .70) + 68 = 160 bpm

    85% TI = (132 × .85) + 68 = 180 bpm

    Cardiovascular training zone: 134 to 180 bpm

The cardiovascular training zone indicates that whenever you exercise to improve the cardiovascular system, you should maintain your heart rate between the 50% and 85% training intensities to obtain adequate development (Figure 6.1). If you have been physically inactive, you should train around the 50% intensity during the first four to six weeks of the exercise program. After the first few weeks, you should exercise between 70% and 85% training intensity.

FIGURE 6.1

Typical cardiovascular or aerobic training pattern.

Following a few weeks of training, you may have a considerably lower resting heart rate (10 to 20 beats in 8 to 12 weeks). Therefore, you should recompute your target zone periodically. Once you have reached an ideal level of cardiovascular endurance, training in the 50% to 85% range will allow you to maintain your fitness level.

You should monitor your exercise heart rate regularly during the first few weeks of an exercise program to make sure you are training in the proper zone. Wait until you are about five minutes into your exercise session before taking your first rate. When you check your heart rate, count your pulse for 10 seconds and then multiply by 6 to get the per-minute pulse rate. Exercise heart rate will remain at the same level for about 15 seconds following exercise. After 15 seconds, your heart rate will drop rapidly. Do not hesitate to stop during your exercise bout to check your pulse. If the rate is too low, increase the intensity of exercise. If the rate is too high, slow down.

Maintain your heart rate between the 50% and 85% training intensity to obtain adequate cardiovascular development.

To develop the cardiovascular system, you do not have to exercise above the 85% rate. From a fitness standpoint, training above this percentage will not produce extra benefits and actually may be unsafe for some individuals. For unconditioned people and older adults, cardiovascular training should be around the 50% rate. This lower rate is recommended to avoid potential problems associated with high-intensity exercise.

Health Fitness Versus Physical Fitness

Training benefits can be obtained by exercising at the 50% training intensity. Training at this lower percentage, however, may place a person in only an average or a "moderately fit" category (see Table 5.8, Chapter 5). As will be discussed under Specific Exercise Considerations, question 1, exercising at this lower intensity lowers the risk for cardiovascular mortality (health fitness) but does not allow the person to achieve a high cardiovascular fitness rating (physical fitness). The latter ratings are obtained by exercising closer to the 85% threshold.

Rate of Perceived Exertion

Because many people do not check their heart rate during exercise, an alternative method of prescribing intensity of exercise has become more popular recently. This method uses a rate of perceived exertion (RPE) scale developed by Gunnar Borg. Using the scale in Figure 6.2, a person subjectively rates the perceived exertion or difficulty of exercise when training in the appropriate target zone. The exercise heart rate then is associated with the corresponding RPE value.

For example, if the training intensity requires a heart rate zone between 150 and 170 bpm, the person associates this with training between "hard" and "very hard." Some individuals, however, may perceive less exertion than others when training in the correct zone. Therefore, you have to associate your own inner perception of the task with the phrases given on the scale. You then may proceed to exercise at that rate of perceived exertion.

You must be sure to cross-check your target zone with your perceived exertion in the first weeks of your exercise program. To help you develop this association, you should keep a regular record of your activities using the form provided in Figure 6.10 at the end of this chapter. After several weeks

6	
7	Very, very light
8	
9	Very light
10	
11	Fairly light
12	
13	Somewhat hard
14	
15	Hard
16	
17	Very Hard
18	
19	Very, very hard
20	

From Borg, G. "Perceived Exertion: A Note on History and Methods." *Medicine and Science in Sports and Exercise* 5:90-93, 1983.

FIGURE 6.2
Rate of Perceived Exertion Scale.

of training, you should be able to predict your exercise heart rate just by your own perceived exertion of the exercise session.

Whether you monitor the intensity of exercise by checking your pulse or through rate of perceived exertion, you should be aware that changes in normal exercise conditions will affect the training zone. For example, exercising on a hot/humid day or at high altitude increases the heart rate response to a given task requiring adjustments in the intensity of your exercise.

MODE OF EXERCISE

The type of exercise that develops the cardiovascular system has to be aerobic in nature. Once you have established your cardiovascular training zone, any activity or combination of activities that will get your heart rate up to that training zone and keep it there for as long as you exercise will give you adequate development. Examples of these activities are walking, jogging, aerobics, swimming, water aerobics, cross-country skiing, rope skipping, cycling, racquetball, stair climbing, and stationary running or cycling (Figure 6.3).

The activity you choose should be based on your personal preferences, what you most enjoy doing, and your physical limitations. The amount of strength or flexibility you develop through various activities differs, but in terms of cardiovascular

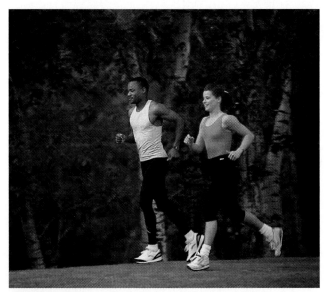

FIGURE 6.3
Aerobic exercise promotes cardiovascular development and helps decrease the risk for chronic diseases.

development, the heart doesn't know whether you are walking, swimming, or cycling. All the heart knows is that it has to pump at a certain rate, and as long as that rate is in the desired range, your cardiovascular fitness will improve.

From a health fitness point of view, training in the lower end of the cardiovascular zone will yield optimal health benefits. The closer the heart rate is to the higher end of the cardiovascular training zone, however, the greater will be the improvements in maximal oxygen uptake (high physical fitness).

Aerobic exercise has to involve the major muscle groups of the body, and it has to be rhythmic and continuous. As the amount of muscle mass involved during exercise increases, so does the effectiveness of the activity in providing cardiovascular development.

Cross-country skiing is regarded as the prime exercise modality for aerobic development. Several major muscle groups are used during this activity because it requires both upper and lower body work. Research has shown that, of all elite athletes, cross-country skiers have the highest maximal oxygen uptake.

Because of the greater amount of muscle mass involved, more oxygen and energy (calories) are used during cross-country skiing than with most other aerobic activities. A limitation of this activity, of course, is the lack of year-round conditions for skiing, and commercially available cross-country skiing simulating equipment is not readily available to most people.

A new mode of aerobic exercise is *Aero-belt exercise*. The Aero-belt* (Aerobic Endurance Resistance Overloader) consists of a belt with an elastic band that freely slides through the belt and attaches to the wrists. The objective of using the Aero-belt is to provide resistance to the arms during lower body physical activity; thereby increasing the person's oxygen consumption, energy expenditure, and upper body strength and endurance development during aerobic exercise. As in cross-country skiing, the Aero-belt provides resistance to the arms while walking, jogging, bounding, stair stepping, riding a stationary bicycle, or doing aerobics (see Figure 6.4)

Using the Aero-belt actually can provide greater upper body conditioning benefits than cross-country skiing. Depending on individual strength and fitness levels, three different tension grades for the elastic

---

* AERO-BELT is a registered trademark of Nurge Fitness Systems, P.O. Box 889, Ketchum, ID 83340 Phone: 1-800-TRY-TO-XL

Aero-belt walking

Aero-belt jogging

Aero-belt step-aerobics (powerobics)

Aero-belt stair climbing

FIGURE 6.4

Aero-belt Exercise: A new exercise modality designed to provide resistance to the arms during lower body physical activity; thereby, increasing the person's oxygen consumption, energy expenditure, and upper body strength development during aerobic exercise.

cord are available. Medium and high tension are mainly for strength conditioning, and low tension is for developing endurance.

The physiologic responses to Aero-belt walking at 4 mph and step-aerobics were investigated recently at Boise State University. Increases in heart rate, oxygen uptake, and caloric expenditure ranged from 32% to 54% from regular walking and step-aerobics to walking and step-aerobics with an Aero-belt.

DURATION OF EXERCISE

The general recommendation is that a person train between 20 and 60 minutes per session. The duration is based on how intensely a person trains. If the training is done around 85%, 20 minutes are sufficient. At 50% intensity, the person should train at least 30 minutes. As mentioned under Intensity of Exercise, unconditioned people and older adults should train at lower percentages; therefore, the activity should be carried out over a longer time.

Although most experts recommend 20 to 30 minutes of aerobic exercise per session, 1990 research published in the *American Journal of Cardiology*[8] indicates that three 10-minute exercise sessions per day (separated by at least 4 hours), at approximately 70% of maximal heart rate, also produce training benefits.

Although the increases in maximal oxygen uptake with the latter program were not as large

(57%) as those found in a group performing a continuous 30-minute bout of exercise per day, the researchers concluded that moderate-intensity exercise training, conducted for 10 minutes, three times per day, benefits the cardiovascular system significantly.

The results of the study are meaningful because people often mention lack of time as the reason for not taking part in an exercise program. Many think they have to exercise at least 20 continuous minutes to get any benefits at all. Even though 20 to 30 minutes are ideal, short, intermittent exercise bouts also are beneficial to the cardiovascular system.

Exercise sessions always should be preceded by a 5-minute warm-up and followed by a 5-minute cool-down period (see Figure 6.1). The warm-up should consist of general calisthenics, stretching exercises, or exercising at a lower intensity level than the actual target zone. The cool-down entails *gradually* decreasing the intensity of exercise. Abruptly stopping causes blood to pool in the exercised body parts, diminishing the return of blood to the heart. Less blood return can cause dizziness and faintness or even bring on cardiac abnormalities.

FREQUENCY OF EXERCISE

Ideally, a person should engage in aerobic exercise three to five times per week. When starting an exercise program, three to five 20- to 30-minute training sessions per week are recommended to improve maximal oxygen uptake. Further improvements are minimal when training is conducted more than 5 days a week.

For individuals on a weight loss program, 45- to 60-minute exercise sessions of low to moderate intensity, conducted five to six days per week, are recommended. Longer exercise sessions increase caloric expenditure for faster weight reduction (see Chapter 4). Three 20- to-30-minute training sessions per week, on nonconsecutive days, will maintain cardiovascular fitness as long as the heart rate is in the appropriate target zone. A summary of the cardiovascular exercise prescription guidelines according to the American College of Sports Medicine is provided in Figure 6.5.

Activity: Aerobic (examples: walking, jogging, cycling, swimming, aerobics, racquetball, soccer, stair climbing)

Intensity: 50–85% heart rate reserve

Duration: 20–60 minutes of continuous aerobic activity

Frequency: 3 to 5 days per week

Source: The recommended quantity and quality of exercise for developing and maintaining cardiorespiratory and muscular fitness in healthy adults by the American College of Sports Medicine. Med. Sci. Sports Exerc. 22:265-274, 1990.

FIGURE 6.5
Cardiovascular exercise prescription guidelines.

RATING THE FITNESS BENEFITS OF AEROBIC ACTIVITIES

The fitness contributions of different aerobic activities to the various health-related components of fitness vary. An accurate assessment of the contributions to each fitness component are difficult to establish, but a summary of likely benefits of several activities is provided in Table 6.1. Instead of a single rating or number, ranges are given for some of the categories. The benefits derived are based on the person's effort while participating in the activity.

The nature of the activity often dictates the potential aerobic development. For example, jogging is much more strenuous than walking. The effort during exercise also has an impact on the amount of physiological development. The training benefits of just going through the motions of a low-impact aerobics routine, as compared to accentuating all motions, are of a different magnitude.

Table 6.1 indicates a starting fitness level for each aerobic activity. Attempting to participate in high-intensity activities without proper conditioning often leads to injuries and discouragement. Beginners should start with low-intensity activities that carry a minimum risk for injuries.

In some cases, such as in high-impact aerobics and rope skipping, the risk for injuries remains high even if the participants have adequate conditioning. These activities should be supplemental only and are not recommended as the sole mode of exercise.

METs are an alternative method of prescribing exercise intensity, frequently used by physicians who work with cardiac patients. The MET range for the various activities is included in Table 6.1. One MET represents the body's energy requirement at rest or the equivalent of an oxygen uptake of 3.5 ml/kg/min. A 10-MET activity requires a ten-fold increase in the resting energy requirement, or approximately 35 ml/kg/min. MET levels for a given activity vary according to the effort expended. The harder a person exercises, the higher the MET level.

The effectiveness of various aerobic activities in weight management also is provided in Table 6.1. As a general rule, the greater the muscle mass involved in exercise, the better the results. Rhythmic and continuous activities that involve large amounts of muscle mass are most effective in burning calories.

Higher intensity activities increase caloric expenditure as well. Exercising longer, however, compensates for lower intensities. If carried out long enough (45 to 60 minutes five to six times per week), even walking can be an excellent exercise mode for weight loss. Additional information on a comprehensive weight management program is given in Chapter 4.

SPECIFIC EXERCISE CONSIDERATIONS

In addition to many of the exercise-related issues discussed to this point, many other concerns require clarification or are somewhat controversial. Let's examine some of these issues.

TABLE 6.1
Ratings for Aerobic Activities

Activity	Recommended Starting Fitness Level[1]	Injury Risk[2]	Potential Cardiovascular Endurance Development (VO_{2max})[3,5]	Upper Body Strength Development[3]	Lower Body Strength Development[3]	Upper Body Flexibility Development[3]	Lower Body Flexibility Development[3]	Weight Control[3]	MET Level[4,5,6]	Caloric Expenditure (cal/hour)[5,6]
Walking	B	L	1–2	1	2	1	1	3	4–6	300–450
Walking/Water/Chest-Deep	I	L	2–4	2	3	1	1	3	6–10	450–750
Hiking	B	L	2–4	1	3	1	1	3	6–10	450–750
Jogging	I	M	3–5	1	3	1	1	5	6–15	450–1125
Jogging/Deep Water	A	L	3–5	2	2	1	1	5	8–15	600–1125
High Impact Aerobics	A	H	3–4	2	4	3	2	4	6–12	450–900
Low Impact Aerobics	B	L	2–4	2	3	3	2	3	5–10	375–750
Step Aerobics	I	M	2–4	2	3–4	3	2	3–4	5–12	375–900
Moderate Impact Aerobics	I	M	2–4	2	3	3	2	3	6–12	450–900
Swimming (front crawl)	B	L	3–5	4	2	3	1	3	6–12	450–900
Water Aerobics	B	L	2–4	3	3	3	2	3	6–12	450–900
Stationary Cycling	B	L	2–4	1	4	1	1	3	6–10	450–750
Road Cycling	I	M	2–5	1	4	1	1	3	6–12	450–900
Cross Training	I	M	3–5	2–3	3–4	2–3	1–2	3–5	6–15	450–1125
Rope Skipping	I	H	3–5	2	4	1	2	3–5	8–15	600–1125
Cross-Country Skiing	B	M	4–5	4	4	2	2	4–5	10–16	750–1200
Aero-belt Exercise	B	M	4–5	4	4	3	2	4–5	10–16	750–1200
In-Line Skating	I	M	2–4	2	4	2	2	3	6–10	450–750
Rowing	B	L	3–5	4	2	3	1	4	8–14	600–1050
Stair Climbing	B	L	3–5	1	4	1	1	4–5	8–15	600–1125
Racquet Sports	I	M	2–4	3	3	3	2	3	6–10	450–750

[1] B = Beginner, I = Intermediate, A = Advanced

[2] L = Low, M = Moderate, H = High

[3] 1 = Low, 2 = Fair, 3 = Average, 4 = Good, 5 = excellent

[4] One MET represents the rate of energy expenditure at rest (3.5 ml/kg/min). Each additional MET is a multiple of the resting value. For example, 5 METs represents an energy expenditure equivalent to five times the resting value or about 17.5 ml/kg/min.

[5] Varies according to the person's effort (exercise intensity) during exercise.

[6] Varies according to body weight.

1. **Does aerobic exercise make a person immune to heart and blood vessel disease?** Although aerobically fit individuals as a whole have a lower incidence of cardiovascular disease, a regular aerobic exercise program by itself does not offer an absolute guarantee against cardiovascular disease. Overall risk factor management is the best way to minimize the risk for cardiovascular disease (see Chapter 12). Many factors can increase the person's risk, including a genetic predisposition. Experts believe, however, that a regular aerobic exercise program not only will delay the onset of cardiovascular problems but that the chances of surviving a heart attack are much better for those who exercise regularly.

   Even moderate increases in aerobic fitness significantly lower the incidences of premature cardiovascular deaths. Data from the Aerobics Research Institute in Dallas, Texas (see Figure 1.7, Chapter 1) indicate that the decrease in cardiovascular mortality is greatest between the unfit (group 1) and the moderately fit (2 and 3) groups. A further decrease in cardiovascular mortality is observed between the moderate and the highly fit groups (4 and 5), but the difference is not as much as that between the unfit and moderate fitness groups.

2. **How much aerobic exercise is required to decrease the risk for cardiovascular disease?** Although research has not yet indicated the exact amount of aerobic exercise required to lower the risk for cardiovascular disease, some general recommendations have been set forth. Dr. Ralph Paffenbarger and co-researchers, in their study "Cause-Specific Death Rates per 10,000 Man-Years of Observation Among 16,936 Harvard Alumni, 1962 to 1968, by Physical Activity Index" showed that 2,000 calories expended per week as a result of physical activity yielded the lowest risk for cardiovascular disease among this group of almost 17,000 Harvard alumni (see Chapter 1, Figure 1.6). Two thousand calories per week represents about 300 calories per daily exercise session.

3. **Do people get a "physical high" during aerobic exercise?** During vigorous exercise, morphine-like substances called *endorphines* are released from the pituitary gland in the brain. These act not only as a pain killer but also can create feelings of euphoria and natural well-being.

Higher levels of endorphines are often seen as a result of aerobic endurance activities and may remain elevated for as long as 30 to 60 minutes following exercise. Many experts believe these higher levels explain the physical high some people experience during and after prolonged exercise.

Endorphine levels also have been shown to be elevated during pregnancy and delivery. As endorphines act as pain killers, these higher levels could explain why a woman has more tolerance for the pain and discomfort of natural childbirth and her pleasant feelings shortly after the baby's birth. Several reports have indicated that well-conditioned women have shorter and easier labor. These women possibly attain higher endorphine levels during delivery, making childbirth less traumatic than it is for untrained women.

4. **Is it safe to exercise during pregnancy?** Women should not forsake exercise during pregnancy. If anything, they should exercise to strengthen the body and prepare for delivery. Moderate exercise during pregnancy helps to prevent excessive weight gain and speed up recovery following birth.

   Pregnant women in Indian tribes continue to carry out all of their difficult work chores up to the very day of delivery, and a few hours after the baby's birth they resume their normal activities. Several women athletes have competed in sports during the early stages of pregnancy. Nevertheless, the woman and her personal physician should make the final decision regarding her exercise program.

   Although starting a new exercise program during pregnancy is not recommended, experts agree that women who have been exercising regularly may continue to carry out an almost similar program through the fourth month of pregnancy. They should take care, however, not to exceed a body (core) temperature of 38.5° C (101.3° F). To ensure adequate oxygen delivery to the baby, exercise heart rates should be kept below 140 beats per minute and training sessions should be limited to 15 minutes.

   After the fourth month, walking, stationary cycling, moderate swimming, and water aerobics are indicated in conjunction with some light strengthening exercises. Exercises that require a woman to lie on her back should be avoided after the fourth month as this position can block blood flow to the uterus and depress the baby's heart rate.

If women have not exercised regularly, 20 to 30 minutes of daily walking and light strengthening exercises are recommended throughout the pregnancy.

5. **Does exercise help relieve dysmenorrhea (painful menstruation)?** Exercise has not been shown to either cure or aggravate painful menstruation, but it has been shown to relieve menstrual cramps because it improves circulation to the uterus. Less severe menstrual cramps also could be related to higher increased levels of endorphines produced during prolonged physical activity, which may counteract pain.

6. **Does participation in exercise hinder menstruation?** In some instances, highly trained athletes may develop amenorrhea (cessation of menstruation) during training and competition. This condition is seen most often in extremely lean women who also engage in sports that require strenuous physical effort over a sustained time, but it is by no means irreversible. At present we do not know whether the condition is caused by physical or emotional stress related to high-intensity training, excessively low body fat, or other factors.

Although, on the average, women have a lower physical capacity during menstruation, medical surveys at the Olympic games have shown that women have broken Olympic and world records at all stages of the menstrual cycle. Menstruation should not keep a woman from participating in athletics, and it will not necessarily have a negative impact on performance.

7. **Does exercise offset the detrimental effects of cigarette smoking?** Physical exercise often motivates toward smoking cessation but does not offset any ill effects of smoking. If anything, smoking greatly decreases the ability of the blood to transport oxygen to working muscles.

Oxygen is carried in the circulatory system by hemoglobin, the iron-containing pigment of the red blood cells. Carbon monoxide, a byproduct of cigarette smoke, has 210 to 250 times greater affinity for hemoglobin over oxygen. Consequently, carbon monoxide combines much faster with hemoglobin, decreasing the oxygen-carrying capacity of the blood.

Chronic smoking also increases airway resistance, requiring the respiratory muscles to work much harder and consume more oxygen just to ventilate a given amount of air. If a person quits smoking, exercise does help increase the functional capacity of the pulmonary system.

8. **What type of clothing should a person wear during exercise?** The type of clothing you wear during exercise is important. Clothing should fit comfortably and allow free movement of the various body parts. Clothes should be geared to air temperature and humidity. Avoid nylon and rubberized materials and tight clothes that will interfere with the cooling mechanism of the human body or obstruct normal blood flow. Properly fitting shoes, manufactured specifically for your choice of activity, will help to prevent lower limb injuries.

9. **How long should a person wait after a meal before exercising strenuously?** The length of time to wait before exercising after a meal depends on the amount of food eaten. On the average, after a regular meal, you should wait about two hours before participating in strenuous physical activity. A walk or some other light physical activity is fine following a meal, though. If anything, it helps burn extra calories and may help the body metabolize fats more efficiently.

10. **What time of the day is best for exercise?** You can do intense exercise almost any time of the day, with the exception of about two hours following a heavy meal, or the noon and early afternoon hours on hot and humid days. Moderate exercise seems to be beneficial shortly after a meal, because exercise enhances the thermogenic response, the amount of energy required to digest food. A walk after a meal burns more calories than a walk several hours after a meal.

Many people enjoy exercising early in the morning because it gives them a boost to start the day. People who exercise in the morning also seem to stick with it more than others. Some prefer the lunch hour for weight control reasons. By exercising at noon, they do not eat as big a lunch, which helps keep daily caloric intake down. Highly stressed people seem to like the evening hours because of the relaxing effects of exercise.

11. **Why is exercising in hot and humid conditions unsafe?** When a person exercises, only 30% to 40% of the energy the body produces is used for mechanical work or movement. The rest of the energy (60% to 70%) is converted into heat. If this heat cannot be dissipated properly because the weather either is too hot or the relative humidity is too high, body temperature increases and, in extreme cases, can result in death.

The specific heat of body tissue (the heat required to raise the temperature of the body by 1°C) is .38 calories per pound of body weight per 1°C (.38 cal/lb/°C). This indicates that if no body heat is dissipated, a 150-pound person needs to burn only 57 calories (150 × .38) to increase total body temperature by 1°C. If this person were to conduct an exercise session requiring 300 calories (about 3 miles running) without any heat dissipation, the inner body temperature would increase by 5.3°C, which is the equivalent of going from 98.6°F to 108.1°F.

This example clearly illustrates the need for caution when exercising in hot or humid weather. If the relative humidity is too high, body heat cannot be lost through evaporation because the atmosphere already is saturated with water vapor. In one instance a football casualty occurred at a temperature of only 64°F, but at a relative humidity of 100%. People must be cautious when air temperature is above 90°F and the relative humidity is above 60%.

The American College of Sports Medicine recommends that individuals should not engage in strenuous physical activity when the readings of a wet bulb globe thermometer exceed 82.4°F. With this type of thermometer, the wet bulb is cooled by evaporation, and on dry days it shows a lower temperature than the regular (dry) thermometer. On humid days the cooling effect is less because of less evaporation; hence, the difference between the wet and dry readings is not as great.

The American Running and Fitness Association offers the following descriptions and first-aid measures for three signs of trouble when exercising in the heat:

■ **Heat cramps.** Symptoms include cramps and spasms and muscle twitching in the legs, arms, and abdomen. To relieve heat cramps, stop exercising, get out of the heat, massage the painful area, slowly stretch, and drink plenty of fluids.

■ **Heat exhaustion.** Symptoms include fainting; dizziness; profuse sweating; cold, clammy skin; weakness; headache and a rapid, weak pulse. If you experience any of these symptoms, stop and find a cool place to rest. Drink plenty of cool fluids. Loosen or remove clothing, and rub your body with a cool, wet towel. Stay out of the heat for the rest of the day, and possibly for the next two or three days.

■ **Heat stroke.** Symptoms include serious disorientation; warm, dry skin; no sweating; rapid, full pulse; vomiting; diarrhea; unconsciousness; and high body temperature. As the temperature climbs, unexplained anxiety sets in. When the body temperature reaches 104°F to 105°F, the individual may get goose bumps, feel a cold sensation in the trunk of the body, nausea, throbbing in the temples, and numbness in the extremities. Most people become incoherent after this stage. When body temperature reaches 105°F to 106°F, disorientation, loss of fine-motor control, and muscular weakness set in. If the temperature exceeds 106°F, serious neurologic injury and death may be imminent.

Heat stroke requires immediate emergency medical attention. Someone should request help (call 911) and get the person out of the sun. While you're waiting for the person to be taken to the hospital's emergency room, spray the person with cool water and rub the body with cool towels. Fan the person and give him or her plenty of cold liquids.

12. **What should a person do to replace fluids lost during prolonged aerobic exercise?** The main objective of fluid replacement during prolonged aerobic exercise is to maintain the blood volume so circulation and sweating can continue at normal levels. Adequate water replacement is the most important factor in preventing heat disorders. Drinking about eight ounces of cool water every 10 to 15 minutes during exercise seems to be ideal to prevent dehydration. Cold fluids seem to be absorbed more rapidly from the stomach.

Commercial fluid replacement solutions (e.g., Take-Five, Gatorade) contain about 5%

glucose, which slows down water absorption when exercising in the heat. During prolonged aerobic exercise in cool environments, commercially prepared solutions may be helpful because not as much water is lost through the sweating mechanism.

Sugar does not become available to the muscles until about 30 minutes after drinking a glucose solution. Drinking solutions with a sugar concentration higher than 5% significantly slows down water absorption from the stomach.

13. **What precautions should be taken when exercising in the cold?** In contrast to hot and humid conditions, exercising in the cold usually does not threaten one's health because clothing for heat conservation can be selected and exercise itself increases the production of body heat. The popular belief that exercising in cold temperatures (32°F and lower) freezes the lungs is totally false, because the air is warmed properly in the air passages before it ever reaches the lungs. Cold is not what poses a threat but, rather, wind velocity, which affects the chill factor greatly.

For example, exercising at a temperature of 25°F with adequate clothing is not too cold, but if the wind is blowing at 25 miles per hour, the chill factor lowers the actual temperature to –5°F. This effect is even worse if a person is wet and exhausted.

Even though the lungs are under no risk when exercising in the cold, the face, head, hands, and feet should be protected, as they are subject to frostbite. In cold temperatures, about 30% of the body's heat is lost through the head's surface area if it is unprotected. Wearing several layers of lightweight clothing is preferable to one single, thick layer because warm air is trapped between layers of clothes, enabling greater heat conservation.

MANAGING EXERCISE-RELATED INJURIES

To enjoy and maintain physical fitness, preventing injury during a conditioning program is essential. Exercise-related injuries, nonetheless, are common in individuals who participate in exercise programs.

Surveys indicate that more than 50% of all new participants suffer injuries during the first six months of the conditioning program.

The three most common causes of injuries are: (a) rapid conditioning programs — doing too much too quick, (b) improper shoes or training surfaces, and (c) anatomical predisposition (body propensity). A significant increase in quantity, intensity, and duration of activities is by far the most common cause of injuries. The body requires time to adapt to more intense activities. Most of these injuries can be prevented through a more gradual and proper conditioning program.

Proper shoes for specific activities are essential (see Figure 6.6). Shoes should be replaced when they show a lot of wear and tear. Softer training surfaces, such as grass and dirt, produce less trauma than asphalt and concrete.

Few people have perfect body alignment, so injuries may occur eventually. These types of injuries often are associated with overtraining. In case of injury, proper treatment can avert a lengthy recovery process. A summary of common exercise-related injuries and how to manage them follows.

ACUTE SPORTS INJURIES

The best treatment always has been prevention itself. If an activity causes unusual discomfort or chronic irritation, you need to treat the cause by decreasing the intensity, switching activities, substituting equipment, or upgrading clothing, such as proper-fitting shoes.

In cases of acute injury, the standard treatment is cold application, compression or splinting (or both), and elevation of the affected body part. This

FIGURE 6.6
Properly fitting shoes for specific activities are recommended to prevent exercise related injuries.

commonly is referred to as ICE. I = Ice application, C = Compression, and E = Elevation. Cold should be applied three to five times a day for 15 to 20 minutes at a time during the first 24 to 36 hours, by submerging the injured area in cold water, using an ice bag, or applying ice massage to the affected part. An elastic bandage or wrap can be used for compression. Elevating the body part decreases blood flow to it.

The purpose of these three types of treatment is to minimize swelling in the area, which hastens recovery time. After the first 36 to 48 hours, heat can be used if there is no further swelling or inflammation. If you have doubts regarding the nature or seriousness of the injury (such as suspected fracture), however, you should seek a medical evaluation.

Obvious deformities (such as in fractures, dislocations, or partial dislocations) call for splinting, cold application with an ice bag, and medical attention. Never try to reset any of these conditions by yourself, as muscles, ligaments, and nerves could be further damaged. Treatment of these injuries always should be in the hands of specialized medical personnel. A quick reference guide for the signs or symptoms and treatment of exercise-related problems is provided in Table 6.2.

TABLE 6.2
Reference Guide for Exercise Related Problems

Injury	Signs/Symptoms	Treatment*
Bruise (contusion)	Pain, swelling, discoloration	Cold application, compression, rest
Dislocations Fractures	Pain, swelling, deformity	Splinting, cold application, seek medical attention
Heat cramps	Cramps, spasms and muscle twitching in the legs, arms, and abdomen	Stop activity, get out of the heat, stretch, massage the painful area, drink plenty of fluids
Heat exhaustion	Fainting, profuse sweating, cold/clammy skin, weak/rapid pulse, weakness, headache	Stop activity, rest in a cool place, loosen clothing, rub body with cool/wet towel, drink plenty of fluids, stay out of heat for 2–3 days
Heat stroke	Hot/dry skin, no sweating, serious disorientation, rapid/full pulse, vomiting, diarrhea, unconsciousness, high body temperature	**Seek immediate medical attention,** request help and get out of the sun, bathe in cold water/spray with cold water/rub body with cold towels, drink plenty of cold fluids
Joint sprains	Pain, tenderness, swelling, loss of use, discoloration	Cold application, compression, elevation, rest, heat after 36 to 48 hours (if no further swelling)
Muscle cramps	Pain, spasm	Stretch muscle(s), use mild exercises for involved area
Muscle soreness and stiffness	Tenderness, pain	Mild stretching, low-intensity exercise, warm bath
Muscle strains	Pain, tenderness, swelling, loss of use	Cold application, compression, elevation, rest, heat after 36 to 48 hours (if no further swelling)
Shin splints	Pain, tenderness	Cold application prior to and following any physical activity, rest, heat (if no activity is carried out)
Side stitch	Pain on the side of the abdomen below the rib cage	Decrease level of physical activity or stop altogether, gradually increase level of fitness
Tendonitis	Pain, tenderness, loss of use	Rest, cold application, heat after 48 hours

* Cold should be applied 3 to 4 times a day for 15 minutes. Heat can be applied 3 times a day for 15 to 20 minutes.

MUSCLE SORENESS AND STIFFNESS

Individuals who begin an exercise program or participate after a long layoff from exercise often develop muscle soreness and stiffness. The acute soreness that sets in the first few hours after exercise is thought to be related to a lack of blood (oxygen) flow and general fatigue of the exercised muscles.

Delayed muscle soreness that appears several hours after exercise (usually about 12 hours later) and lasts for two to four days may be related to actual tiny tears in muscle tissue, muscle spasms that increase fluid retention stimulating the pain nerve endings, and overstretching or tearing of connective tissue in and around muscles and joints.

Mild stretching before and adequately stretching after exercise helps to prevent soreness and stiffness. Gradually progressing into an exercise program is important, too. A person should not attempt to do too much too quickly. To relieve pain, mild stretching, low-intensity exercise to stimulate blood flow, and a warm bath might help.

EXERCISE INTOLERANCE

When starting an exercise program, participants should stay within the safe limits. The best method to determine whether you are exercising too strenuously is to check your heart rate and make sure it does not exceed the limits of your target zone. Exercising above this target zone may not be safe for unconditioned or high-risk individuals. You do not need to exercise beyond your target zone to gain the desired cardiovascular benefits.

Several physical signs will tell you when you are exceeding your functional limitations. A rapid or irregular heart rate, difficult breathing, nausea, vomiting, lightheadedness, headaches, dizziness, pale skin, flushness, extreme weakness, lack of energy, shakiness, sore muscles, cramps, and tightness in the chest are all signs of exercise intolerance. You should learn to listen to your body. If you notice any of these symptoms, you should seek medical attention before continuing your exercise program.

Recovery heart rate is another indicator of overexertion. To a certain extent, recovery heart rate is related to fitness level. The higher your cardiovascular fitness level, the faster your heart rate will decrease following exercise. As a rule of thumb, heart rate should be below 120 beats per minute five minutes into recovery. If your heart rate is above 120, you most likely have overexerted yourself or possibly could have some other cardiac abnormality. If you lower the intensity or duration of exercise, or both, and you still have a fast heart rate five minutes into recovery, you should consult your physician.

SIDE STITCH

The exact cause of this sharp pain that sometimes occurs during exercise is unknown. Some experts suggest that it could be related to a lack of blood flow to the respiratory muscles during strenuous physical exertion. Side stitch seems to occur only in unconditioned beginners or trained individuals when they exercise at higher intensities than usual. This stitch is encountered primarily in the early stages of exercise participation. As you improve your physical condition, this problem will disappear unless you start training at a higher intensity. If it occurs, slow down, and if it persists, stop altogether.

SHIN SPLINTS

The shin splint, one of the most common injuries to the lower limbs, is characterized by pain and irritation in the shin region of the leg and usually results from one or more of the following: (a) lack of proper and gradual conditioning, (b) doing physical activities on hard surfaces (wooden floors, hard tracks, cement, and asphalt), (c) fallen arches in the feet, (d) chronic overuse, (e) muscle fatigue, (f) faulty posture, (g) improper shoes, and (h) participating in weight-bearing activities when excessively overweight.

Shin splints are managed by: (a) removing or reducing the cause (exercising on softer surfaces, wearing better shoes and/or arch supports, or completely stopping exercise until the shin splints heal); (b) doing mild stretching exercises before and after physical activity; (c) using ice massage for 10 to 20 minutes before and after physical exercise; and (d) applying active heat (whirlpool and hot baths) for 15 minutes, two to three times a day. In addition, supportive taping during physical activity is helpful (the proper taping technique can be learned readily from a qualified athletic trainer).

MUSCLE CRAMPS

Muscle cramps are caused by the body's depletion of essential electrolytes or a breakdown in the coordination between opposing muscle groups. If you have a muscle cramp, you should first attempt to stretch the muscles involved. For example, in the case of the calf muscle, pull your toes up toward the knees. After stretching the muscles, gently rub them down, and finally do some mild exercises requiring the use of those muscles.

In pregnant and lactating women, muscle cramps often are related to a lack of calcium. If women get cramps during these times, calcium supplements usually relieve the problem. Tight clothing also can cause cramps, by decreasing blood flow to active muscle tissue.

LEISURE-TIME PHYSICAL ACTIVITY

Although individuals have notable differences, the average person in developed countries has about 3.5 hours of "free" or leisure-time daily. Unfortunately, in the current automated society, most of this time is spent in sedentary living.

Leisure-time physical activity usually is viewed as any activity undertaken during an individual's discretionary time that helps to increase resting energy or caloric expenditure. These activities are selected based on personal interests. Motivational factors for participation include health, aesthetics, weight control, competition and challenge, fun, social interaction, mental arousal, relaxation, and stress management.

Frequently, leisure-time physical activity does not include exercise performed during a regular exercise program. It consists of activities such as walking, hiking, gardening, yard work, occupational work and chores, and moderate sports such as tennis, table tennis, badminton, golf, or croquet.

Every small increase in daily physical activity contributes to the development of health and wellness. Small increases in physical activity have a large impact in decreasing early risk for disease and premature death. Therefore, a new, concerted effort must be made to spend leisure-time in activities that will promote energy expenditure, provide a break from daily tasks, and contribute to health-related fitness.

GETTING STARTED AND ADHERING TO A LIFETIME EXERCISE PROGRAM

Having learned the basic principles of cardiovascular exercise prescription, you can proceed to Lab 6C and fill out your own prescription. This exercise prescription calls for a gradual increase in intensity, duration, and frequency.

If you have not been exercising regularly, you could go ahead and attempt to train five or six times a week for 30 minutes at a time. You may find this discouraging, however, and may drop out before getting too far because you probably will develop some muscle soreness and stiffness, and possibly incur minor injuries.

Muscle soreness and stiffness, and the risk for injuries, can be lessened or eliminated by increasing the intensity, duration, and frequency of exercise progressively as outlined in Lab 6C. Or, if using the computer software available with this book you can obtain a printout of your personalized cardiovascular exercise prescription (see Figure 6.7). You also can create and regularly update a computer file to keep a record of your activity program (see Figure 6.8). This file is based on the EXLOG computer program.

Once you have determined your exercise prescription, the difficult part begins: starting and sticking to a lifetime exercise program. Although you may be motivated after reading the benefits to be gained from physical activity, lifelong dedication and perseverance are necessary to reap and maintain good fitness.

The first few weeks are probably the most difficult, but, where there's a will, there's a way. Once you begin to see positive changes, it won't be as hard. Soon you will develop a habit for exercise that will be deeply satisfying and will bring about a sense of self-accomplishment. The following suggestions have been used successfully by others:

1. **Select aerobic activities you enjoy.** If you pick an activity you don't enjoy, you will be less likely to keep exercising. Don't be afraid to try out a new activity, even if that means learning new skills.

2. **Combine different activities.** You can train by doing two or three different activities the same

```
         PERSONALIZED CARDIOVASCULAR EXERCISE PRESCRIPTION
                      Fitness & Wellness Series
                      Morton Publishing Company


     Jim R. Davis              Age: 19           Date: 01-08-1992
     Est. maximal heart rate: 201 bpm    Resting heart rate: 76 bpm
     Present cardiovascular fitness level: average

     The following is your personal program for cardiovascular fit-
     ness development and/or maintenance.  If you have been exer-
     cising regularly and you are in the average  or good category,
     you may start at week five.  If you are in the excellent cate-
     gory, you can start at week nine.
```

Week	Time (min.)	Frequency (per week)	Heart Rate Range (beats per minute)	Pulse (10 sec. count)
1	15	3	141 to 151	24 to 25
2	15	4	141 to 151	24 to 25
3	20	4	141 to 151	24 to 25
4	20	5	141 to 151	24 to 25
5	20	4	151 to 164	25 to 27
6	20	5	151 to 164	25 to 27
7	30	4	151 to 164	25 to 27
8	30	5	151 to 164	25 to 27
9	30	4	164 to 176	27 to 29
10	30	5	164 to 176	27 to 29
11	30—40	5	164 to 176	27 to 29
12	30—40	5-6	164 to 176	27 to 29

```
     You may participate in any combination of activities which are
     aerobic  and continuous in nature,  such as walking,  jogging,
     swimming, cross country skiing, rope skipping, cycling, aero-
     bic dancing, racquetball,  stair climbing, stationary  running
     or cycling, etc. As long as the heart rate reaches the desired
     range, and it stays in that range for the period of time indi-
     cated, the cardiovascular system will improve its capacity.

     Following the twelve week program,  in order to maintain  your
     fitness level, you should exercise between 164 and 176 bpm for
     about 30 minutes, a minimum of three times per week on noncon-
     secutive days.

     When you exercise, allow about 5 minutes for a gradual warm-up
     period and another  5 for gradual  cool-down.   Also, when you
     check your exercise heart rate,  only count your pulse for  10
     seconds (start counting with 0) and then refer to the above 10
     sec. pulse count.  You may also multiply by  6 to obtain  your
     rate in beats per minute.

     Good cardiovascular fitness will greatly contribute toward the
     enhancement and maintenance of good health.   It is especially
     important in the prevention of coronary heart disease.  We en-
     courage you to be persistent  in your exercise program and  to
     participate regularly.  Best of luck Jim.
```

FIGURE 6.7
Sample computerized exercise prescription.

FITNESS & WELLNESS SERIES
By Werner W.K. Hoeger
Morton Publishing Company — Englewood, Colorado

MONTHLY EXERCISE LOG

Jim R. Davis
1234 Veterans Park
Los Escondidos, CA   99222

Month of January 1992

Date	Body Weight	Type of Exercise	Exercise Heart Rate	Duration of Exercise	Distance (miles)	Calories Burned
1	179.5	Walking (4.5 mph)	120	30 min.	2.0	242
		Running 11 min/mile	156	34 min.	3.0	426
		Golf	102	90 min.		483
4	179.0	Running 11 min/mile	156	33 min.	3.0	413
		Tennis (moderate)	126	60 min.		483
6	178.5	Running 11 min/mile	162	38 min.	3.5	475
8	178.0	Running 8.5 min/mile	180	12 min.	1.5	192
		Calisthenics	96	30 min.		176
9	178.0	Water Aerobics (vig)	150	30 min.		534
11	177.5	Running 8.5 min/mile	174	28 min.	3.0	439
		Racquetball	144	60 min.		692
13	176.5	Running 8.5 min/mile	174	29 min.	3.0	453
14	177.0	Swimming 25 yrds/min	138	25 min.	0.5	177
16	177.5	Running 8.5 min/mile	174	26 min.	3.0	415
17	176.5	Dance (moderate)	102	120 min.		635
18	176.0	Basketball (mod)	144	60 min.		486
		Skiing (downhill)	96	60 min.		634
20	176.0	Running 7 min/mile	172	18 min.	2.5	323
22	176.0	Running 7 min/mile	174	23 min.	3.0	404
24	175.5	Running 7 min/mile	168	23 min.	3.0	412
25	175.0	Soccer	150	90 min.		929
27	176.0	Running 7 min/mile	174	23 min.	3.0	404
28	175.0	Aerobic Dance (vig)	156	30 min.		499
		Volleyball	120	45 min.		236
30	175.0	Strength Training	108	60 min.		525
31	174.5	Running 7 min/mile	168	22 min.	3.0	383
		Bowling	102	90 min.		471

MONTHLY SUMMARY

Average body weight:	176.7 lbs.
Average exercise heart rate:	144 bpm
Total number of days exercised:	19 days
Average exercise time/day:	62 min.
Total number of calories burned:	11,943
Average number of calories per day exercised:	629
Total number of miles run:	35
Total number of miles swum:	1
Total number of miles walked:	2

FIGURE 6.8
Sample monthly exercise record using the EXLOG (Exercise Log) computer program.

FIGURE 6.9
Cross training enhances fitness, decreases the rate of injuries, and eliminates the monotony of single-activity programs.

week. This cross-training may deter the monotony of repeating the same activity every day. Try lifetime sports (Figure 6.9). Many endurance sports such as racquetball, basketball, soccer, badminton, roller skating, cross-country skiing, and surfing (paddling the board) provide a nice break from regular workouts.

3. **Set aside a regular time for exercise.** If you don't plan ahead, it is a lot easier to skip. Holding your exercise hour "sacred" helps you adhere to the program.

4. **Obtain the proper equipment for exercise.** A poor pair of shoes, for example, can make you more prone to injury, discouraging you right from the beginning.

5. **Find a friend or group of friends to exercise with.** Social interaction will make exercise more fulfilling. Besides, it's harder to skip if someone else is waiting for you.

6. **Set goals and share them with others.** Quitting is tougher when someone else knows what you are trying to accomplish. When you reach a targeted goal, reward yourself with a new pair of shoes or a jogging suit.

7. **Don't become a chronic exerciser.** Learn to listen to your body. Overexercising can lead to chronic fatigue and injuries. Exercise should be

enjoyable, and in the process you should *stop and smell the roses.*

8. **Exercise in different places and facilities.** This will add variety to your workouts.

9. **Keep a regular record of your activities.** Keeping a record allows you to monitor your progress and compare it against previous months and years.

10. **Conduct periodic assessments.** Improving to a higher fitness category is a reward in itself.

11. **See a physician if health problems arise.** When in doubt, it's better to be safe than sorry.

PREDICTING OXYGEN UPTAKE AND CALORIC EXPENDITURE

As pointed out in Chapter 5, oxygen uptake can be expressed in liters per minute (L/min) or milliliters per kilogram per minute (ml/kg/min). The latter is used to classify individuals into the various cardiovascular fitness categories (see Table 5.8 in Chapter 5).

Oxygen uptake expressed in L/min is valuable in determining the caloric expenditure of physical activity. *The human body burns about five calories for each liter of oxygen consumed.* During aerobic exercise the average person trains between 50% and 70% of maximal oxygen uptake.

A person with a maximal oxygen uptake of 3.5 L/min who trains at 60% of maximum uses 2.1 (3.5 × .60) liters of oxygen per minute of physical activity. This indicates that 10.5 calories are burned each minute of exercise (2.1 × 5). If the activity is carried out for 30 minutes, 315 calories (10.5 × 30) have been burned.

Applying the principle of five calories burned per liter of oxygen consumed, you can determine with reasonable accuracy your own caloric output for walking and jogging. Table 6.3 contains the oxygen requirement (uptake) for walking speeds between 50 and 100 meters per minute and for jogging speeds in excess of 80 meters per minute.

There is a transition period from walking to jogging for speeds in the range of 80 to 134 meters per minute. Consequently, the person must be truly jogging at these lower speeds to use the estimated oxygen uptakes for jogging in Table 6.3. Because these uptakes are expressed in ml/kg/min, you will need to convert this figure to L/min to predict caloric output. This is done by multiplying the oxygen uptake in ml/kg/min by your body weight in kilograms (kg) and then dividing by 1,000.

For example, let's estimate the caloric cost for an individual who weighs 145.5 pounds and runs 3 miles in 21 minutes. Each mile is about 1,600 meters, or four laps around a 400-meter (440-yard) track. Three miles then would be 4,800 meters (1,600 × 3). Therefore, 3 miles (4,800 meters) at a speed of 21 minutes represents a pace of 228.6 meters per minute (4,800 ÷ 21).

Table 6.3 indicates an oxygen requirement (uptake) of 49.5 ml/kg/min for a speed of 228.6 meters per minute. A weight of 145.5 pounds equals 66 kilograms (145.5 ÷ 2.2046). The oxygen uptake in L/min now can be calculated by multiplying the value in ml/kg/min by body weight in kg and dividing by 1,000. In our example it is 49.5 by 66 and divided by 1,000, which equals 3.3 L/min. This oxygen uptake in 21 minutes represents a total of 347 calories (3.3 × 5 × 21).

In Lab 6D you have an opportunity to determine your own oxygen uptake and caloric expenditure for walking and jogging. Using your oxygen uptake information in conjunction with exercise heart rates allows you to estimate your caloric expenditure for almost any activity, as long as the heart rate ranges from 110 to 180 beats per minute. To make an accurate estimate, you have to be skilled in assessing exercise heart rate. Also, as your level of fitness improves, you will need to reassess your exercise heart rate because it will drop (at the same workload) with improved physical condition.

TABLE 6.3
Oxygen Uptake (VO₂) Estimates (ml/kg/min) for Selected Walking and Jogging Speeds (meters/min)*

WALKING		JOGGING			
Speed	VO₂	Speed	VO₂	Speed	VO₂
50	8.5	80	19.5	210	45.5
52	8.7	85	20.5	215	46.5
54	8.9	90	21.5	220	47.5
56	9.1	95	22.5	225	48.5
58	9.3	100	23.5	230	49.5
60	9.5	105	24.5	235	50.5
62	9.7	110	25.5	240	51.5
64	9.9	115	26.5	245	52.5
66	10.1	120	27.5	250	53.5
68	10.3	125	28.5	255	54.5
70	10.5	130	29.5	260	55.5
72	10.7	135	30.5	265	56.5
74	10.9	140	31.5	270	57.5
76	11.1	145	32.5	275	58.5
78	11.3	150	33.5	280	59.5
80	11.5	155	34.5		
82	11.7	160	35.5		
84	11.9	165	36.5		
86	12.1	170	37.5		
88	12.3	175	38.5		
90	12.5	180	39.5		
92	12.7	185	40.5		
94	12.9	190	41.5		
96	13.1	195	42.5		
98	13.3	200	43.5		
100	13.5	205	44.5		

*Table developed using the metabolic calculations contained in Guidelines for Exercise Testing and Exercise Prescription by the American College of Sports Medicine. Philadelphia: Lea & Febiger, 1991.

A LIFETIME COMMITMENT TO FITNESS

The benefits of fitness can be maintained only through a regular lifetime program. Exercise is not like putting money in the bank. It does not help to exercise four or five hours on Saturday and not do anything else the rest of the week. If anything, exercising only once a week is unsafe for unconditioned adults.

Even the greatest athletes on earth, if they were to stop exercising, would be, after just a few years, at a similar risk for disease as someone who has never done any physical activity. Staying with a physical fitness program long enough brings about positive physiological and psychological changes, and once you are there, you will not want to have it any other way.

The time involved in losing the benefits of exercise varies among the different components of physical fitness and also depends on the person's condition before the interruption. In regard to cardiovascular endurance, it has been estimated that four weeks of aerobic training are completely reversed in two consecutive weeks of physical inactivity. On the other hand, if you have been exercising regularly for months or years, two weeks of inactivity will not hurt you as much as it will someone who has exercised only a few weeks.

As a rule of thumb, after 48 to 62 hours of aerobic inactivity, the cardiovascular system starts to lose some of its capacity. Flexibility can be maintained with two or three stretching sessions per week. Strength is easily retained with just one maximal training session per week.

To maintain fitness, you should maintain a regular exercise program, even during vacations. If you have to interrupt your program for reasons beyond your control, you should not attempt to resume training at the same level you left off but, rather, build up gradually again.

LABORATORY EXPERIENCE

LAB 6A
Advantages and Disadvantages of Adding Exercise to Your Lifestyle

Lab Preparation
None required.

LAB 6B
Exercise Readiness Questionnaire

Lab Preparation
None required.

LAB 6C
Cardiovascular Exercise Prescription

Lab Preparation
None required.

LAB 6D
Exercise Heart Rate and Caloric Cost of Physical Activity

Lab Preparation
Wear exercise clothing, including jogging shoes. Do not engage in vigorous physical activity before the lab. Bring your own stopwatch or a watch with a second hand. Prior to this lab, read the information on predicting caloric expenditure from exercise heart rate in this chapter.

REFERENCES

1. American College of Sports Medicine. *Guidelines for Exercise Testing and Prescription*. Philadelphia: Lea & Febiger, 1991.
2. American College of Sports Medicine. "The Recommended Quantity and Quality of Exercise for Developing and Maintaining Cardiorespiratory and Muscular Fitness in Healthy Adults." *Medicine and Science in Sports and Exercise* 22:265-274, 1990.
3. Arnheim, D. D. *Modern Principles of Athletic Training*. St. Louis, MO: Times Mirror/Mosby College Publishing, 1988.

4. Borg, G. "Perceived Exertion: A Note on History and Methods." *Medicine and Science in Sports and Exercise* 5:90 93, 1973.
5. DeBusk, R. F., U. Stenestrand, M. Sheehan, and W. L. Haskell. "Training Effects of Long Versus Short Bouts of Exercise in Healthy Subjects." *The American Journal of Cardiology* 65:1010-1013, 1990.
6. Fox, E. L., R. W. Bowers, and M. L. Fossand. *The Physiological Basis for Exercise and Sport*. Philadelphia: Saunders College Publishing, 1993.

7. Teitz, C. C. "Overuse Injuries," in *Scientific Foundations of Sports Medicine* (C.C. Teitz Editor, pp. 299-328). Philadelphia: B.C. Deckerm, 1989.
8. Wilmore, J. H., and D. L. Costill. *Training for Sport and Activity*. Dubuque, IA: Wm. C. Brown Publishers, 1988.

Month _____

Date	Body Weight	Exercise Heart Rate	Type of Exercise	Distance In Miles	Time Hrs/Min	RPE*
1						
2						
3						
4						
5						
6						
7						
8						
9						
10						
11						
12						
13						
14						
15						
16						
17						
18						
19						
20						
21						
22						
23						
24						
25						
26						
27						
28						
29						
30						
31						
Total						

*Rate of perceived exertion.

Month _____

Date	Body Weight	Exercise Heart Rate	Type of Exercise	Distance In Miles	Time Hrs/Min	RPE*
1						
2						
3						
4						
5						
6						
7						
8						
9						
10						
11						
12						
13						
14						
15						
16						
17						
18						
19						
20						
21						
22						
23						
24						
25						
26						
27						
28						
29						
30						
31						
Total						

*Rate of perceived exertion.

FIGURE 6.10
Cardiovascular exercise record form.

Month ___

Date	Body Weight	Exercise Heart Rate	Type of Exercise	Distance In Miles	Time Hrs/Min	RPE*
1						
2						
3						
4						
5						
6						
7						
8						
9						
10						
11						
12						
13						
14						
15						
16						
17						
18						
19						
20						
21						
22						
23						
24						
25						
26						
27						
28						
29						
30						
31						
Total						

*Rate of perceived exertion.

Month ___

Date	Body Weight	Exercise Heart Rate	Type of Exercise	Distance In Miles	Time Hrs/Min	RPE*
1						
2						
3						
4						
5						
6						
7						
8						
9						
10						
11						
12						
13						
14						
15						
16						
17						
18						
19						
20						
21						
22						
23						
24						
25						
26						
27						
28						
29						
30						
31						
Total						

*Rate of perceived exertion.

FIGURE 6.10 (Continued) Cardiovascular exercise record form.

MUSCULAR STRENGTH AND ENDURANCE ASSESSMENT

7

Evidence of the benefits of strength training in enhancing health and well-being is well-documented. Nevertheless, many people are still under the impression that strength is necessary only for highly trained athletes and other individuals who hold jobs that require heavy muscular work.

Strength, however, is a basic component of fitness and wellness and is crucial for optimal performance in daily activities such as sitting, walking, running, lifting and carrying objects, doing housework, and even enjoying recreational activities. Strength also is of great value in improving posture, personal appearance and self-image, in developing sports skills, and in meeting certain emergencies in life in which strength is necessary to cope effectively. From a health standpoint, strength helps to maintain muscle tissue and a higher resting metabolism, decreases the risk for injury, helps to prevent and eliminate chronic low back pain, and is an important factor in childbearing.

Perhaps one of the most significant benefits of maintaining a good strength level is its relationship to human metabolism. *Metabolism* is defined as *all energy and material transformations within living cells*. A primary outcome of a strength-training program is an increase in muscle mass or size (lean body mass), known as *muscle hypertrophy*.

Muscle tissue uses energy even at rest. In contrast, fatty tissue uses very little energy and may be considered metabolically inert from the point of view of caloric use. As muscle size increases, so does the resting metabolism or the amount of energy (calories) an individual requires during resting conditions to sustain proper cell function. Even small increases in muscle mass may affect resting metabolism.

As indicated in Chapter 4, each additional pound of muscle tissue is estimated to increase resting metabolism by 30 to 50 calories per day. All other factors being equal, if two individuals both weigh 150 pounds but have different amounts of muscle mass, let's say five pounds, the one with more muscle mass will have a higher resting metabolic rate, allowing this person to ingest more calories to maintain the muscle tissue.

AGING AND METABOLIC RATE

Loss of lean tissue also is thought to be the main reason for the decrease in metabolism as people grow older. Contrary to some beliefs, metabolism does not have to slow down significantly with aging. It is not so much that metabolism slows down. It's that we slow down.

Lean body mass decreases with sedentary living, which, in turn, slows down the resting metabolic rate. If people continue eating at the same rate, body fat increases. The average decrease in resting metabolism for a 60-year-old person is about 360 calories per day, as compared to a 26-year-old person. Hence, participating in a strength-training program is important in preventing and reducing excess body fat.

GENDER DIFFERENCES

One of the most common misconceptions about physical fitness is related to women and strength training. Because of the increase in muscle mass commonly seen in men, some women think that strength-training programs are counterproductive because they, too, will develop large musculature.

Even though the quality of muscle in men and women is the same, endocrinological differences do not allow women to achieve the same amount of muscle hypertrophy (size) as men. Men also have more muscle fibers, and because of the male sex-specific hormones, each individual fiber has more potential for hypertrophy.

The idea that strength training allows women to develop muscle hypertrophy to the same extent as men do is as false as the notion that playing basketball will turn women into giants. Masculinity and femininity are established by genetic inheritance, not by the amount of physical activity.

Variations in the extent of masculinity and femininity are determined by individual differences in hormonal secretions of androgen, testosterone, estrogen, and progesterone. Women with a bigger-than-average build often are inclined to participate in sports because of their natural physical advantage. As a result, many women have associated sports and strength participation with large muscle size.

As the number of women who participate in sports has increased steadily during the last few years, the myth that strength training in women leads to large increases in muscle size has been disappearing gradually. For example, per pound of body weight, women gymnasts are considered to be among the strongest athletes in the world. These athletes engage regularly in serious strength-training programs. Yet, female gymnasts have some of the most well-toned and graceful figures of all women (Figure 7.1). In recent years, improved body appearance has become the rule rather than the exception for women who participate in strength-training programs. Some of the most attractive women movie stars also train with weights to further improve their personal image. In his textbook *Weight Training for Life*, Dr. James Hesson points out that many beauty pageant participants engage in some sort of strength-training program as they prepare for the pageant. A survey at a recent state beauty pageant revealed that 86% of the participants (38 of 44 contestants) exercised with weights!

On the other hand, you may ask yourself, "If weight training does not masculinize women, why do so many women body builders develop such heavy musculature?" In the sport of body building, the athletes follow intense training routines consisting of two or more hours of constant weight lifting with short rest intervals between sets. Many times body building training routines call for back-to-back exercises using the same muscle groups. The objective of this type of training is to "pump" extra blood into the muscles, which makes the muscles appear much bigger than they really are in resting conditions. Based on the intensity and the length of the

FIGURE 7.1
Female gymnast performing a strength skill on the floor exercise event. Contrary to some beliefs, high levels of strength do not masculinize women.

training session, the muscles can remain filled with blood, appearing measurably larger for several hours after completing the training session. Therefore, in real life, these women are not as muscular as they seem when they are "pumped up" for a contest.

In the sport of body building, a big point of controversy is the use of anabolic steroids and human growth hormones, even among women participants. *Anabolic steroids* are synthetic versions of the male sex hormone testosterone, which promotes muscle development and hypertrophy. These hormones, however, produce detrimental and undesirable side effects, which some women deem tolerable (e.g., hypertension, fluid retention, decreased breast size, deepening of the voice, facial whiskers, and body hair growth). Anabolic steroid use in general, except for medical reasons and when carefully monitored by a physician, can lead to serious health consequences. A summary of detrimental effects of steroid use is provided in Figure 7.2.

Anabolic steroid use among women body builders is widespread. According to several sports medicine physicians and women body builders, about 80% of women body builders have used steroids. Furthermore, according to several women's track-and-field coaches, as many as 95% of women athletes around the world in this sport had used anabolic steroids to remain competitive at the international level.

Women who take steroids undoubtedly will build heavy musculature, and, if the steroids are taken long enough, will produce masculinizing effects. As a result, the International Federation of Body Building instituted a mandatory steroid-testing program for women participating in the Miss Olympia contest. When drugs are not used to promote development, improved body image is the rule rather than the exception among women who participate in body building, strength training, or sports in general.

Another benefit of strength training, accentuated even more when combined with aerobic exercise, is a decrease in adipose or fatty tissue around the muscle fibers themselves. The decrease in fatty tissue often is greater than the amount of muscle hypertrophy (see Figure 7.3). Therefore, losing inches but not body weight is common.

Because muscle tissue is more dense than fatty tissue, and despite the fact that inches are lost during a combined strength-training and aerobic program, people, especially women, often become discouraged because they cannot see the results readily on the scale. They can offset this discouragement by determining body composition regularly to monitor changes in percent body fat rather than simply measure changes in total body weight.

- Liver tumors
- Hepatitis
- Hypertension
- Reduction of high density lipoprotein (HDL)
- Elevation of low density lipoprotein (LDL)
- Hyperinsulinism
- Impaired pituitary function
- Impaired thyroid function
- Mood swings
- Aggressive behavior
- Increased irritability
- Acne
- Fluid retention
- Decreased libido
- HIV infection (via injectable steroids)
- Prostate problems (men)
- Testicular atrophy (men)
- Reduced sperm count (men)
- Clitoral enlargement (women)
- Decreased breast size (women)
- Increased body and facial hair (nonreversible in women)
- Deepening of the voice (nonreversible in women)

FIGURE 7.2
Selected detrimental effects of anabolic steroid use.

MUSCULAR STRENGTH AND ENDURANCE ASSESSMENT

Although muscular strength and endurance are interrelated, there is a basic difference.

1. *Strength* is defined as *the ability to exert maximum force against resistance.*
2. *Endurance* is *the ability of a muscle to exert submaximal force repeatedly over a period of time.*

Muscular endurance (also referred to as localized muscular endurance) depends to a large extent on muscular strength and to a much lesser extent on cardiovascular endurance. Weak muscles cannot repeat an action several times or sustain it for a long time. Keeping these principles in mind, strength tests

PRE-TRAINING   **POST-TRAINING**

Skin

Adipose tissue (fat)

Muscle tissue

FIGURE 7.3
Changes in body composition as a result of a combined aerobic and strength training program.

and training programs have been designed to measure and develop absolute muscular strength, muscular endurance, or a combination of both.

Muscular strength usually is determined by the maximal amount of resistance (one repetition maximum or 1 RM) an individual is able to lift in a single effort. This assessment yields a good measure of absolute strength, but it does require a considerable amount of time, as the 1 RM is determined through trial and error. For example, strength of the chest muscles frequently is measured through the bench press exercise. If the individual has not trained with weights, he or she may try 100 pounds and lift this resistance quite easily. Then 50 pounds are added, and the person fails to lift the resistance. The resistance then is decreased by 10 or 20 pounds and, finally, after several trials the 1 RM is established.

A true 1 RM might be difficult to obtain the first time an individual is tested, because fatigue becomes a factor. By the time the 1 RM is established, the person already has made several maximal, or near-maximal attempts.

Muscular endurance commonly is established by the number of repetitions an individual can perform against a submaximal resistance or by the length of time a given contraction can be sustained. For example, how many push-ups can an individual perform, or how many times can he or she lift 50 pounds, or how long can a person hold the chin above a bar while holding on to it?

A key concept in strength testing is that several body sites should be tested. Because different body parts have different strength levels, no single strength test provides a good assessment of overall body strength. As a minimum, a strength profile should include the upper body, the lower body, and the abdominal muscles.

If time is a factor and only one test item can be done, the Hand Grip Test commonly is used to assess strength (see Figure 7.4). Even this test, though, provides only a weak correlation with overall body strength. A description of this test is provided in Figure 7.7.

Lab 7A provides the opportunity to assess your own level of muscular strength or endurance, through three tests. You may take one or more of these tests according to your time and the facilities available.

Muscular strength and endurance are both highly specific. A high degree of strength or endurance in one body part does not necessarily indicate a high degree in other parts. Accordingly, exercises for the strength tests in Lab 7A were selected to obtain a profile including the upper body, lower body, and mid-body regions.

Before taking the strength test, you should become familiar with the procedures for the respective tests (Figures 7.5, 7.6, and 7.7). For safety reasons, you always should take a friend or group of

FIGURE 7.4
The hand grip strength test.

friends with you when you train with weights or conduct any type of strength assessment. Also, because these are different tests, the same test should be used to make valid pre- to post-test comparisons. The following are the strength assessment options.

MUSCULAR STRENGTH AND ENDURANCE TEST

On this test, you will lift a submaximal resistance as many times as possible on five different strength-training exercises, and you will also perform an abdominal crunch test. The resistance for each lift is determined according to selected percentages of body weight (see Figure 7.5). If you are not familiar with the different lifts, graphic illustrations are provided in Chapter 8.

A strength/endurance rating is determined according to the maximum number of repetitions you are able to perform on each exercise. *A 16-station, fixed-resistance, Universal Gym apparatus is necessary to administer all but the abdominal curls exercise on this test* (see Chapter 8, Mode of Training, for an explanation on fixed-resistance equipment).

For individuals who do only a few repetitions, the test will primarily measure absolute strength. For those who are able to do a lot of repetitions, the test will be an indicator of muscular endurance. A percentile rank for each exercise is given based on the number of repetitions performed (see Table 7.1), and an overall muscular strength/endurance rating can be determined by taking an average of the percentile ranks obtained for each exercise.

If no fixed resistance Universal Gym equipment is available, you can still perform the test using different equipment. In that case, though, the percentile rankings and strength fitness categories may not be accurate because a certain resistance (for example, 50 pounds) is seldom the same on two different weight machines. The industry has no standard calibration procedure for strength equipment. Consequently, if you lift a certain weight on one machine, you may or may not be able to lift the same amount on a different piece of equipment.

Even though the percentile ranks may not be valid when using different equipment, test results still can be used to evaluate changes in fitness. For example, you may be able to do 7 repetitions on the equipment available to you (whereas you might have done 10 on Universal Gym fixed resistance), but if you can perform 14 repetitions after 12 weeks of training, that's a measure of improvement. When performing this test on different equipment, you should disregard the percentile ranks and use the test to assess *changes* in fitness only.

MUSCULAR STRENGTH AND ENDURANCE TEST

1. A sixteen-station, fixed resistance, Universal Gym apparatus is required to perform this test.

2. Familiarize yourself with the six lifts used for this test: bench press, arm curl, lateral pull-down, leg extension (quad lift), leg curl, and sit-up. Graphic illustrations for each lift are given in Chapter 8. For the leg curl exercise, the knees should be flexed to ninety degrees. A description and illustration of the abdominal crunch exercise is provided in Figure 7.6. For the lateral pull-down exercise, use a sitting position and have your partner hold you down by the waist or shoulders. On the leg extension lift, maintain the trunk in an upright position.

3. Determine your body weight in pounds.

4. Determine the amount of resistance to be used on each lift. To obtain this number, multiply your body weight by the percent given below for each lift.

Lift	Percent of Body Weight	
	Men	**Women**
Lat Pull-Down	.70	.45
Leg Extension	.65	.50
Bench Press	.75	.45
Abdominal Crunch	NA*	NA*
Leg Curl	.32	.25
Arm Curl	.35	.18

*NA = not applicable — *see* Figure 7.6

5. Perform the maximum continuous number of repetitions possible.

6. Based on the number of repetitions performed, look up the percentile rank for each lift in the far left column of Table 7.1.

7. An overall strength fitness category can be obtained by determining an average percentile score for all six lifts. Determine your overall muscular endurance fitness category according to the following ratings:

Average Score	Fitness Classification
≥81	Excellent
61–80	Good
41–60	Average
21–40	Fair
≤20	Poor

FIGURE 7.5

Procedure for the Muscular Strength and Endurance Test.

TABLE 7.1
Muscular Strength and Endurance Scoring Table

			MEN			
Percentile Rank	Lat. Pull-Down	Leg Extension	Bench Press	Abdominal Crunch	Leg Curl	Arm Curl
99	30	25	26	100	24	25
95	25	20	21	100	20	21
90	19	19	19	100	19	19
80	16	15	16	66	15	15
70	13	14	13	45	13	12
60	11	13	11	38	11	10
50	10	12	10	33	10	9
40	9	10	7	29	8	8
30	7	9	5	26	6	7
20	6	7	3	22	4	5
10	4	5	1	18	3	3
5	3	3	0	16	1	2

			WOMEN			
Percentile Rank	Lat. Pull-Down	Leg Extension	Bench Press	Abdominal Crunch	Leg Curl	Arm Curl
99	30	25	27	100	20	25
95	25	20	21	100	17	21
90	21	18	20	69	12	20
80	16	13	16	49	10	16
70	13	11	13	37	9	14
60	11	10	11	34	7	12
50	10	9	10	31	6	10
40	9	8	5	27	5	8
30	7	7	3	24	4	7
20	6	5	1	21	3	6
10	3	3	0	15	1	3
5	2	1	0	0	0	2

▨ High physical fitness standard
▨ Health fitness standard
See Chapter 1, Fitness Standards: Health vs Physical Fitness, p. 6.

MUSCULAR ENDURANCE TEST

Three exercises were selected to assess the endurance of the upper body, lower body, and mid-body muscle groups (see Figure 7.6). The advantage of this test is that it does not require strength-training equipment.

For this test you will need a stopwatch, a metronome, a bench or gymnasium bleacher 16¼″ high, a cardboard strip 3½″ wide by 30″ long, and a partner. As with the Muscular Strength and Endurance Test, a percentile rank is given for each exercise according to the number of repetitions performed (see Table 7.2). An overall endurance rating can be obtained through the average percentile rank for the three exercises.

MUSCULAR ENDURANCE TEST

1. Three exercises are conducted on this test: bench-jumps, modified dips (men) or modified push-ups (women), and abdominal crunches. All exercises should be conducted with the aid of a partner. The correct procedures for performing each exercise are as follows:

Bench-jumps. Using a bench or gymnasium bleacher 16¼ inches high, attempt to jump up and down the bench as many times as possible in a one-minute period. If you cannot jump the full minute, you may step up and down. A repetition is counted each time both feet return to the floor.

Modified dips. This upper-body exercise is performed by men only. Using a bench or gymnasium bleacher, place the hands on the bench with the fingers pointing forward. Have a partner hold your feet in front of you. The hips should be bent at approximately 90 degrees (you may also use three sturdy chairs, put your hands on two chairs placed by the sides of your body, and the feet on the third chair in front of you). Lower your body by flexing the elbows until you reach a ninety-degree angle at this joint, then return to the starting position (see Exercise 6 in Chapter 8).

Modified push-ups. Women will perform the modified push-up exercise instead of the chair-dip exercise. Lie down on the floor (face down), bend the knees (feet up in the air), and place the hands on the floor by the shoulders with the fingers pointing forward. The lower body will be supported at the knees (as opposed to the feet) throughout the test (see Exercise 3 in Chapter 8). The chest must touch the floor on each repetition. As with the chair-dip exercise, the repetitions are performed to a two-step cadence (up-down) regulated with a metronome set at fifty-six beats per minute. Perform as many continuous repetitions as possible. You cannot count any more repetitions if you fail to follow the metronome cadence.

Abdominal crunch. Tape a 3½ x 30" strip of cardboard onto the floor. Lie down on the floor in a supine position (face up) with the knees bent at approximately 100-degrees and the legs slightly apart. The feet should be on the floor and you must hold them in place yourself throughout the test. Straighten out your arms and place them on the floor alongside the trunk with the palms down and the fingers fully extended. The fingertips of both hands should barely touch the closest edge of the cardboard (see Figure 7.6a). Bring the head off the floor until the chin is 1 to 2" away from your chest. The head should remain in this position during the entire test (do not move the head by flexing or extending the neck). You are now ready to begin the test.

The repetitions are performed to a two-step cadence (up-down) regulated with a metronome set at sixty beats per minute. As you curl up, slide the fingers over the cardboard until the fingertips reach the far end (3½") of

the board (see Figure 7.6b), then return to the starting position.

FIGURE 7.6a

FIGURE 7.6b

Allow a brief practice period of five to ten seconds to familiarize yourself with the cadence. The up movement is initiated with the first beat, and the down movement with the next beat. One repetition is accomplished every two beats of the metronome. Count as many repetitions as you are able to perform following the proper cadence. You may not count a repetition if the fingertips fail to reach the distant end of the cardboard.

The test is terminated if: (a) you fail to maintain the appropriate cadence, (b) the heels come off the floor, (c) the chin is not kept close to the chest, (d) you accomplish 100 repetitions, or (e) you can no longer perform the test. Have your partner check the angle at the knees throughout the test to make sure that the 100-degree angle is maintained as close as possible.

For this test you may also use a Crunch-Ster Curl-Up Tester available from Novel Products.* An illustration of the test performed with this equipment is provided in Figures 7.6c and 7.6d.

FIGURE 7.6c

FIGURE 7.6d

2. According to your results, look up your percentile rank for each exercise in the far left column of Table 7.2.

3. Total the percentile scores obtained for each exercise, and divide by three to obtain an average score. Determine your overall muscular endurance fitness category according to the following ratings:

Average Score	Fitness Classification
≥81	Excellent
61-80	Good
41-60	Average
21-40	Fair
≤20	Poor

*Novel Products, Inc. Figure Finder Collection. P.O. Box 408, Rockton, IL 61072-0408. 1-800-323-5143.

FIGURE 7.6
Procedure for the Muscular Endurance Test.

TABLE 7.2
Muscular Endurance Scoring Table

Percentile Rank	MEN			WOMEN		
	Bench Jumps	Modified Dips	Abdominal Crunch	Bench Jumps	Modified Push-ups	Abdominal Crunch
99	66	54	100	58	95	100
95	63	50	100	54	70	100
90	62	38	100	52	50	69
80	58	32	66	48	41	49
70	57	30	45	44	38	37
60	56	27	38	42	33	34
50	54	26	33	39	30	31
40	51	23	29	38	28	27
30	48	20	26	36	25	24
20	47	17	22	32	21	21
10	40	11	18	28	18	15
5	34	7	16	26	15	0

▨ High physical fitness standard
▨ Health fitness standard
See Chapter 1, Fitness Standards: Health vs Physical Fitness, p. 6.

HAND GRIP TEST

As indicated earlier, when time is a factor, the Hand Grip test can be used to provide a rough estimate of strength. Unlike the previous two tests, this is an isometric (static contraction, see Chapter 8) test. If the proper grip is used, no visible finger or body movement should occur during the test. A description of the test procedure is given in Figure 7.7.

Changes in strength may be more difficult to evaluate with this test. Most strength-training programs are isotonic in nature, and this test

HAND GRIP STRENGTH TEST

1. Adjust the width of the dynamometer* so the middle bones (middle phalanges) of your fingers rest on the distant end of the dynamometer grip (see Figure 7.7a).

FIGURE 7.7a
Proper grip size for the hand grip test.

2. Use your dominant hand for this test. Place your elbow at a 90° angle and about 2" away from the body (see Figure 7.4).

3. Now grip as hard as you can for a few seconds. Do not move any other body part as you perform the test (do not flex or extend the elbow, do not move the elbow away or toward the body, and do not lean forward or backward during the test).

4. Record the dynamometer reading in pounds (if reading is in kilograms, multiply by 2.2046).

5. Three trials are allowed for this test. Use the highest reading for your final test score.

6. The hand grip strength fitness category is obtained according to the following guidelines:

Percentile Rank	Fitness Classification
≥81	Excellent
61–80	Good
41–60	Average
21–40	Fair
≤20	Poor

*A Lafayette model 78010 dynamometer is recommended for this test. Lafayette Instruments Co., Sagamore and North 9th Street, Lafayette, IN 47903.

FIGURE 7.7
Procedure for the Hand Grip Strength Test.

provides an isometric assessment. Further, grip strength exercises seldom are used in strength training, and increases in strength are specific to the body parts exercised. This test also can be used to

supplement the Muscular Strength and Endurance or the Muscular Endurance tests.

TABLE 7.3
Grip Strength Scoring Table

Percentile Ranks	Men	Women
99	153	101
95	145	94
90	141	91
80	139	86
70	132	80
60	124	78
50	122	74
40	114	71
30	110	66
20	100	64
10	91	60
5	76	58

■ High physical fitness standard
■ Health fitness standard
See Chapter 1, Fitness Standards: Health vs Physical Fitness, p. 6.

STRENGTH TRAINING PROGRAMS

After assessing your own level of strength, and now that you realize the contributions of a strength-training program in improving your quality of life, you can proceed to Chapter 8, which introduces the basic principles and programs for strength development.

LABORATORY EXPERIENCE

LAB 7A
Muscular Strength and Endurance Assessment

Lab Preparation
Wear exercise clothing and be prepared to take the Muscular Strength and Endurance Test, the Muscular Endurance Test, or the Hand Grip Test. Avoid strenuous strength training 48 hours before doing this lab.

REFERENCES

1. Bowers, R. W. and Fox, E. L. *Sports Physiology*. Dubuque, IA: Wm. C. Brown Publishers, 1992.
2. Fox, E. L., R. W. Bowers, and M. L. Fossand. *The Physiological Basis for Exercise and Sport*. Philadelphia: Saunders College Publishing, 1993.
3. Hesson, J. L. *Weight Training for Life*. Englewood, Colorado: Morton Publishing Company, 1991.
4. Hoeger, W. W. K., and S. A. Hoeger. *Lifetime Physical Fitness and Wellness: A Personalized Program*. Englewood, Colorado: Morton Publishing Company, 1992.
5. Hoeger, W. W. K., D. R. Hopkins, S. L. Barette, & D. F. Hale. "Relationship between repetitions and selected percentages of one repetition maximum: a comparison between untrained and trained males and females. *Journal of Applied Sport Science Research*, 4(2):47-51, 1990.
6. McArdle, W. D., F. I. Katch, and V. L. Katch. *Exercise Physiology: Energy, Nutrition and Human Performance*. Philadelphia: Lea & Febiger, 1991.
7. O'Shea, J. P. *Scientific Principles and Methods of Strength Fitness*. Reading, MA: Addison-Wesley Publishing Co., 1976.
8. Silvester, L. J. *Weight Training for Strength and Fitness*. Boston, MA: Jones and Bartlett Publishers, 1992.

PRINCIPLES OF STRENGTH TRAINING

8

L A B S

Muscle cells increase and decrease their capacity to exert force according to the demands placed upon the muscular system. If muscle cells are overloaded beyond their normal use, such as in strength-training programs, the cells increase in size (hypertrophy) and strength. If the demands placed on the muscle cells decrease, such as in sedentary living or required rest because of illness or injury, the cells decrease in size (atrophy) and lose strength. A good level of muscular strength is important to develop and maintain fitness, health, and total well-being. Helping you develop a lifetime strength-training program is the focus of this chapter.

OBJECTIVES

- Identify the factors that affect strength.
- Become acquainted with the different types of muscle fibers.
- Understand the overload principle for strength development.
- Recognize the principles that govern the development of muscular strength and muscular endurance (mode, resistance, sets, and frequency).
- Introduce three distinct strength-training programs.

FACTORS THAT AFFECT STRENGTH

Several physiological factors are related to muscle contraction and subsequent strength gains: neural stimulation, type of muscle fiber, the overload principle, and specificity of training. Basic knowledge of these factors is important in understanding the principles involved in strength training.

NEURAL STIMULATION

Within the neuromuscular system single motor *neurons* (nerves traveling from the central nervous system to the muscle) branch and attach to multiple muscle fibers. The combination of the motor neuron and the fibers it innervates is called a *motor unit*. The number of fibers a motor neuron can innervate varies from just a few in muscles that require precise control (eye muscles, for example) to as many as 1,000 or more in large muscles that do not perform refined or precise movements.

Stimulation of a motor neuron causes the muscle fibers to contract maximally or not at all. Variations in the number of fibers innervated and the frequency of their stimulation determine the strength of the muscle contraction. As the number of fibers innervated and frequency of stimulation increase, so does the strength of the muscular contraction.

TYPES OF FIBER

Two basic types of muscle fibers determine muscle response: (a) slow-twitch or red fibers, and (b) fast-twitch or white fibers. *Slow-twitch fibers* have a greater capacity for aerobic work. *Fast-twitch fibers* have a greater capacity for anaerobic work and produce a greater overall force. The latter are important for quick and powerful movements commonly used in strength-training activities.

> *To improve muscular strength and endurance, the load placed on a muscle must be progressively increased over time.*

The proportion of slow- and fast-twitch fibers is determined genetically, and consequently varies from one person to another. Nevertheless, training increases the functional capacity of both types of fiber, and more specifically, strength training increases their ability to exert force.

During muscular contraction, slow-twitch fibers always are recruited first. As the force and speed of muscle contraction increase, the relative importance of the fast-twitch fibers also increases. An activity must be intense and powerful to activate the fast-twitch fibers.

OVERLOAD PRINCIPLE

Strength gains are achieved in two ways:

1. Through increased ability of individual muscle fibers to generate a stronger contraction.
2. By recruiting a greater proportion of the total available fibers for each contraction.

These two factors combine in the overload principle.

The overload principle states that, for strength to improve, the demands placed on the muscle must be increased systematically and progressively over time, and the resistance must be of a magnitude significant enough to cause physiologic adaptation. In simpler terms, just like all other organs and systems of the human body, muscles have to be taxed beyond their accustomed loads to increase in physical capacity. Because of this principle, strength training also is called *progressive resistance training*.

SPECIFICITY OF TRAINING

The principle of specificity of training indicates that, for a muscle to increase in strength or endurance, the training program must be specific to obtain the desired effects. In like manner, to increase static (isometric) versus dynamic (isotonic) strength, an individual must use static against dynamic training procedures to achieve the desired results.

PRINCIPLES INVOLVED IN STRENGTH TRAINING

Because muscular strength and endurance are important in developing and maintaining overall fitness and well-being, the principles necessary to develop a strength-training program have to be followed, as in the prescription of cardiovascular exercise. These principles are: mode, resistance, sets, and frequency of training.

MODE OF TRAINING

Two basic types of training methods are used to improve strength: isometric (static) and isotonic (dynamic).

1. *Isometric training* refers to a muscle contraction producing little or no movement, such as pushing or pulling against immovable objects (see Figure 8.1).
2. *Isotonic training* refers to a muscle contraction with movement (see Figure 8.2), such as extending the elbows with resistance (weight) on the hands (triceps extension exercise).

Isometric training does not require much equipment. It was commonly used several years ago, but its popularity has waned. Because strength gains with isometric training are specific to the angle of muscle contraction, this type of training is beneficial in a sport such as gymnastics, which requires regular static contractions during routines.

Isotonic training programs can be conducted without weights or with free weights (barbells and

and angle of pull as the joint moves through its range of motion.

As strength training became more popular, new strength-training machines were developed. This technology brought about *isokinetic* and *variable resistance* training. These training programs require special machines equipped with mechanical devices that provide differing amounts of resistance, with the intent of overloading the muscle group maximally through the entire range of motion. A distinction of isokinetic training (see Figure 8.3) is that the speed of the muscle contraction is kept constant because the machine provides resistance to match the user's force through the range of motion. The mode of training an individual selects depends mainly on the type of equipment available and the specific objective the training program is attempting to accomplish.

Isotonic training is the most popular mode for strength training. The primary advantage is that strength is gained through the full range of motion. Most daily activities are isotonic in nature. We are constantly lifting, pushing, and pulling objects, and strength is needed through a complete range of motion. Another advantage is that improvements are measured easily by the amount lifted.

The benefits of isokinetic and variable resistance training are similar to the other isotonic training methods. Theoretically, strength gains should be

FIGURE 8.1
Isometric training.

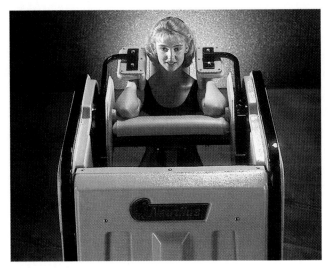

FIGURE 8.2
Isotonic training.

dumbbells), fixed resistance machines, variable resistance machines, and isokinetic equipment. When performing isotonic exercises without weights (for example, pull-ups, push-ups), with free weights, or with *fixed resistance* machines, a constant resistance is moved through a joint's full range of motion. The greatest resistance that can be lifted equals the maximum weight that can be moved at the weakest angle of the joint. This is due to changes in muscle length

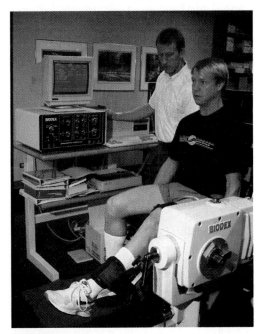

FIGURE 8.3
Isokinetic training.

better because maximum resistance is applied at all angles. Research, however, has not shown this type of training to be more effective than other modes of isotonic training. A possible advantage, though, is that specific speeds used in various sport skills can be duplicated more closely with isokinetic strength-training, which may enhance performance (specificity of training). A disadvantage is that the equipment is not readily available to many people.

RESISTANCE

Resistance in strength training is the equivalent of intensity in cardiovascular exercise prescription. The amount of resistance, or weight lifted, depends on whether the individual is trying to develop muscular strength or muscular endurance.

To stimulate strength development, a resistance of approximately 80% of the maximum capacity (1 RM) is recommended. For example, a person who can press 150 pounds should work with at least 120 pounds (150 × .80). Less than 80% will help increase muscular endurance rather than strength.

From a health-fitness point of view, training with 8 to 12 repetitions maximum is ideal for strength development.

Because of the time factor involved in constantly determining the 1 RM on each lift to ensure that the person is indeed working above 80%, a rule of thumb widely accepted by many authors and coaches is that individuals should perform between 3 and 12 repetitions maximum (3 to 12 RM) for adequate strength gains. For example, if a person is training with a resistance of 120 pounds and cannot lift it more than 12 times, the training stimulus is adequate for strength development.

Once the person can lift weight more than 12 times, the resistance should be increased by 5 to 10 pounds and the person again should build up to 12 repetitions. If training is conducted with more than 12 repetitions, primarily muscular endurance will be developed.

Strength research indicates that the closer a person trains to the 1 RM, the greater are the strength gains. A disadvantage of constantly working at or near the 1 RM is that it increases the risk for injury.

Highly trained athletes seeking maximum strength development often use 1 to 6 repetitions maximum.

Working around 10 repetitions maximum seems to produce the best results in terms of muscular hypertrophy.

Body builders tend to work with moderate resistance levels (60% to 85% of the 1 RM) and perform 8 to 20 repetitions to near fatigue. A foremost objective of body building is to increase muscle size. Moderate resistance promotes blood flow to the muscles, "pumping up the muscles" (also known as "the pump") and making them look much larger than they are in a relaxed state.

From a health-fitness point of view, 8 to 12 repetitions maximum are ideal for adequate development. We live in an "isotonic world" in which muscular strength and endurance are both required to lead an enjoyable life. Therefore, working near a 10 repetition threshold seems best to improve overall performance.

SETS

In strength training a set has been defined as *the number of repetitions performed for a given exercise.* For example, a person lifting 120 pounds eight times has performed one set of eight repetitions (1 × 8 × 120).

When working with 8 to 12 repetitions maximum, three sets per exercise are recommended. Because of the characteristics of muscle fiber, the number of sets that can be done is limited. As the number of sets increases, so does the amount of muscle fatigue and subsequent recovery time. Therefore, strength gains may be lessened by performing too many sets.

Most people perform three sets of 8 to 12 exercises three times per week.

A recommended program for beginners in their first year of training is three heavy sets, up to the maximum number of repetitions, preceded by one or two light warm-up sets using about 50% of the 1 RM (no warm-up sets are necessary for subsequent exercises that use the same muscle group). Because of the lower resistances used in body building, four to eight sets can be done for each exercise.

To avoid muscle soreness and stiffness, new participants ought to build up gradually to the three sets of maximal repetitions. This can be done by performing only one set of each exercise with a lighter resistance on the first day, two sets of each exercise on the second day — one light and the second with the regular resistance — and three sets on the third day — one light and two heavy. After that, a person should be able to do all three heavy sets.

The time necessary to recover between sets depends predominantly on the resistance used during each set. In strength training, the energy to lift heavy weights is derived primarily from the ATP-CP or *phosphagen system* (also see the Chapter 2 discussion on energy production, page 31). Ten seconds of maximal exercise pretty much depletes the CP stores in the exercised muscle(s). These stores are replenished in about three minutes of recovery.

> *Alternating two or three exercises that require different muscle groups makes a training program more time-effective.*

Based on this principle, about three minutes of rest between sets are necessary for people who are trying to maximize their strength gains. Individuals training for health-fitness purposes might allow two minutes. Body builders should rest no more than a minute to maximize the "pumping" effect.

The exercise program will be more time-effective by alternating two or three exercises that require different muscle groups. In this way, an individual will not have to wait two to three minutes before proceeding to a new set on a different exercise. For example, bench press, leg extensions, and sit-ups may be combined so the person can go almost directly from one set to the next.

FREQUENCY OF TRAINING

Strength training should be done either through a total body workout three times per week, or more frequently if using a split-body routine (upper body one day, lower body the next). After a maximum strength workout, the muscles should be rested for about two to three days to allow adequate recovery. If not completely recovered in two to three days, the person most likely is overtraining and therefore not reaping the full benefits of the program. In that case,

the person should do fewer sets or exercises than in the previous workout. A summary of strength training guidelines for health-fitness purposes is provided in Figure 8.4.

To achieve significant strength gains, a minimum of eight weeks of consecutive training is needed. Once an ideal level of strength is achieved, one training session per week will be sufficient to maintain the new strength level.

Frequency of strength training for body builders varies from person to person. Because they use moderate resistances, daily or even two-a-day workouts are common. The frequency depends on the amount of resistance, number of sets performed per session, and the person's ability to recover from the previous exercise bout (see Table 8.1). The latter often is dictated by level of conditioning.

Mode:	8 to 10 isotonic strength-training exercises involving the body's major muscle groups.
Resistance:	Enough resistance to perform 8 to 12 repetitions to near fatigue.
Sets:	A minimum of one set.
Frequency:	At least two times per week.

Source: The recommended quantity and quality of exercise for developing and maintaining cardiorespiratory and muscular fitness in healthy adults by the American College of Sports Medicine. Med. Sci. Sports Exerc. 22:265–274, 1990.

FIGURE 8.4
Strength-training guidelines.

TABLE 8.1
Guidelines for Various Strength-Training Programs

Strength Training Program	Resistance	Sets	Rest Between Sets*	Frequency (workouts per week)**
Health fitness	8–12 reps max.	3	2 min.	2–3
Maximal strength	1–6 reps max.	3–6	3 min.	2–3
Muscular endurance	10–30 reps	3–6	2 min.	3–6
Body building	8–20 reps near max.	3–8	0–1 min.	4–12

*Recovery between sets can be decreased by alternating exercises that use different muscle groups.

**Weekly training sessions can be increased by using a split body routine.

PLYOMETRICS

Strength, speed, and explosiveness are all crucial for success in athletics. All three of these factors are enhanced with a progressive resistance training program, but greater increases in speed and explosiveness are thought possible with plyometric training.

Plyometric exercise is best defined as *explosive jump training* (see Figure 8.5). It attempts to incorporate speed and strength training to enhance explosiveness. The objective is to generate the greatest amount of force in the shortest time. A sound strength base is necessary before attempting plyometric exercises.

Plyometric training is popular in sports that require powerful movements, such as basketball, volleyball, sprinting, jumping, and tumbling. A typical plyometric exercise involves jumping off and back onto a box, attempting to rebound as quickly as possible on each jump. Box heights are increased progressively from about 12" to 22".

The bounding action during plyometrics attempts to take advantage of the stretch-recoil and stretch reflex characteristics of muscle. The rapid stretch applied to the muscle during ground contact is thought to augment muscle contraction, leading to more explosiveness.

A drawback of plyometric training is the higher risk for injuries, compared to conventional modes of progressive resistance training. The potential for injury escalates as box height increases.

Plyometrics also can be used for strengthening upper body muscles. An example is push-ups with a forceful extension of the arms to drive the hands (and body) completely off the floor during each repetition.

STRENGTH-TRAINING EXERCISES

The three strength-training programs introduced next provide a complete body workout. The major muscles of the human body referred to in the exercises are pointed out at the end of this chapter, in Figure 8.6.

Only a minimum of equipment is required for the first program, Strength-Training Exercises Without Weights (Exercises 1 through 10). This program can be conducted within the walls of your own home. Your body weight is used as the primary resistance for most exercises. A few call for a friend's help or some basic implements from around your house, to provide greater resistance.

The second program, Universal Gym Equipment Strength-Training Exercises (Exercises 11 through 27), requires machines such as those shown in the accompanying photographs. These exercises can be conducted on either fixed resistance or variable resistance equipment. Many of these exercises also can be performed with free weights. The first eight exercises (11 to 18) are recommended to get a complete workout. The rest are optional. If one of the optional exercises involves the same body parts, however, the person may substitute the latter for one of the basic nine (Exercise 21 for 11, 19 or 20 for 12, 26 for 13, 23 or 24 for 14, 22 for 16, and 25 for 18).

Nautilus Strength-Training Exercises (Exercises 28 through 39) make up the third program. These also require machines, as illustrated in the photographs. All of these machines use variable resistance. In this last program, Exercises 28 through 38

FIGURE 8.5
Plyometric training.

are recommended for a complete body workout, and Exercise 39 may be substituted for Exercise 31.

SETTING UP YOUR OWN STRENGTH-TRAINING PROGRAM

Depending on the facilities available, you can choose one of the three training programs outlined in this chapter. Once you begin your strength-training program, you may use the form provided in Figure 8.7 to keep a record of your training sessions.

The resistance and the number of repetitions you use with your program should be based on whether you want to increase muscular strength or muscular endurance. Do up to 12 repetitions maximum for strength gains, and more than 12 for muscular endurance. For most people, three training sessions per week on nonconsecutive days is an ideal arrangement for proper development.

Because both strength and endurance are required in daily activities, three sets of about 12 repetitions maximum for each exercise are enough. In doing this, you will obtain good strength gains and yet be close to the endurance threshold. If you are training for reasons other than health fitness, a summary of the guidelines is provided in Table 8.1.

Perhaps the only exercise that calls for more than 12 repetitions is the abdominal group of exercises. The abdominal muscles are considered primarily anti-gravity or postural muscles. Hence, a little more endurance may be required. When doing abdominal work, most people perform about 20 repetitions.

If time is a concern in completing a strength-training exercise program, the American College of Sports Medicine, in *The Recommended Quantity and Quality of Exercise for Developing and Maintaining Cardiorespiratory and Muscular Fitness in Healthy Adults* (see Appendix B), recommends as a minimum: (a) one set of 8 to 12 repetitions performed to near fatigue, and (b) 8 to 10 exercises involving the major muscle groups of the body, conducted twice a week. The recommendation is based on research showing that this training generates 70% to 80% of the improvements reported in other programs using three sets of about 10 RM.

L A B O R A T O R Y E X P E R I E N C E

LAB 8A
Sample Strength-Training Program

Lab Preparation
Wear exercise clothing and prepare to participate in a sample strength-training exercise session.

R E F E R E N C E S

1. Allsen, P.E. *Strength Training: Beginners, Bodybuilders, and Athletes.* Glenview, IL: Scott, Foresman and Company, 1987.
2. American College of Sports Medicine. "The Recommended Quantity and Quality of Exercise for Developing and Maintaining Cardiorespiratory and Muscular Fitness in Healthy Adults." *Medicine and Science in Sports and Exercise* 22:265-274, 1990.
3. Bowers, R. W., and E. L. Fox, *Sports Physiology.* Dubuque, IA: Wm. C. Brown Publishers, 1992.
4. Fox, E.L., R.W. Bowers, and M.L. Fossand. *The Physiological Basis for Exercise and Sport.* Philadelphia: Saunders College Publishing, 1993.
5. Getchell, B. *Physical Fitness: A Way of Life.* New York: Macmillan Publishing Company, 1992.
6. Hesson, J.L. *Weight Training for Life.* Englewood, CO: Morton Publishing Company, 1991.
7. Heyward, V.H. *Advanced Fitness Assessment & Exercise Prescription.* Champaign, IL: Human Kinetic, 1991.
8. Hoeger, W.W.K., and S.A. Hoeger. *Lifetime Physical Fitness and Wellness: A Personalized Program.* Englewood, CO: Morton Publishing Company, 1992.
9. Hoeger, W.W.K., D.R. Hopkins, S.L. Barette, & D.F. Hale. "Relationship between repetitions and selected percentages of one repetition maximum: a comparison between untrained and trained males and females." *Journal of Applied Sport Science Research* 4(2):47-51, 1990.
10. McArdle, W.D., F.I. Katch, and V.L. Katch. *Exercise Physiology: Energy, Nutrition and Human Performance.* Philadelphia: Lea and Febiger, 1991.
11. O'Shea, J.P. *Scientific Principles and Methods of Strength Fitness.* Reading, MA: Addison-Wesley Publishing Co., 1976.
12. Silvester, L.J. *Weight Training for Strength and Fitness.* Boston, MA: Jones and Bartlett Publishers, 1992.

Temporalis
(closes jaw)

Masseter
(flexes jaw)
(closes)

Sterno-cleido-mastoid
(rotates head)

Intercostals
(breathing)

Pectoralis minor
(abducts ribs)

Biceps brachii
(flexes elbow)

Serratus
(adducts shoulder)

Rectus abdominus

Deep flexors
(flexes fingers)

Internal oblique
(flattens abdomen)

Tendons from
forearm flexors
to fingers

Sartorius
(rotates thigh)

Rectus femoris
(extends knee)

Gastrocnemius
(points toe, flexes knee)

Soleus
(points toe)

Tendons of toes

Frantalis
(raises eyebrow)

Orbicularis oculi
(closes eye)

Orbicularis oris
(purses lips)

Throat muscles
(aids swallowing)

Pectoralis major
(adducts arm)

Deltoid
(abducts arm)

Brachialis
(flexes arm)

External oblique
(flattens abdomen)

Superficial flexors
(flex fingers)

Vastus lateralis
(extends knee)

Vastus medialis
(extends knee)

Tibialis anterior
(raises feet)

Splenius capitus

Sternomastoid

Trapezius

Deltoid

Triceps

Latissimus dorsi

Serratus posterior
inferior

Extensors
of forearm

Gluteus
maximus

Tendons
from forearm,
extensors
to fingers

Biceps femoris

Semitendonosus

Gastrocnemius

Tendon of Achilles

THE MUSCULAR SYSTEM

From Chaffee, E., and F. Lytle, *Basic Physiology and Anatomy*, Philadelphia: Lippincott Co., 1980. Reproduced with permission.

FIGURE 8.6
Major muscles of the human body.

Name

Date										
Exercise	St/Reps/Res*	St/Reps/Res*	St/Reps/Res*	St/Reps/Res*	St/Reps/Res*	St/Reps/Res*	St/Reps/Res*	St/Reps/Res*	St/Reps/Res*	St/Reps/Res*

*St/Reps/Res = Sets, Repetitions, and Resistance (e.g., 1/6/125 = 1 set of 6 repetitions with 125 pounds)

FIGURE 8.7
Strength training record form .

Name_____

Date									
Exercise	St/Reps/Res*	St/Reps/Res*	St/Reps/Res*	St/Reps/Res*	St/Reps/Res*	St/Reps/Res*	St/Reps/Res*	St/Reps/Res*	St/Reps/Res*

*St/Reps/Res = Sets, Repetitions, and Resistance (e.g., 1/6/125 = 1 set of 6 repetitions with 125 pounds)

FIGURE 8.7 (Continued)
Strength training record form.

Step-Up

ACTION Step up and down using a box or chair approximately twelve to fifteen inches high. Conduct one set using the same leg each time you go up and then conduct a second set using the other leg. You could also alternate legs on each step-up cycle. You may increase the resistance by holding a child or some other object in your arms (hold the child or object close to the body to avoid increased strain in the lower back).

MUSCLES DEVELOPED Gluteal muscles, quadriceps, gastrocnemius, and soleus.

High-Jumper

ACTION Start with the knees bent at approximately 150° and jump as high as you can, raising both arms simultaneously.

MUSCLES DEVELOPED Gluteal muscles, quadriceps, gastrocnemius, and soleus.

Photographs for Exercises 11, 13, 16, and 17 are courtesy of Universal Gym® Equipment, Inc., 930 27th Avenue, S.W., Cedar Rapids, IA 52406. Photographs for Exercises 12, 14, and 15 are courtesy of Nautilus®, a registered trademark of Nautilus® Sports/Medical Industries, Inc., P.O. Box 809014, Dallas, TX 75380-9014.

E X E R C I S E **3**

Push-Up

ACTION   Maintaining your body as straight as possible, flex the elbows, lowering the body until you almost touch the floor, then raise yourself back up to the starting position. If you are unable to perform the push-up as indicated, you can decrease the resistance by supporting the lower body with the knees rather than the feet (see illustration c) or using an incline plane and supporting your hands at a higher point than the floor (see illustration d). If you wish to increase the resistance, have someone else add resistance to your shoulders as you are coming back up (see illustration e).

MUSCLES DEVELOPED   Triceps, deltoid, pectoralis major, erector spinae, and abdominals.

a

b

c

d

e

E X E R C I S E **4**

Abdominal Crunch and Abdominal Curl-Up

ACTION   Start with your head and shoulders off the floor, arms crossed on your chest, and knees slightly bent (the greater the flexion of the knee, the more difficult the curl-up). Now curl up to about 30° (abdominal crunch — see illustration b) or curl all the way up (abdominal curl-up), then return to the starting position without letting the head or shoulders touch the floor, or allowing the hips to come off the floor. If you allow the hips to raise off the floor and the head and shoulders to touch the floor, you will most likely "swing up" on the next sit-up, which minimizes the work of the abdominal muscles. If you cannot curl up with the arms on the chest, place the hands by the side of the hips or even help yourself up by holding on to your thighs (illustrations d and e). Do not perform the sit-up exercise with your legs completely extended, as this will cause strain on the lower back.

MUSCLES DEVELOPED   Abdominal muscles and hip flexors.

a

b

c

d

e

Leg Curl

ACTION Lie on the floor face down. Cross the right ankle over the left heel. Apply resistance with your right foot, while you bring the left foot up to 90° at the knee joint. (Apply enough resistance so that the left foot can only be brought up slowly.) Repeat the exercise, crossing the left ankle over the right heel.

MUSCLES DEVELOPED   Hamstrings (and quadriceps).

Modified Dip

ACTION Place your hands and feet on opposite chairs with knees slightly bent (make sure that the chairs are well stabilized). Dip down at least to a 90° angle at the elbow joint, then return to the initial position. To increase the resistance, have someone else hold you down by the shoulders on the way up (see illustration c). You may also perform this exercise using a gymnasium bleacher or box and with the help of a partner, as illustrated in photo d.

MUSCLES DEVELOPED Triceps, deltoid, and pectoralis major.

E X E R C I S E **7**

Pull-Up

ACTION   Suspend yourself from a bar with a pronated grip (thumbs in). Pull your body up until your chin is above the bar, then lower the body slowly to the starting position. If you are unable to perform the pull-up as described, either have a partner hold your feet to push off and facilitate the movement upward (illustrations c and d) or use a lower bar and support your feet on the floor (illustration e).

MUSCLES DEVELOPED   Biceps, brachioradialis, brachialis, trapezius, and latissimus dorsi.

a

b

c

d

e

Arm Curl

ACTION   Using a palms-up grip, start with the arm completely extended, and with the aid of a sandbag or bucket filled (as needed) with sand or rocks, curl up as far as possible, then return to the initial position. Repeat the exercise with the other arm.

MUSCLES DEVELOPED   Biceps, brachioradialis, and brachialis.

Heel Raise

ACTION   From a standing position with feet flat on the floor, raise and lower your body weight by moving at the ankle joint only (for added resistance, have someone else hold your shoulders down as you perform the exercise).

MUSCLES DEVELOPED   Gastrocnemius and soleus.

Leg Abduction and Adduction

ACTION   Both participants sit on the floor. The subject on the left places the feet on the inside of the other participant's feet. Simultaneously, the subject on the left presses the legs laterally (to the outside — abduction), while the subject on the right presses the legs medially (adduction). Hold the contraction for five to ten seconds. Repeat the exercise at all three angles, and then reverse the pressing sequence. The subject on the left places the feet on the outside and presses inward, while the subject on the right presses outward.

MUSCLES DEVELOPED

Hip abductors (rectus femoris, sartori, gluteus medius and minimus), and adductors (pectineus, gracilis, adductor magnus, adductor longus, and adductor brevis).

Universal Gym® Equipment Strength-Training Exercises*

Arm Curl

ACTION   Use a supinated or palms-up grip, and start with the arms almost completely extended. Now curl up as far as possible, then return to the starting position.

MUSCLES DEVELOPED   Biceps, brachioradialis, and brachialis.

Leg Press

ACTION From a sitting position with the knees flexed at about 90 degrees and both feet on the footrest, fully extend the legs, then return slowly to the starting position.

MUSCLES DEVELOPED Quadriceps and gluteal muscles.

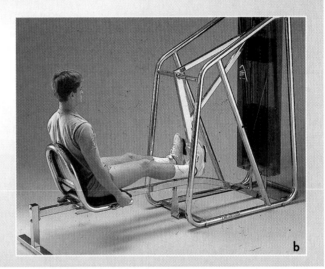

Abdominal Curl-Up or Abdominal Crunch

See exercise 4 in this chapter.

Bench Press

ACTION Lie down on the bench with the head by the weight stack, the bench press bar above the chest, and keep the feet on the floor. Grasp the bar handles and press upward until the arms are completely extended, then return to the original position. Do not arch the back during this exercise. CAUTION: If you are susceptible to low back pain, place your feet on the bench.

MUSCLES DEVELOPED Pectoralis major, triceps, and deltoid.

E X E R C I S E

15

Leg Curl

ACTION Lie with the face down on the bench, legs straight, and place the back of the feet under the padded bar. Curl up to at least 90°, and return to the original position.

MUSCLES DEVELOPED Hamstrings.

E X E R C I S E

16

Lat Pull-Down

ACTION Start from a sitting position, and hold the exercise bar with a wide grip. Pull the bar down until it touches the base of the neck, then return to the starting position (if a heavy resistance is used, stabilization of the body may be required by either using equipment as shown or by having someone else hold you down by the waist or shoulders).

MUSCLES DEVELOPED Latissimus dorsi, pectoralis major, and biceps.

Heel Raise

ACTION   Start with your feet either flat on the floor or the front of the feet on an elevated block, then raise and lower yourself by moving at the ankle joint only. If additional resistance is needed, you can use a squat strength-training machine.

MUSCLES DEVELOPED
Gastrocnemius and soleus.

Triceps Extension

ACTION   Using a palms-down grip, grasp the bar slightly closer than shoulder width, and start wth the elbows almost completely bent. Fully extend the arms, then return to starting position.

MUSCLES DEVELOPED   Triceps.

EXERCISE **19**

Squat

ACTION Sit in an upright position with the feet under the padded bar and grasp the handles at the sides. Extend the legs until they are completely straight, then return to the starting position.

MUSCLES DEVELOPED
Quadriceps.

EXERCISE **20**

Leg Extension

ACTION   Sit in an upright position with the feet under the padded bar and grasp the handles at the sides. Extend the legs until they are completely straight, then return to the starting position.

MUSCLES DEVELOPED
Quadriceps.

Upright Rowing

ACTION   Start with the arms extended and grip the handles with the palms down. Pull all the way up to the chin, then return to the starting position.

MUSCLES DEVELOPED   Biceps, brachioradialis, brachialis, deltoid, and trapezius.

Bent-arm Pullover

ACTION   Sit back into the chair and grasp the bar behind your head. Pull the bar over your head all the way down to your abdomen and slowly return to the original position.

MUSCLES DEVELOPED
Latissimus dorsi, pectoral muscles, deltoid, and serratus anterior.

Chest Press

ACTION   Start with the arms to the side and elbows bent at 90 degrees. Press your arms forward until the padded bars touch in front of your chest, then return to the starting position.

MUSCLES DEVELOPED   Pectoralis major and deltoid.

Shoulder Press

ACTION   Sit in an upright position and grasp the bar wider than the shoulder width. Press the bar all the way up until the arms are fully extended, then return to the initial position.

MUSCLES DEVELOPED   Triceps, deltoid, and pectoralis major.

25

Dip

ACTION   Start with the elbows flexed then fully extend the arms and slowly return to the initial position.

MUSCLES DEVELOPED
Triceps, deltoid, and pectoralis major.

26

Abdominal Crunch

ACTION   Sit back into the machine and place the hands inside the straps as illustrated. Slowly crunch forward to a seated upright position, then return to the starting position.

MUSCLES DEVELOPED
Abdominals.

Seated Back

ACTION Sit in the machine with your trunk flexed and the upper back against the shoulder pad. Place the feet under the padded bar and hold on with your hands to the bars on the sides. Start the exercise by pressing backward, simultaneously extending the trunk and hip joints. Slowly return to the original position.

MUSCLES DEVELOPED Erector spinae and gluteus maximus.

a

b

Nautilus® Strength-Training Exercises*

Multi-Biceps (Arm Curl)

ACTION Sit into the machine and grasp the bar with the arms completely extended using a supinated or palms up grip. Curl up as far as possible and then return to the starting position.

MUSCLES DEVELOPED Biceps, brachioradialis, and brachialis.

a

b

Abdominal Crunch

ACTION   Sit in an upright position and grasp the handles over your shoulders and crunch forward. Slowly return to the original position.

MUSCLES DEVELOPED   Abdominals.

Leg Extension

ACTION   Sit in an upright position with the feet under the padded bar and grasp the handles at the sides. Extend the legs until they are completely straight, then return to the starting position.

MUSCLES DEVELOPED   Quadriceps.

a

b

Bench Press

ACTION   Lie down on the bench with the head by the weight stack, the bench press bar above the chest, and the knees bent so the feet rest on the far end of the bench. Grasp the bar handles and press upward until the arms are completely extended, then return to the original position. Do not arch the back during this exercise

MUSCLES DEVELOPED   Pectoralis major, triceps, and deltoid.

 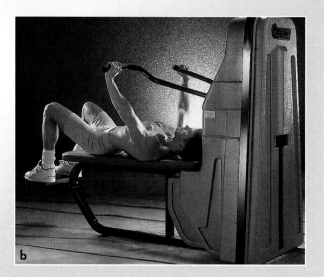

Seated Leg Curl

ACTION   Sit in the unit and place the strap over the upper thighs. With legs extended place the back of the feet over the padded rollers. Flex the knees until you reach a 90 to 100 degree angle. Slowly return to the starting position.

MUSCLES DEVELOPED   Hamstrings.

Lower Back

ACTION   Place yourself in the machine so that the front of the thigh and the upper back rest against the padded bars as illustrated. Slowly press backward against the padded bar until the back is fully extended. Slowly return to the original position.

MUSCLES DEVELOPED   Erector spinae and gluteus maximus.

Rowing Torso

ACTION   Sit in the machine with your arms in front of you, elbows bent and resting against the padded bars. Press back as far as possible, drawing the shoulder blades together. Return to the original position.

MUSCLES DEVELOPED   Posterior deltoid, rhomboids, and trapezius.

Leg Press

ACTION From a sitting position with the knees flexed at about 90 degrees and both feet on the footrest, fully extend the legs, then return slowly to the starting position.

MUSCLES DEVELOPED Quadriceps and gluteal muscles.

Pullover

ACTION Sit back into the chair, arms bent, place the elbows against the padded end of the movement arm, and grasp the bar behind your head. Press forward and downward with your arms, pulling the bar over your head all the way down to your abdomen. Slowly return to the starting position.

MUSCLES DEVELOPED
Latissimus dorsi, pectoral muscles, deltoid, and serratus anterior.

Rotary Torso

ACTION Sit upright into the machine and place the elbows behind the padded bars. Rotate the torso as far as possible to one side and then slowly return to the starting position. Repeat the exercise to the opposite side.

MUSCLES DEVELOPED
Internal and external obliques (abdominal muscles).

Triceps Extension

ACTION Sit in an upright position, arms up, elbows bent, and place the little finger side of the hands and wrists against the pads (palms of the hands facing each other). Fully extend one arm at a time and then return to the original position. Repeat with the other arm.

MUSCLES DEVELOPED
Triceps.

Chest Press

ACTION   Start with the arms up to the side, hands resting against the handle bars, and elbows bent at 90 degrees. Press the movement arms forward as far as possible, leading with the elbows. Slowly return to the starting position.

MUSCLES DEVELOPED   Pectoralis major and deltoid.

MUSCULAR FLEXIBILITY ASSESSMENT

9

Flexibility is defined as the ability of a joint to move freely through its full range of motion. Health care professionals and practitioners generally have underestimated and overlooked the contribution of good muscular flexibility to overall fitness and preventive health care. Sports medicine specialists believe that many muscular/skeletal problems and injuries, especially in adults, may be related to a lack of flexibility. Improving and maintaining good range of motion in the joints is important to enhance the quality of life.

Approximately 80% of all low back problems in the United States stems from improper alignment of the vertebral column and pelvic girdle — a direct result of inflexible and weak muscles. This backache syndrome costs American industry more than $1 billion each year in lost productivity and services alone, and an extra $225 million in worker's compensation.

In daily life we often have to make rapid or strenuous movements we are not accustomed to making, which may cause injury. Physical therapists have indicated that improper body mechanics often are the result of poor flexibility.

Participating in a regular flexibility program will help a person maintain good joint mobility, increase resistance to muscle injury and soreness, prevent low-back and other spinal column problems, improve and maintain good postural alignment, promote proper and graceful body movement, improve personal appearance and self-image, and help to develop and maintain motor skills throughout life. In addition, flexibility exercises have been prescribed successfully to treat dysmenorrhea (painful menstruation) and general neuromuscular tension (stress).

Further, stretching exercises, in conjunction with calisthenics, are helpful in warm-up routines to prepare the human body for more vigorous aerobic or strength-training exercises, as well as cool-down routines following exercise to help the person return to a normal resting state. Fatigued muscles tend to contract to a shorter than average resting length, and stretching exercises help fatigued muscles reestablish their normal resting length.

FACTORS AFFECTING FLEXIBILITY

Total range of motion around a joint is highly specific and varies from one joint to another (hip, trunk, shoulder), as well as from one individual to the next. Muscular flexibility relates primarily to genetic factors and to physical activity. Beyond that, factors such as joint structure, ligaments, tendons, muscles, skin, tissue injury, adipose tissue (fat), body temperature, age, and gender influence range of motion about a joint.

Because of the specificity of flexibility, it is difficult to indicate what constitutes an ideal level of flexibility. Nevertheless, flexibility is important to everyone's health, and even more so during the aging process.

The range of motion about a given joint depends mostly on the structure of that joint. Greater range of motion, however, can be attained through plastic and elastic elongation. Plastic elongation is permanent lengthening of soft tissue. Even though joint capsules, ligaments, and tendons are primarily nonelastic, they can undergo plastic elongation. This permanent lengthening, accompanied by increases in range of motion, is best attained through slow-sustained stretching exercises.

Plastic elongation is permanent lengthening of soft tissue. Elastic elongation refers to temporary lengthening of soft tissue.

Elastic elongation refers to temporary lengthening of soft tissue. Muscle tissue has elastic properties and responds to stretching exercises by undergoing elastic or temporary lengthening. Elastic elongation increases the extensibility of the muscles.

Changes in muscle temperature can increase or decrease flexibility by as much as 20%. Properly warmed-up individuals have better flexibility than non-warmed-up people. Cool temperatures have the opposite effect, impeding joint range of motion.

Because of the effects of temperature on muscular flexibility, many people prefer to do their stretching exercises after the aerobic phase of their workout. Aerobic activities raise body temperature, facilitating plastic elongation.

Another factor that influences flexibility is the amount of adipose tissue in and around joints and muscle tissue. A lot of adipose tissue not only increases resistance to movement, but the added bulk also hampers joint mobility because of the contact between body surfaces.

On the average, women have more flexibility than men do, and they seem to retain this advantage throughout life. Aging does decrease the extensibility of soft tissue, though, resulting in less flexibility in both genders.

The two most significant contributors to lower flexibility levels are sedentary living and lack of physical activity. With less physical activity, muscles lose their elasticity and tendons and ligaments tighten and shorten. Inactivity also tends to be accompanied by an increase in adipose tissue, which further decreases joint range of motion. Finally, injury to muscle tissue and tight skin from excessive scar tissue has a negative effect on joint range of motion.

ASSESSMENT OF FLEXIBILITY

Most of the flexibility tests developed over the years are specific to certain sports and are not practical for the general population. Their application in health and fitness programs is limited. For example, the Front-to-Rear Splits Test, and the Bridge-Up Test (see Figure 9.1) may have applications in sports such as gymnastics and several track and field events, but they do not represent actions most people encounter in daily life.

Because of the lack of practical flexibility tests, most health/fitness centers have relied strictly on the Sit and Reach Test as an indicator of overall flexibility (see Figure 9.2). This test measures flexibility of the hamstring muscles (back of the thigh) and, to a lesser extent, the lower back muscles.

Because flexibility is joint-specific and a high degree of flexibility in one joint does not necessarily indicate the same is true in other joints, two additional tests — indicators of everyday movements such as reaching, bending, and turning — are included to determine your flexibility profile. These tests are the Total Body Rotation Test and the Shoulder Rotation Test.

FIGURE 9.1
Front-to-Rear Splits Test (left), and Bridge-Up Test (right). These tests are not practical for use with the general population because they are not indicative of actions most people encounter in daily life.

FIGURE 9.2
Sit and Reach Test.

The Sit and Reach Test has been modified from the traditional test. Unlike the traditional Sit and Reach Test, arm and leg lengths are taken into consideration to determine the score (see Figure 9.3).

In the original sit and reach test, the 15″ mark of the yardstick used to measure flexibility always is set at the edge of the box where the feet are placed. This procedure does not take into consideration an individual with long arms and/or short legs or one with short arms and/or long legs, or both.[7, 8, 9] All other factors being equal, an individual with longer arms or shorter legs, or both, receives a better rating because of the structural advantage.

The procedures and norms for the battery of flexibility tests are described in Figures 9.3 through 9.5 and Tables 9.1 through 9.3. You will be able to assess your flexibility profile in Lab 9A.

After obtaining your scores and fitness ratings for each test, you can determine the fitness category for each flexibility test using the guidelines given in Table 9.4. The overall flexibility fitness classification is obtained by computing an average percentile rank from all three tests and using the same guidelines given in Table 9.4.

EVALUATING BODY POSTURE

Posture tests are used to detect deviations from normal body alignment and prescribe corrective exercises or procedures to improve alignment. These analyses preferably are conducted early in life, because certain postural deviations are more complex to correct in older people. If deviations are allowed to go uncorrected, they usually become more serious as the person grows older. Consequently, corrective exercises or other medical procedures should be used to stop or slow down postural degeneration.

Faulty posture and weak and inelastic muscles are the leading causes for chronic low back problems in the United States. An estimated 75 million Americans have low back problems each year. About 80% of low back pain is caused by a combination of poor flexibility and improper postural alignment in the lower back and a weak abdominal wall.

A battery of tests to evaluate these areas becomes crucial in preventing and rehabilitating low back pain. The results of these tests can be used to prescribe corrective exercises.

MODIFIED SIT-AND-REACH TEST

1. To perform this test, you will need the Acuflex I* Sit-and-Reach Flexibility Tester, or you may simply place a yardstick on top of a box approximately twelve inches high.

2. Be sure that the person is properly warmed up prior to the first trial.

3. All participants should remove their shoes for the test. Have the person sit on the floor with the hips, back, and head against a wall; the legs fully extended; and the bottom of the feet against the Acuflex I or sit-and-reach box.

4. Have the person place the hands one on top of the other, and have him/her reach forward as far as possible without letting the head and back come off the wall (the shoulders may be rounded as much as possible, but neither the head nor back should come off the wall at this time). The technician can then slide the reach indicator on the Acuflex I (or yardstick) along the top of the box until the end of the indicator touches the participant's fingers (see Figure 9.3a). The indicator must then be held firmly in place throughout the rest of the test.

5. The person's head and back can now come off the wall. He/she should then gradually reach forward three times, the third time stretching forward as far as possible on the indicator (or yardstick), and holding the final position for at least two seconds (see Figure 9.2). Be sure that during the test the backs of the knees are kept

FIGURE 9.3a
Determining the starting position for the Sit-and-Reach Test.

flat against the floor. Record the final number of inches reached to the nearest one-half inch.

6. The person is allowed two trials and an average of the two scores is used as the final test score. The respective percentile ranks and fitness categories for this test are given in Tables 9.1 and 9.4.

* The Acuflex I Flexibility Tester for the Modified Sit-and-Reach Test can be obtained from Figure Finder Collection, Novel Products, Inc. P.O. Box 408, Rockton, Illinois 61072-0408. Phone 800-323-5143, Fax 815-624-4866.

FIGURE 9.3
Procedure for the Modified Sit-and-Reach Test.

TABLE 9.1
Percentile Ranks for the Modified Sit and Reach Test

	Percentile Rank	Age Category					Percentile Rank	Age Category			
		≤18	19–35	36–49	≥50			≤18	19-35	36–49	≥50
	99	20.8	20.1	18.9	16.2		99	22.6	21.0	19.8	17.2
	95	19.6	18.9	18.2	15.8		95	19.5	19.3	19.2	15.7
	90	18.2	17.2	16.1	15.0		90	18.7	17.9	17.4	15.0
	80	17.8	17.0	14.6	13.3		80	17.8	16.7	16.2	14.2
	70	16.0	15.8	13.9	12.3		70	16.5	16.2	15.2	13.6
	60	15.2	15.0	13.4	11.5		60	16.0	15.8	14.5	12.3
Men	50	14.5	14.4	12.6	10.2	Women	50	15.2	14.8	13.5	11.1
	40	14.0	13.5	11.6	9.7		40	14.5	14.5	12.8	10.1
	30	13.4	13.0	10.8	9.3		30	13.7	13.7	12.2	9.2
	20	11.8	11.6	9.9	8.8		20	12.6	12.6	11.0	8.3
	10	9.5	9.2	8.3	7.8		10	11.4	10.1	9.7	7.5
	05	8.4	7.9	7.0	7.2		05	9.4	8.1	8.5	3.7
	01	7.2	7.0	5.1	4.0		01	6.5	2.6	2.0	1.5

■ High physical fitness standard
■ Health fitness standard
See Chapter 1, Fitness Standards: Health vs Physical Fitness, p. 6.

TOTAL BODY ROTATION TEST

1. An Acuflex II* Total Body Rotation Flexibility Tester or a measuring scale with a sliding panel is needed to administer this test. The Acuflex II or scale is placed on the wall at shoulder height and should be adjustable to accommodate individual differences in height. If you need to build your own scale, use two measuring tapes and glue them above and below the sliding panel centered at the fifteen-inch mark. Each tape should be at least thirty inches long. If no sliding panel is available, simply tape the measuring tapes onto a wall. A line must also be drawn on the floor and centered with the fifteen-inch mark (see Figures 9.4a, 9.4b, 9.4c, and 9.4d).

2. Be sure that the person is properly warmed up prior to initiating this test.

3. Have the person stand sideways, an arm's length away from the wall, with the feet straight ahead, slightly separated, and the toes right up to the corresponding line drawn on the floor. The arm opposite to the wall is held out horizontally from the body, making a fist with the hand. The Acuflex II, measuring scale, or tapes should be shoulder height at this time.

4. The participant can now rotate the trunk, the extended arm going backward (always maintaining a horizontal plane) and making contact with the panel, gradually sliding it forward as far as possible. If no panel is available, slide the fist alongside the tapes as far as possible. The final position must be held for at least two seconds. The hand should be positioned with the little finger side forward during the entire sliding movement as illustrated in Figure 9.4e. **It is crucial to use proper hand position. Many people will attempt to open the hand, or push with extended fingers, or slide the panel with the knuckles — none of which is an acceptable test procedure.** During the test, the knees can be slightly bent, but **the feet cannot be moved, always pointing straight forward.** The body must be kept as straight (vertical) as possible.

5. The test is conducted on either the right or the left side of the body. Each participant is allowed two trials on the selected side. The farthest point reached, measured to the nearest one-half inch, and held for at least two seconds is recorded. The average of the two trials is used as the final test score. Using Tables 9.2 and 9.4, determine the percentile rank and flexibility fitness classification for this test.

FIGURE 9.4a
Acuflex II measuring device for the Total Body Rotation Test.

FIGURE 9.4b
Homemade measuring device for the Total Body Rotation Test.

*The Acuflex II Flexibility Tester for the Total Body Rotation Test can be obtained from Figure Finder Collection, Novel Products, Inc., P.O. Box 408, Rockton, Illinois 61072-0408. Phone: (800) 323-5143, FAX 815-624-4866.

FIGURE 9.4c
Measuring tapes for the Total Body Rotation Test.

FIGURE 9.4d
Total Body Rotation Test.

FIGURE 9.4e
Proper hand position for the Total Body Rotation Test.

FIGURE 9.4
Procedure for the Total Body Rotation Test.

TABLE 9.2
Percentile Ranks for the Total Body Rotation Test

	Percentile Rank	Left Rotation				Right Rotation			
		≤18	19–35	36–49	≥50	≤18	19–35	36–49	≥50
	99	29.1	28.0	26.6	21.0	28.2	27.8	25.2	22.2
	95	26.6	24.8	24.5	20.0	25.5	25.6	23.8	20.7
	90	25.0	23.6	23.0	17.7	24.3	24.1	22.5	19.3
	80	22.0	22.0	21.2	15.5	22.7	22.3	21.0	16.3
	70	20.9	20.3	20.4	14.7	21.3	20.7	18.7	15.7
	60	19.9	19.3	18.7	13.9	19.8	19.0	17.3	14.7
Men	50	18.6	18.0	16.7	12.7	19.0	17.2	16.3	12.3
	40	17.0	16.8	15.3	11.7	17.3	16.3	14.7	11.5
	30	14.9	15.0	14.8	10.3	15.1	15.0	13.3	10.7
	20	13.8	13.3	13.7	9.5	12.9	13.3	11.2	8.7
	10	10.8	10.5	10.8	4.3	10.8	11.3	8.0	2.7
	05	8.5	8.9	8.8	0.3	8.1	8.3	5.5	0.3
	01	3.4	1.7	5.1	0.0	6.6	2.9	2.0	0.0
	99	29.3	28.6	27.1	23.0	29.6	29.4	27.1	21.7
	95	26.8	24.8	25.3	21.4	27.6	25.3	25.9	19.7
	90	25.5	23.0	23.4	20.5	25.8	23.0	21.3	19.0
	80	23.8	21.5	20.2	19.1	23.7	20.8	19.6	17.9
	70	21.8	20.5	18.6	17.3	22.0	19.3	17.3	16.8
	60	20.5	19.3	17.7	16.0	20.8	18.0	16.5	15.6
Women	50	19.5	18.0	16.4	14.8	19.5	17.3	14.6	14.0
	40	18.5	17.2	14.8	13.7	18.3	16.0	13.1	12.8
	30	17.1	15.7	13.6	10.0	16.3	15.2	11.7	8.5
	20	16.0	15.2	11.6	6.3	14.5	14.0	9.8	3.9
	10	12.8	13.6	8.5	3.0	12.4	11.1	6.1	2.2
	05	11.1	7.3	6.8	0.7	10.2	8.8	4.0	1.1
	01	8.9	5.3	4.3	0.0	8.9	3.2	2.8	0.0

█ High physical fitness standard

█ Health fitness standard

See Chapter 1, Fitness Standards: Health vs Physical Fitness, p. 6.

SHOULDER ROTATION TEST

1. This test can be performed using the Acuflex III* Flexibility Tester, which consists of a shoulder caliper and a measuring device for shoulder rotation. If unavailable, you can quite easily construct your own device. The caliper can be built with three regular yardsticks. Nail and glue two of the yardsticks at one end at a ninety degree angle, and use the third one as the sliding end of the caliper. The rotation device is constructed by placing a sixty-inch measuring tape on an aluminum or wood stick, starting at about six or seven inches from the end of the stick.

2. Be sure that the person is properly warmed up prior to the test.

3. Using the shoulder caliper, measure the biacromial width to the nearest one-fourth inch (use the red scale on the Acuflex III). Biacromial width is measured between the lateral edges of the acromion processes of the shoulders, as shown in Figure 9.5a.

4. Place the Acuflex III or homemade device behind the participant's back and use a reverse grip (thumbs out) to hold on to the device (see Figure 9.5b). The right hand is placed next to the zero point of the scale or tape (blue scale on the Acuflex III) and is held firmly in place throughout the test. The left hand is placed on the other end of the measuring device, as wide as needed.

5. Standing straight up and extending both arms to full length, **with elbows locked,** the individual slowly brings the measuring device over the head until it reaches forehead level (Figure 9.5c). For succeeding trials, depending on the resistance encountered when rotating the shoulders, the left grip may be moved in one-half to one inch at a time, and the task repeated until the person can no longer rotate the shoulders without undue strain or starts bending the elbows to do so. The right-hand grip is always kept against the zero point of the scale. Measure the last successful trial to the nearest one-half inch. This measurement should be taken right at the inner edge of the left hand on the side of the little finger.

6. The final score for this test is determined by subtracting the biacromial width from the best score (shortest distance) between both hands on the rotation test. For example, if the best score is thirty-five inches and the biacromial width is fifteen inches, the final score would be twenty inches (35 – 15 = 20). Using Tables 9.3 and 9.4, determine the percentile rank and flexibility fitness classification for this test.

FIGURE 9.5a
Measuring biacromial width.

FIGURE 9.5b
Starting position for the Shoulder Rotation Test (note the reverse grip used for this test).

FIGURE 9.5c
Shoulder Rotation Test.

*The Acuflex III Flexibility Tester for the Shoulder Rotation Test can be obtained from Figure Finder Collection, Novel Products, Inc., P.O. Box 408, Rockton, Illinois 61072-0408. Phone: (800) 323-5143, FAX 815-624-4866.

FIGURE 9.5
Procedure for the Shoulder Rotation Test.

TABLE 9.3
Percentile Ranks for the Shoulder Rotation Test

	Percentile Rank	Age Category			
		≤18	19-35	36-49	≥50
Men	99	2.2	-1.0	18.1	21.5
	95	15.2	10.4	20.4	27.0
	90	18.5	15.5	20.8	27.9
	80	20.7	18.4	23.3	28.5
	70	23.0	20.5	24.7	29.4
	60	24.2	22.9	26.6	29.9
	50	25.4	24.4	28.0	30.5
	40	26.3	25.7	30.0	31.0
	30	28.2	27.3	31.9	31.7
	20	30.0	30.1	33.3	33.1
	10	33.5	31.8	36.1	37.2
	05	34.7	33.5	37.8	38.7
	01	40.8	42.6	43.0	44.1
Women	99	2.6	-2.4	11.5	13.1
	95	8.0	6.2	15.4	16.5
	90	10.7	9.7	16.8	20.9
	80	14.5	14.5	19.2	22.5
	70	16.1	17.2	21.5	24.3
	60	19.2	18.7	23.1	25.1
	50	21.0	20.0	23.5	26.2
	40	22.2	21.4	24.4	28.1
	30	23.2	24.0	25.9	29.9
	20	25.0	25.9	29.8	31.5
	10	27.2	29.1	31.1	33.1
	05	28.0	31.3	33.4	34.1
	01	32.5	37.1	34.9	35.4

■ High physical fitness standard
■ Health fitness standard

See Chapter 1, Fitness Standards: Health vs Physical Fitness, p. 6.

TABLE 9.4
Flexibility Fitness Categories

Percentile Rank	Fitness Category
≥81	Excellent
61-80	Good
41-60	Average
21-40	Fair
≤20	Poor

Adequate body mechanics also aid in reducing chronic low back pain. Proper body mechanics means using correct positions in all the activities of daily life, including sleeping, sitting, standing, walking, driving, working, and exercising. Because of the high incidence of low back pain, a series of corrective and preventive exercises, along with illustrations of proper body mechanics, are given in Chapter 10.

Most people are unaware of how faulty their posture is until they see themselves in a photograph, such as shown in Figure 9.6. This can be quite a shock to many people and often is enough to motivate change.

Faulty posture and weak and inelastic muscles are the leading causes of chronic low back problems in the United States.

Besides engaging in the recommended exercises, to elicit changes in postural alignment, people need to be continually aware of the corrections they are trying to make. As their posture improves, people frequently become motivated to change other aspects such as improving muscular strength and flexibility and decreasing body fat.

Proper body alignment has been difficult to evaluate because most experts still don't know exactly what constitutes good posture. To objectively analyze a person's posture, an observer either must be adequately trained or have some guidelines to identify abnormalities and give ratings according to the amount of deviation from "normal" posture.

FIGURE 9.6
Photographic technique for posture evaluation.

A posture rating chart, such as given in Lab 9B (Figure 9B.1), provides simple guidelines for evaluating posture. Assuming the drawings in the left column as proper alignment and the drawings in the right column as extreme deviations from normal, an observer is able to rate each body segment on a scale from 1 to 5.

Postural analysis can be done with more precision with the aid of a plumb line, two mirrors, and a Polaroid camera. The mirrors are placed at an 80° to 85° angle, and the plumb line is centered in front of the mirrors. Another line is drawn down the center of the mirror on the right. The person should stand with the left side to the plumb line (see Figure 9.6). The plumb line is used as a reference to divide the body into front and back halves (try to center the line with the hip joint and the shoulder). The line on the back mirror should divide the body into right and left sides. A picture then is taken that can be compared to the rating chart given in Lab 9B.

The photographic procedure allows for a better comparison of the different body segment alignments and a more objective analysis. If no mirrors and camera are available, the participant should stand with his or her side to the line, and then repeat with the back to the line, while the evaluator does the assessment.

A final posture score is determined according to the sum of the ratings obtained for each body segment. Table 9.5 contains the various categories as determined by the final posture score.

TABLE 9.5
Posture Evaluation Standards

Total Points	Classification
≥45	Excellent
40-44	Good
30-39	Average
20-29	Fair
≤19	Poor

Source: Hoeger, W. W. K. *The Complete Guide for the Development and Implementation of Health Promotion Programs.* Englewood, CO: Morton Publishing, 1987. Reproduced with permission.

LABORATORY EXPERIENCE

LAB 9A
Muscular Flexibility Assessment

Lab Preparation
Wear loose exercise clothing.

LAB 9B
Posture Evaluation

Lab Preparation
For the posture analysis, men should wear shorts only, and women should wear shorts and a tank top. Study the posture analysis form given in Lab 9B, and review the section on Posture Evaluation in this chapter prior to the lab.

REFERENCES

1. Billing, H., and E. Loewendahl. *Mobilization of the Human Body.* Palo Alto, CA: Stanford University Press, 1949.

2. Chapman, E. A., H. A. deVries, and R. Swezey. "Joint Stiffness: Effects of Exercise on Young and Old Men." *Journal of Gerontology* 27:218-221, 1972.

3. Dickerson, R. V. "The Specificity of Flexibility." *Research Quarterly* 33:222-229, 1962.

4. Fleishman, E. A. *Examiners Manual for Basic Fitness Tests.* Englewood Cliffs, NJ: Prentice Hall, Inc., 1964.

5. Hoeger, W. W. K., S. Button, D. R. Hopkins, and T. A. Palmer. "Relationship Among Four Selected Flexibility Tests for High School-Age Students." *Northwest Journal for Health, Physical Education, Recreation and Dance,* 1(2):6-10, 1989.

6. Hoeger, W. W. K., and D. R. Hopkins. "Assessing Muscular Flexibility." *Fitness Management,* 6(2):34-36, 42, 1990.

7. Hoeger, W. W. K., and D. R. Hopkins. "A Comparison Between The Sit and Reach and The Modified Sit and Reach in the Measurement of Flexibility in Women." *Research Quarterly for Exercise and Sport,* 63:191-195, 1992.

8. Hoeger, W. W. K, D. R. Hopkins, S. Button, and T. A. Palmer. "Comparing The Sit and Reach with the Modified Sit and Reach in Measuring Flexibility in Adolescents." *Pediatric Exercise Science,* 2:156-162, 1990.

9. Hopkins, D. R., and W. W. K. Hoeger. "A Comparison of the Sit and Reach and the Modified Sit and Reach in the Measurement of Flexibility for Males." *Journal of Applied Sports Science Research,* 6:7-10, 1992.

10. Holt, L. E., T. M. Travis, and T. Okita. "Comparative Study of Three Stretching Techniques." *Perceptual and Motor Skills* 31:611-616, 1970.

11. Johnson, B. L., and J. K. Nelson. *Practical Measurements for Evaluation in Physical Education.* Minneapolis, MN: Burgess Publishing Co., 1979.

12. Sapega, A. A., T. C. Quedenfeld, R. A. Moyer, and R. A. Butler. "Biophysical Factors in Range-of-Motion Exercise." *Physician and Sportsmedicine* 9:57-65, 1981.

13. Wright, V., and R. J. Johns. "Physical Factors Concerned with Stiffness of Normal and Diseased Joints." *Bulletin of Johns Hopkins Hospital* 106:215-231, 1960.

PRINCIPLES OF MUSCULAR FLEXIBILITY PRESCRIPTION

Developing and maintaining good joint range of motion (flexibility) is important to enhance health and quality of life. Even though genetics play a crucial role in body flexibility, range of joint mobility can be increased and maintained through a regular flexibility exercise program. Because range of motion is highly specific to each body part (ankle, trunk, shoulder), a comprehensive stretching program should include all body parts and follow the basic guidelines for flexibility development.

KEY CONCEPTS

Ballistic stretching
Slow-sustained stretching
Proprioceptive neuromuscular facilitation (PNF)

OBJECTIVES

- Define ballistic stretching, slow-sustained stretching, and proprioceptive neuromuscular facilitation stretching.
- Explain the factors that contribute to the development of muscular flexibility.
- Learn a complete set of exercises for an overall body flexibility-development program.
- Be aware of a program for the prevention and rehabilitation of low back pain.

GUIDELINES FOR FLEXIBILITY DEVELOPMENT

The overload and specificity of training principles discussed in conjunction with strength development in Chapter 8 apply as well to the development of muscular flexibility. To increase the total range of motion of a joint, the specific muscles surrounding that joint have to be stretched progressively beyond their accustomed length. The principles of mode, intensity, repetitions, and frequency of exercise also can be applied to flexibility programs.

MODE OF TRAINING

Three modes of stretching exercises can increase flexibility:

1. Ballistic stretching.
2. Slow-sustained stretching.
3. Proprioceptive neuromuscular facilitation stretching.

Although research has indicated that all three types of stretching are effective in improving flexibility, each technique has certain advantages.

Ballistic or dynamic stretching exercises are done with jerky, rapid, and bouncy movements that provide the necessary force to

L A B S

lengthen the muscles. This type of stretching helps to develop flexibility, but the ballistic actions may cause muscle soreness and injury from small tears to the soft tissue.

Precautions must be taken not to overstretch ligaments, because they undergo plastic or permanent elongation. If the stretching force cannot be controlled, as in fast, jerky movements, ligaments easily can be overstretched. This, in turn, leads to excessively loose joints, increasing the risk for injuries, including joint dislocation and subluxation (partial dislocation). Most authorities, therefore, do not recommend ballistic exercises for development of flexibility.

With the *slow-sustained stretching* technique, muscles are lengthened gradually through a joint's complete range of motion, and the final position is held for a few seconds. A slow-sustained stretch causes the muscles to relax so greater length can be achieved. This type of stretch causes little pain and has a low risk for injury. Slow-sustained stretching exercises are the most frequently used and recommended for flexibility development programs.

Proprioceptive neuromuscular facilitation (PNF) stretching has become more popular in the last few years. This technique, based on a "contract and relax" method, requires the assistance of another person (see Figure 10.1). The procedure is as follows:

1. The person assisting with the exercise provides initial force by slowly pushing in the direction of the desired stretch. This first stretch does not cover the entire range of motion.
2. The person being stretched then applies force in the opposite direction of the stretch, against the assistant, who tries to hold the initial degree of stretch as close as possible. An isometric contraction is being performed at that angle.
3. After four or five seconds of isometric contraction, the muscle being stretched is completely relaxed. The assistant then slowly increases the degree of stretch to a greater angle.
4. The isometric contraction then is repeated for another four or five seconds, following which the muscle is relaxed again. The assistant then can slowly increase the degree of stretch one more time. Steps one to four are repeated two to five times, until the exerciser feels mild discomfort. On the last trial the final stretched position should be held for several seconds.

Theoretically, with the PNF technique, the isometric contraction helps relax the muscle being stretched, which results in greater muscle length. Some fitness leaders believe PNF is more effective than slow-sustained stretching. Disadvantages, however, are more pain with PNF, a second person is required to assist, and more time is necessary to conduct each session.

INTENSITY OF EXERCISE

The intensity, or degree of stretch when doing flexibility exercises, should be only to a point of mild discomfort. Pain does not have to be a part of the stretching routine. Excessive pain is an indication that the load is too high and may lead to injury.

All stretching should be done to slightly below the pain threshold. As participants reach this point, they should try to relax the muscle being stretched as much as possible. After completing the stretch, the body part is brought back gradually to the starting point.

FIGURE 10.1
Proprioceptive Neuromuscular Facilitation (PNF) Stretching Technique: (a) isometric phase, (b) stretching phase.

REPETITIONS

The time required for an exercise session for flexibility development is based on the number of repetitions performed and the length of time each repetition (final stretched position) is held. The general recommendation is that each exercise be done four or five times, holding the final position each time for about 20 seconds.

As flexibility increases, a person can gradually increase the time each repetition is held, to a maximum of one minute. Individuals who are susceptible to flexibility injuries, however, should limit each stretch to 20 seconds.

FREQUENCY OF EXERCISE

Flexibility exercises should be conducted five to six times a week in the early stages of the program. After a minimum of six to eight weeks of almost daily stretching, flexibility levels can be maintained with only two or three sessions per week, using about three repetitions of 10 to 15 seconds each. Figure 10.2 provides a summary of flexibility development guidelines.

WHEN TO STRETCH?

Many people do not differentiate a warm-up from stretching. Warming up means starting a workout slowly with walking, slow jogging, or light calisthenics. Stretching implies movement of joints through their range of motion.

■ **Mode**

   Static stretching or proprioceptive neuromuscular facilitation (PNF)

■ **Intensity**

   Stretch to the point of mild discomfort

■ **Repetitions**

   Repeat each exercise four to five times and hold the final stretched position for 10 to 60 seconds

■ **Frequency**

   Two to six days per week

FIGURE 10.2
Guidelines for flexibility development.

Before performing flexibility exercises, the muscles should be properly warmed up. Failing to warm up increases the risk for muscle pulls and tears. Surveys have shown that individuals who stretch before workouts without an adequate warm-up actually have a higher rate of injuries than those who do not stretch at all.

A good time to do flexibility exercises is after aerobic workouts. Higher body temperature in itself helps to increase joint range of motion. Muscles also are fatigued following exercise. A fatigued muscle tends to shorten, which can lead to soreness and spasms. Stretching exercises help fatigued muscles reestablish their normal resting length and prevent unnecessary pain.

FLEXIBILITY EXERCISES

To improve body flexibility, each major muscle group should be subjected to at least one stretching exercise. A complete set of exercises for developing muscular flexibility is presented at the end of this chapter.

You may not be able to hold a final stretched position with some of these exercises (examples: lateral head tilts and arm circles), but you should still perform the exercise through the joint's full range of motion. Depending on the number and length of the repetitions, a complete workout will last between 15 and 30 minutes.

PREVENTING AND REHABILITATING LOW BACK PAIN

Few people make it through life without having low back pain at some point. An estimated 75 million Americans currently suffer from chronic low back pain each year. About 80% of the time, backache syndrome is preventable and is caused by: (a) physical inactivity, (b) poor postural habits and body mechanics, and (c) excessive body weight.

Lack of physical activity is the most common factor contributing to chronic low back pain. Deterioration or weakening of the abdominal and gluteal muscles, along with tightening of the lower back (erector spine) muscles, brings about an unnatural forward tilt of the pelvis (see Figure 10.3). This tilt puts extra pressure on the spinal vertebrae, causing pain in the lower back. Accumulation of fat around the midsection of the body contributes to the forward tilt of the pelvis, which further aggravates the condition.

Low back pain frequently is associated with faulty posture and improper body mechanics (body positions in all of life's daily activities, including sleeping, sitting, standing, walking, driving, working, and exercising). Incorrect posture and poor mechanics, as explained in Figure 10.4, increase strain not only on the lower back but on many other bones, joints, muscles, and ligaments as well.

The incidence and frequency of low back pain episodes can be reduced greatly by including some specific stretching and strengthening exercises in the regular fitness program. In most cases, back pain is present only with movement and physical activity. If the pain is severe and persists even at rest, the first step is to consult a physician, who can rule out any disc damage and most likely will prescribe proper bed rest using several pillows under the knees for leg support (see Figure 10.4). This position helps release muscle spasms by stretching the muscles involved. In addition, a physician may prescribe a muscle relaxant or anti-inflammatory medication (or both) and some type of physical therapy.

Once a person is pain-free in the resting state, he or she needs to start correcting the muscular imbalance by stretching the tight muscles and strengthening the weak ones. Stretching exercises always are performed first.

Several exercises for preventing and rehabilitating the backache syndrome are given at the end of this chapter. These exercises can be done twice or more daily when a person has back pain. Under normal circumstances, doing these exercises three to four times a week is sufficient to prevent the syndrome.

FIGURE 10.3
A comparison of incorrect (left) and correct (right) pelvic alignment.

LABORATORY EXPERIENCE

LAB 10A
Sample Flexibility Development Program

Lab Preparation
Wear exercise clothing and be prepared to participate in a sample flexibility development session.

LAB 10B
Exercises for the Prevention and Rehabilitation of Low Back Pain

Lab Preparation
Wear exercise clothing and prepare to perform all of the exercises for the prevention and rehabilitation of low back pain outlined in this chapter.

REFERENCES

1. Heyward, V. H. *Advanced Methods for Physical Fitness Assessment and Exercise Prescription.* Champaign, IL: Human Kinetic Publishers, 1991.

2. Hoeger, W. W. K. *The Complete Guide for the Development & Implementation of Health Promotion Programs.* Englewood, CO: Morton Publishing Company, 1987.

3. "Your Back and How to Care For It." Kenilworth, NJ: Schering Corporation, 1965.

Your back and how to care for it

Whatever the cause of low back pain, part of its treatment is the correction of faulty posture. But good posture is not simply a matter of "standing tall." It refers to correct use of the body at all times. In fact, for the body to function in the best of health it must be so used that no strain is put upon the muscles, joints, bones, and ligaments. To prevent low back pain, avoiding strain must become a way of life, practiced while lying, sitting, standing, walking, working, and exercising. When body position is correct, internal organs have enough room to function normally and blood circulates more freely.

With the help of this guide, you can begin to correct the positions and movements which bring on or aggravate backache. Particular attention should be paid to the positions recommended for resting, since it is possible to strain the muscles of the back and neck even while lying in bed. By learning to live with good posture, under all circumstances, you will gradually develop the proper carriage and stronger muscles needed to protect and support your hard-working back.

HOW TO STAY ON YOUR FEET WITHOUT TIRING YOUR BACK

To prevent strain and pain in everyday activities, it is restful to change from one task to another before fatigue sets in. Housewives can lie down between chores; others should check body position frequently, drawing in the abdomen, flattening the back, bending the knees slightly.

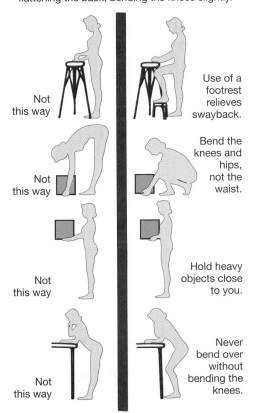

Not this way / Use of a footrest relieves swayback.

Not this way / Bend the knees and hips, not the waist.

Not this way / Hold heavy objects close to you.

Not this way / Never bend over without bending the knees.

CHECK YOUR CARRIAGE HERE

In correct, fully erect posture, a line dropped from the ear will go through the tip of the shoulder, middle of hip, back of kneecap, and front of anklebone.

Incorrect
Lower back is arched or hollow.

Incorrect
Upper back is stooped, lower back is arched, abdomen sags.

Incorrect
Note how, in strained position pelvis tilts forward, chin is out, and ribs are down, crowding internal organs.

Correct
In correct position, chin is in, head up back flattened, pelvis held straight.

To find the correct standing position: Stand one foot away from wall. Now sit against wall, bending knees slightly. Tighten abdominal and buttock muscles. This will tilt the pelvis back and flatten the lower spine. Holding this position, inch up the wall to standing position, by straightening the legs. Now walk around the room, maintaining the same posture. Place back against wall again to see if you have held it.

HOW TO SIT CORRECTLY

A back's best friend is a straight, hard chair. If you can't get the chair you prefer, learn to sit properly on whatever chair you get. To correct sitting position from forward slump: Throw head well back, then bend it forward to pull in the chin. This will straighten the back. Now tighten abdominal muscles to raise the chest. Check position frequently.

Relieve strain by sitting well forward, flatten back by tightening abdominal muscles, and cross knees.

Use of footrest relieves swayback. Aim is to have knees higher than hips.

Correct way to sit while driving, close to pedals. Use seat belt or hard backrest, available commercially.

TV slump leads to "dowager's hump," strains neck and shoulders.

If chair is too high, swayback is increased.

Keep neck and back in as straight a line as possible with the spine. Bend forward from hips.

Driver's seat too far from pedals emphasizes curve in lower back.

Strained reading position. Forward thrusting strains muscles of neck and head.

FIGURE 10.4

HOW TO PUT YOUR BACK TO BED

For proper bed posture, a firm mattress is essential. Bedboards, sold commercially, or devised at home, may be used with soft mattresses. Bedboards, preferably, should be made of 3/4 inch plywood. Faulty sleeping positions intensify swayback and result not only in backache but in numbness, tingling, and pain in arms and legs.

Incorrect:

Lying flat on back makes swayback worse.

Use of high pillow strains neck, arms, shoulders.

Sleeping face down exaggerates swayback, strains neck and shoulders.

Bending one hip and knee does not relieve swayback.

Correct:

Lying on side with knees bent effectively flattens the back. Flat pillow may be used to support neck, especially when shoulders are broad.

Sleeping on back is restful and correct when knees are properly supported.

Raise the foot of the mattress eight inches to discourage sleeping on the abdomen.

Proper arrangement of pillows for resting or reading in bed.

A straight-back chair used behind a pillow makes a serviceable backrest.

WHEN DOING NOTHING, DO IT RIGHT

Rest is the first rule for the tired, painful back. The following positions relieve pain by taking all pressure and weight off the back and legs.

Note pillows under knees to relieve strain on spine.

For complete relief and relaxing effect, these positions should be maintained from 5 to 25 minutes.

FIGURE 10.4 *(Continued)*

EXERCISE — WITHOUT GETTING OUT OF BED

Exercises to be performed while lying in bed are aimed not so much at strengthening muscles as at teaching correct positioning. But muscles used correctly become stronger and in time are able to support the body with the least amount of effort.

Do all exercises in this position. Legs should not be straightened.

Bring knee up to chest. Lower slowly but do not straighten leg. Relax. Repeat with each leg 10 times.

Bring both knees slowly up to chest. Tighten muscles of abdomen, press back flat against bed. Hold knees to chest 20 seconds, then lower slowly. Relax. Repeat 5 times. This exercise gently stretches the shortened muscles of the lower back, while strengthening abdominal muscles. Clasp knees, bring them up to chest, at the same time coming to a sitting position. Rock back and forth.

EXERCISE — WITHOUT ATTRACTING ATTENTION

Use these inconspicuous exercises whenever you have a spare moment during the day, both to relax tension and improve the tone of important muscle groups.

1. Rotate shoulders, forward and backward.
2. Turn head slowly side to side.
3. Watch an imaginary plane take off, just below the right shoulder. Stretch neck, follow it slowly as it moves up, around and down, disappearing below the other shoulder. Repeat, starting on left side.
4. Slowly, slowly, touch left ear to left shoulder, right ear to right shoulder. Raise both shoulders to touch ears, drop them as far down as possible.
5. At any pause in the day — waiting for an elevator to arrive, for a specific traffic light to change — pull in abdominal muscles, tighten, hold it for the count of eight without breathing. Relax slowly. Increase the count gradually after the first week, practice breathing normally with the abdomen flat and contracted. Do this sitting, standing, and walking.

RULES TO LIVE BY - FROM NOW ON

1. Never bend from the waist only; bend the hips and knees.
2. Never lift a heavy object higher than your waist.
3. Always turn and face the object you wish to lift.
4. Avoid carrying unbalanced loads; hold heavy objects close to your body.
5. Never carry anything heavier than you can manage with ease.
6. Never lift or move heavy furniture. Wait for someone to do it who knows the principles of leverage.
7. Avoid sudden movements, sudden "overloading" of muscles. Learn to move deliberately, swinging the legs from the hips.
8. Learn to keep the head in line with the spine, when standing, sitting, lying in bed.
9. Put soft chairs and deep couches on your "don't sit" list. During prolonged sitting, cross your legs to rest your back.
10. Your doctor is the only one who can determine when low back pain is due to faulty posture. He is the best judge of when you may do general exercises for physical fitness. when you do, omit any exercise which arches or overstrains the lower back: backward bends, or forward bends, touching the toes with the knees straight.
11. Wear shoes with moderate heels, all about the same height. Avoid changing from high to low heels.
12. Put a footrail under the desk, and a footrest under the crib.
13. Diaper the baby sitting next to him or her on the bed.
14. Don't stoop and stretch to hand the wash; raise the clothesbasket and lower the washline.
15. Beg or buy a rocking chair. Rocking rests the back by changing the muscle groups used.
16. Train yourself vigorously to use your abdominal muscles to flatten your lower abdomen. In time, this muscle contraction will become habitual, making you the envied possessor of a youthful body-profile!
17. Don't strain to open windows or doors.
18. For good posture, concentrate on strengthening "nature's corset" — the abdominal and buttock muscles. The pelvic roll exercise is especially recommended to correct the postural relation between the pelvis and the spine.

Flexibility Exercises

EXERCISE 1

Lateral Head Tilt

ACTION   Slowly and gently tilt the head laterally. Repeat several times to each side.

AREAS STRETCHED   Neck flexors and extensors and ligaments of the cervical spine.

EXERCISE 2

Arm Circles

ACTION   Gently circle your arms all the way around. Conduct the exercise in both directions.

AREAS STRETCHED   Shoulder muscles and ligaments.

EXERCISE 3

Side Stretch

ACTION   Stand straight up, feet separated to shoulder width, and place your hands on your waist. Now move the upper body to one side and hold the final stretch for a few seconds. Repeat on the other side.

AREAS STRETCHED   Muscles and ligaments in the pelvic region.

EXERCISE 4

Body Rotation

ACTION   Place your arms slightly away from your body and rotate the trunk as far as possible, holding the final position for several seconds. Conduct the exercise for both the right and left sides of the body. You can also perform this exercise by standing about two feet away from the wall (back toward the wall), and then rotate the trunk, placing the hands against the wall.

AREAS STRETCHED
Hip, abdominal, chest, back, neck, and shoulder muscles; hip and spinal ligaments.

EXERCISE 5

Chest Stretch

ACTION   Kneel down behind a chair and place both hands on the back of the chair. Gradually push your chest downward and hold for a few seconds.

AREAS STRETCHED   Chest (pectoral) muscles and shoulder ligaments.

EXERCISE 7

Shoulder Rotation Stretch

ACTION   With the aid of surgical tubing or an aluminum or wood stick, place the tubing or stick behind your back and grasp the two ends using a reverse (thumbs-out) grip. Slowly bring the tubing or stick over your head, keeping the elbows straight. Repeat several times (bring the hands closer together for additional stretch).

AREAS STRETCHED   Deltoid, latissimus dorsi, and pectoral muscles; shoulder ligaments.

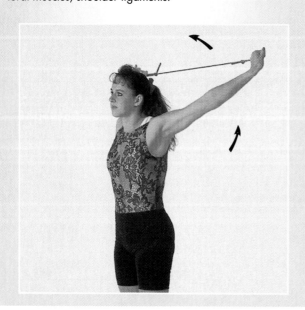

EXERCISE 6

Shoulder Hyperextension Stretch

ACTION   Have a partner grasp your arms from behind by the wrists and slowly push them upward. Hold the final position for a few seconds.

AREAS STRETCHED   Deltoid and pectoral muscles, and ligaments of the shoulder joint.

EXERCISE 8

Quad Stretch

ACTION   Lie on your side and move one foot back by flexing the knee. Grasp the front of the ankle and pull the ankle toward the gluteal region. Hold for several seconds. Repeat with the other leg.

AREAS STRETCHED   Quadriceps muscle, and knee and ankle ligaments.

EXERCISE 9

Heel Cord Stretch

ACTION   Stand against the wall or at the edge of a step and stretch the heel downward, alternating legs. Hold the stretched position for a few seconds.

AREAS STRETCHED   Heel cord (Achilles tendon), gastrocnemius, and soleus muscles.

EXERCISE 10

Adductor Stretch

ACTION   Stand with your feet about twice shoulder width and place your hands slightly above the knee. Flex one knee and slowly go down as far as possible, holding the final position for a few seconds. Repeat with the other leg.

AREAS STRETCHED   Hip adductor muscles.

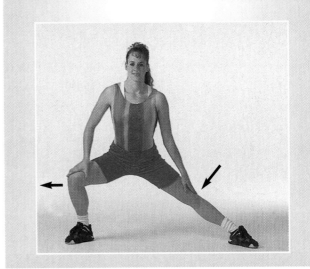

EXERCISE 11

Sitting Adductor Stretch

ACTION   Sit on the floor and bring your feet in close to you, allowing the soles of the feet to touch each other. Now place your forearms (or elbows) on the inner part of the thigh and push the legs downward, holding the final stretch for several seconds.

AREA STRETCHED
Hip adductor muscles.

EXERCISE 12

Sit-and-Reach Stretch

ACTION   Sit on the floor with legs together and gradually reach forward as far as possible. Hold the final position for a few seconds. This exercise may also be performed with the legs separated, reaching to each side as well as to the middle.

AREAS STRETCHED   Hamstrings and lower back muscles, and lumbar spine ligaments.

EXERCISE **13**

Triceps Stretch

ACTION   Place the right hand behind your neck. Grasp the right arm above the elbow with the left hand. Gently pull the elbow backward. Repeat the exercise with the opposite arm.

AREAS STRETCHED   Back of upper arm (triceps muscle) and shoulder joint.

Exercises for the Prevention and Rehabilitation of Low Back Pain

EXERCISE **14**

Single-Knee to Chest Stretch

ACTION   Lie down flat on the floor. Bend one leg at approximately 100° and gradually pull the opposite leg toward your chest. Hold the final stretch for a few seconds. Switch legs and repeat the exercise.

AREAS STRETCHED   Lower back and hamstring muscles, and lumbar spine ligaments.

EXERCISE **15**

Double-Knee to Chest Stretch

ACTION   Lie flat on the floor and then slowly curl up into a fetal position. Hold for a few seconds.

AREAS STRETCHED   Upper and lower back and hamstring muscles; spinal ligaments.

EXERCISE
EXERCISE 16

Upper and Lower Back Stretch

ACTION Sit in a chair with feet separated greater than shoulder width. Place your arms to the inside of the thighs and bring your chest down toward the floor. At the same time, attempt to reach back as far as you can with your arms.

AREAS STRETCHED Upper and lower back muscles and ligaments

EXERCISE 17

Sit-and-Reach Stretch

(see Exercise 12 in this chapter)

EXERCISE 18

Gluteal Stretch

ACTION Sit on the floor, bend the right leg and place your right ankle slightly above the left knee. Grasp the left thigh with both hands and gently pull the leg toward your chest. Repeat the exercise with the opposite leg.

AREAS STRETCHED Buttock area (gluteal muscles).

EXERCISE 19

Back Extension

ACTION Lie face down on the floor with the elbows by the chest, forearms on the floor, and the hands beneath the chin. Gently raise the trunk by extending the elbows until you reach an approximate 90° angle at the elbow joint. Be sure that the forearms remain in contact with the floor at all times. DO NOT extend the back beyond this point. Hyperextension of the lower back may lead to or aggravate an already existing back problem. Hold the stretched position for about ten seconds.

AREA STRETCHED
Abdominal region.

ADDITIONAL BENEFIT
Restore lower back curvature.

EXERCISE 20

Trunk Rotation and Lower Back Stretch

ACTION Sit on the floor and bend the left leg, placing the left foot on the outside of the right knee. Place the right elbow on the left knee and push against it. At the same time, try to rotate the trunk to the left (counterclockwise). Hold the final position for a few seconds. Repeat the exercise with the other side.

AREAS STRETCHED Lateral side of the hip and thigh; trunk, and lower back.

Pelvic Tilt

ACTION　Lie flat on the floor with the knees bent at about a 70° angle. Tilt the pelvis by tightening the abdominal muscles, flattening your back against the floor, and raising the lower gluteal area ever so slightly off the floor (see illustration b). Hold the final position for several seconds. The exercise can also be performed against a wall (as shown in illustration c).

AREAS STRETCHED　Low back muscles and ligaments.

AREAS STRENGTHENED　Abdominal and gluteal muscles.

NOTE:

This is perhaps the most important exercise for the care of the lower back. It should be included as a part of the your daily exercise routine and should be performed several times throughout the day when pain in the lower back is present as a result of muscle imbalance.

Abdominal Crunch and Abdominal Curl-Up

(see Exercise 4 in Chapter 8)

It is important that you do not stabilize your feet when performing either of these exercises, because doing so decreases the work of the abdominal muscles. Also, remember not to "swing up" but rather to curl up as you perform these exercises.

SKILL-RELATED COMPONENTS OF PHYSICAL FITNESS

11

OBJECTIVES

■ Learn the benefits of good skill-related fitness.

■ Identify and define the six components of skill-related fitness.

■ Become familiar with performance tests to assess skill-related fitness.

Skill-related fitness is important for successful motor performance in athletic events and in lifetime sports and activities such as basketball, racquetball, golf, hiking, soccer, and water skiing. Good skill-related fitness also enhances overall quality of life by helping people cope more effectively in emergency situations. The components of skill-related fitness are agility, balance, coordination, power, reaction time, and speed. All are important to a certain extent in sports and athletics.

For example, outstanding gymnasts must achieve good skill-related fitness in all components. A significant amount of agility is necessary to perform a double back somersault with a full twist — a skill during which the athlete must simultaneously rotate around one axis and twist around a different one. Static balance is essential for maintaining a handstand or a scale. Dynamic balance is needed to perform many of the gymnastics routines (e.g., balance beam, parallel bars, pommel horse). Coordination is important to successfully integrate various skills requiring varying degrees of difficulty into one routine. Power and speed are needed to propel the body into the air, such as when tumbling or vaulting. Reaction time is necessary in determining when to end rotation upon a visual clue, such as spotting the floor on a dismount.

As with the health-related fitness components, the principle of *specificity of training* also applies to skill-related components. This principle states that *to develop a given component, the training program must be specific to the type of development the individual is trying to achieve.*

In the case of agility, balance, coordination, and reaction time, research indicates that development of these components is highly task-specific. That is, to develop a certain task or skill, the individual must practice that same specific task many times. There seems to be very little crossover learning effect.

For instance, proper practice of a handstand (balance) eventually will lead to successful performance of the skill, but complete mastery of this skill does not ensure that the person will have immediate success when attempting to perform other static

L A B S

balance positions in gymnastics. Power and speed may be improved with a specific strength-training program or frequent repetition of the specific task to be improved, or both.

The rate of learning in skill-related fitness varies from person to person, mainly because these components seem to be determined to a large extent by hereditary factors. Individuals with good skill-related fitness tend to do better and learn faster when performing a wide variety of skills. Nevertheless, few individuals enjoy complete success in all skill-related components. Furthermore, though skill-related fitness can be enhanced with practice, improvements in reaction time and speed are limited and seem to be related primarily to genetic endowment.

> *To develop a given component, the training program must be specific to the type of development the individual is trying to achieve.*

Although we do not know how much skill-related fitness is desirable, everyone should attempt to develop and maintain a better than average level. As pointed out earlier, this type of fitness is crucial for athletes, and it also is important to lead a better and happier life. Improving skill-related fitness not only affords an individual more enjoyment and success in lifetime sports (e.g., tennis, racquetball, basketball), but it also can help a person cope more effectively in emergency situations. For example:

1. Good reaction time, balance, coordination, and agility can help you avoid a fall or break a fall and thereby minimize injury.
2. The ability to generate maximum force in a short time (power) may be crucial to ameliorate injury or even preserve life in a situation in which you may be called upon to lift a heavy object that has fallen on another person or even on yourself.
3. In our society, where the average lifespan continues to expand, maintaining speed can be especially important for elderly people. Many of these individuals and, for that matter, many unfit/overweight young people no longer have the speed they need to cross an intersection safely before the light changes for oncoming traffic.

Regular participation in a health-related fitness program can heighten performance of skill-related components and vice versa. For example, significantly overweight people do not have good agility or speed. Because participating in aerobic and strength-training programs helps take off body fat, an overweight individual who loses weight through such an exercise program can improve agility and speed. A sound flexibility program decreases resistance to motion about body joints, which may increase agility, balance, and overall coordination. Improvements in strength definitely help develop power. On the other hand, people who have good skill-related fitness usually participate in lifetime sports and games, which in turn helps develop health-related fitness.

PERFORMANCE TESTS FOR SKILL-RELATED FITNESS

Several performance tests have been developed over the years to assess the various components of skill-related fitness. Results of the performance tests, expressed in percentile ranks, are given in Tables 11.1 (men) and 11.2 (women), at the end of the chapter. Fitness categories for skill-fitness components are established according to percentile rankings only. The categories are similar to those given for muscular strength and endurance, and flexibility (see Table 11.3).

AGILITY

Agility is defined as *the ability to quickly and efficiently change body position and direction.* Agility is important in sports such as basketball, soccer (Figure 11.1), and racquetball, in which the participant must change direction rapidly and also maintain proper body control.

AGILITY TEST
SEMO Agility Test[4]

Objective
To measure general body agility

Procedure
The free throw area of a basketball court or any other smooth area 12 by 19 feet with adequate

FIGURE 11.1
Successful soccer players demonstrate high levels of skill-fitness.

running space around it can be used for this test. Four plastic cones or similar objects are placed on each corner of the free throw lane, as shown in Figure 11.2.

Start on the outside of the free throw lane at point A, with your back to the free throw line. When given the "go" command, sidestep from A to B (do not make crossover steps), backpedal from B to D, sprint forward from D to A, again backpedal from A to C, sprint forward from C to D, and sidestep from B to the finish line at A.

During the test, always go around (outside) each corner cone. (The stopwatch is to be started at the "go" command and stopped when crossing the finish line.) Use the best of two trials, preceded by a practice trial, as the final test score. Record the time to the nearest tenth of a second.

BALANCE

The ability to maintain the body in proper equilibrium, balance is vital in activities such as gymnastics, diving, ice skating, skiing (Figure 11.3), or even football and wrestling, in which the athlete attempts to upset the opponent's equilibrium.

BALANCE TEST
One-Foot Stand Test (preferred foot, without shoes)

Objective
To measure static balance.

Procedure
A flat, smooth floor, not carpeted, is used for this test. Remove your shoes and socks, and stand on your preferred foot, placing the other foot on the inside of the supporting knee and the hands on the sides of the hips. When the "go" command is given, raise your heel off the floor and balance yourself as long as possible without moving the ball of the foot from its initial position (see Figure 11.4).

The test is terminated when any of the following conditions occur:

1. The supporting foot moves (shuffles).
2. The raised heel touches the floor.

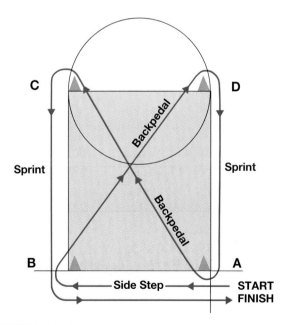

FIGURE 11.2
Graphic description of the SEMO (agility) test.

FIGURE 11.3
Nordic skiing requires good balance, a skill-related component of fitness.

FIGURE 11.4
Balance test.

3. The hands are moved from the hip.
4. A minute has elapsed.

The test is scored by recording the number of seconds balance is maintained on the selected foot, starting with the "go" command. The best of two trials, preceded by a practice trial, is used as the final performance score. Record the time to the nearest tenth of a second.

COORDINATION

Coordination can be defined as *the integration of the nervous and the muscular systems to produce correct, graceful, and harmonious body movements.* This component is important in a wide variety of motor activities such as golf, baseball, karate, soccer, and racquetball, in which hand-eye or foot-eye movements, or both, must be integrated.

COORDINATION TEST
"Soda Pop" Test (see Figure 11.5)

Objective
To assess overall motor/muscular control and movement time

Procedure
Administrator: Homemade equipment is necessary to perform this test. Draw a straight line lengthwise through the center of a piece of cardboard approximately 32″ long by 5″ wide. Draw six marks exactly 5″ away from each other on this line (draw the first mark about 2½″ from the edge of the cardboard). Using a compass, draw six circles 3¼″ in diameter (a radius of 1 centimeter larger than a can of soda pop), which must be centered on the six marks along the line.

For purpose of this test, each circle is assigned a number starting with 1 for the first circle on the right of the subject, all the way to 6 for the last circle on the left. The cardboard, three unopened (full) cans of soda pop, a table, a chair, and a stopwatch are needed to perform the test.

Place the cardboard on a table and have the person sit in front of it with the center of the cardboard bisecting the body. The preferred hand is used for this test. If the right hand is used, place the three cans of pop on the cardboard in the following manner: can 1 centered in circle 1 (farthest to the right), can 2 in circle 3, and can 3 in circle 5.

Participant: To start the test, place the right hand, with the thumb up, on can 1 and the elbow joint at about 100–120°. When the tester gives the signal and the stopwatch is started, proceed to turn the cans of soda pop upside down, placing can 1 inside circle 2, followed by can 2 inside circle 4, and then can 3 inside circle 6. Immediately return all three cans, starting with can 1 (see Figure 11.6), then can

FIGURE 11.5
"Soda pop" (coordination) test.

2, and can 3, turning them right side up to their original placement. On this "return trip," grasp the cans with the hand in a thumb-down position.

The entire procedure is done twice, without stopping, and is counted as one trial. Two "trips" down and up are required to complete one trial. The watch is stopped when the last can of soda pop is returned to its original position, following the second trip back. The preferred hand (in this case, the right hand) is used throughout the entire task, and the object of the test is to perform the task as fast as possible, making sure the cans always are placed within each circle. If the person misses a circle at any time during the test (a can placed on a line or outside a circle), the trial must be repeated from the start. A graphic illustration of this test is provided in Figure 11.6.

If the participant chooses to use the left hand, the same procedure is followed, except the cans are placed starting from the left, with can 1 in circle 6, can 2 in circle 4, and can 3 in circle 2. The procedure is initiated by turning can 1 upside down onto circle 5, can 2 onto circle 3, and so on.

Two practice trials are allowed prior to initiating the test. Two test trials then are administered, and the best time, recorded to the nearest tenth of a second, is used as the test score. If the person has a mistrial (misses a circle), the test is repeated until two successful trials are accomplished.

POWER

Power is defined as *the ability to produce maximum force in the shortest time*. The two components of power are *speed* and *force* (strength). An effective combination of these two components allows a person to produce explosive movements such as in jumping, putting the shot, and spiking/throwing/hitting a ball.

POWER TEST
Standing Long Jump Test[1]

Objective
To measure leg power

Procedure
Administrator: Draw a takeoff line on the floor, and place a 10-foot-long tape measure perpendicular to this line. Have the participant stand with feet several inches apart, centered with the tape measure and toes just behind the takeoff line (see Figure 11.7).

Participant: Prior to the jump, swing your arms backward and bend your knees. Perform the jump by extending your knees and swinging your arms forward at the same time.

The distance is recorded from the takeoff line to the heel or other body part that touches the floor nearest the takeoff line. Three trials are allowed, and the best trial, measured to the nearest inch, becomes the final test score.

FIGURE 11.6
Graphic illustration of the "Soda Pop" (coordination) test.

FIGURE 11.7
Correct placement of the feet for the start of the standing broad jump (power test).

REACTION TIME

Reaction time can be defined as *the time required to initiate a response to a given stimulus.* Good reaction time is important for starts in track and swimming, to react quickly when playing tennis at the net, or in sports such as ping pong, boxing, and karate.

REACTION TIME TEST

"Yardstick" Test (preferred hand)

Objective

To measure hand reaction time in response to a visual stimulus

Procedure

Administrator: For this test you will need a regular yardstick with a shaded "concentration zone" marked on the first 2″ of the stick. Administer the test with the participant sitting in a chair adjacent to a table and the preferred forearm and hand resting on the table.

Participant: As illustrated in Figure 11.8, hold the tips of the thumb and fingers in a "ready to pinch" position, about 1″ apart and 3″ beyond the edge of the table, with the upper edges of the thumb and index finger parallel to the floor. With the person administering the test holding the yardstick near the end and the zero point of the stick even with the upper edge of your thumb and index finger (the administrator may steady the middle of the stick with the other hand), look at the "concentration zone" and react by catching the stick when it is dropped. Do not look at the administrator's hand or move it up or down while trying to catch the stick.

Twelve trials comprise the test, each preceded by the preparatory command "ready." The administrator makes a random 1– to 3–second count between the "ready" command and each drop of the stick. Each trial is scored to the nearest half inch, read just above the upper edge of the thumb. Three practice trials are given before the actual test to be sure the person understands the procedure. The three lowest and the three highest scores are discarded, and the average of the middle six is used as the final test score. The testing area should be as free from distractions as possible.

SPEED

Speed is *the ability to rapidly propel the body or a part of the body from one point to another.* Sprints in track, stealing a base in baseball, soccer, and basketball are examples of activities that require good speed for success.

SPEED TEST

50-Yard Dash[1]

Objective

To measure speed

Procedure

Two participants are preferable. Take your positions behind the starting line. The starter raises one arm and says "Are you ready?" followed by the command "go," simultaneously swinging an arm downward as a signal for the timer (or timers) who stands at the finish line to start the stopwatch (or stopwatches).

The score is the time that elapses between the starting signal and the moment the participant crosses the finish line, recorded to the nearest tenth of a second.

FIGURE 11.8
"Yard Stick" (reaction time) test.

TABLE 11.1
Percentile Ranks and Fitness Classification for Skill-Related Fitness Components — Men

	Agility*	Balance*	Coordination*	Power**	Reaction Time*	Speed**
99	9.5	59.8	5.8	9'10"	3.5	5.4
95	10.3	46.9	7.5	8'5"	4.2	5.9
90	10.6	41.1	7.7	8'2"	4.5	6.0
80	11.1	24.9	8.5	7'10"	4.9	6.3
70	11.5	15.4	8.9	7'7"	5.3	6.4
60	11.7	12.0	9.3	7'5"	5.5	6.5
50	11.9	9.2	9.6	7'2"	5.8	6.6
40	12.1	7.3	9.9	7'0"	6.1	6.8
30	12.4	5.8	10.2	6'8"	6.5	7.0
20	12.9	4.3	10.7	6'4"	6.7	7.1
10	13.7	3.1	11.3	5'10"	7.2	7.5
5	14.0	2.6	11.8	5'3"	7.4	7.9

* Norms developed at Boise State University, Department of Physical Education. Research conducted by Werner W. K. Hoeger, Sherman G. Button, and Troy A. Palmer.
** From *AAHPERD Youth Fitness: Test Manual.* Reproduced with permission.

TABLE 11.2
Percentile Ranks and Fitness Classification for Skill-Related Fitness Components — Women

	Agility*	Balance*	Coordination*	Power**	Reaction Time*	Speed**
99	11.1	59.9	7.5	7'6"	3.3	6.4
95	12.0	39.1	8.0	6'9"	4.5	6.8
90	12.2	25.8	8.2	6'6"	4.7	7.0
80	12.5	16.7	8.6	6'2"	5.1	7.3
70	12.9	11.9	9.0	5'11"	5.3	7.5
60	13.2	9.8	9.2	5'9"	5.9	7.6
50	13.4	7.6	9.5	5'5"	6.1	7.9
40	13.9	6.2	9.6	5'3"	6.4	8.0
30	14.2	5.0	9.9	5'0"	6.7	8.2
20	14.8	4.2	10.3	4'9"	7.2	8.5
10	15.5	2.9	10.7	4'4"	7.8	9.0
5	16.2	1.8	11.2	4'1"	8.4	9.5

* Norms developed at Boise State University, Department of Physical Education. Research conducted by Werner W. K. Hoeger, Sherman G. Button, and Troy A. Palmer.
** From *AAHPERD Youth Fitness: Test Manual.* Reproduced with permission.

TABLE 11.3
Skill-Fitness Categories

Percentile Rank	Fitness Category
≥81	Excellent
61-80	Good
41-60	Average
21-40	Fair
≤20	Poor

L A B O R A T O R Y
E X P E R I E N C E

LAB 11A
Assessment of Skill-Related Components of Fitness

Lab Preparation
Bring exercise clothing, including running shoes. Do not exercise strenuously several hours prior to this lab.

REFERENCES

1. AAHPERD. *Youth Fitness: Test Manual.* Reston, VA: AAHPERD, 1976.
2. Corbin, C. B., and R. Lindsey. *Concepts of Physical Fitness with Laboratories.* Dubuque, IA: Wm. C. Brown Publishers, 1991.
3. Johnson, B. L., and J. K. Nelson. *Practical Measurements for Evaluation in Physical Education.* Minneapolis: Burgess Publishing, 1979.
4. Kirby, R. F. "A Simple Test of Agility." *Coach and Athlete* (June 1971): 30–31.
5. Lepanto, J. D., and F. Compton. *Exercise: For the Health of It.* Dubuque, IA: Kendall/Hunt, 1986.
6. Stokes, R., and A. C. Moore, and C. Moore. *Fitness: The New Wave.* Winston-Salem, NC: Hunter Textbooks, 1986.

PREVENTING CARDIOVASCULAR DISEASE

12

Cardiovascular disease is the leading cause of death in the United States, accounting for nearly half of the total mortality rate in 1990. The disease encompasses any pathological condition that affects the heart and the circulatory system (blood vessels). Some examples of cardiovascular disease are coronary heart disease, peripheral vascular disease, congenital heart disease, rheumatic heart disease, strokes, high blood pressure, congestive heart failure, and atherosclerosis (fatty/cholesterol deposits in the walls of the arteries leading to plaque formation). Cardiovascular disease alone now costs the nation well over $135 billion annually.

Although heart and blood vessel disease is still the number-one health problem in the United States, the incidence has declined by 36% in the last two decades, mainly because of health education. More people now are aware of the risk factors for cardiovascular disease and are changing their lifestyles to lower their own potential risk for this disease.

The major form of cardiovascular disease is **coronary heart disease (CHD)**, a condition in which *the arteries that supply the heart muscle with oxygen and nutrients are narrowed by fatty deposits such as cholesterol and triglycerides.* Narrowing of the coronary arteries diminishes the blood supply to the heart muscle, which can precipitate a heart attack (see Figure 12.1).

> *Almost all of the risk factors for coronary heart disease are preventable and reversible, and risk reduction can be accomplished by the individual.*

CHD is the single leading cause of death in the United States, accounting for approximately a third of all deaths and more than half of all cardiovascular deaths. Oddly enough, almost all of the risk factors for CHD are preventable and reversible, and risk reduction can be accomplished by the individual.

Each year, more than 330,000 coronary bypass operations and 190,000 coronary angioplasty procedures are performed in

THE HEART AND ITS BLOOD VESSELS

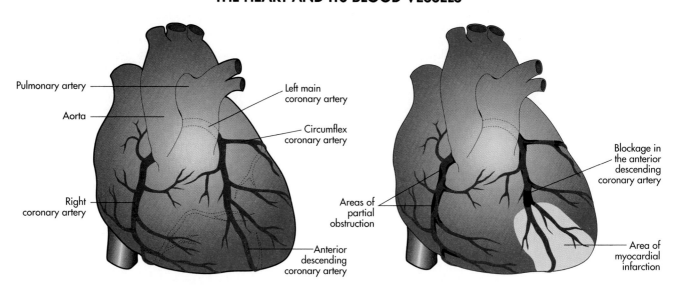

FIGURE 12.1.
Left: a normal/healthy heart. Right: myocardial infarction (heart attack) as a result of acute reduction in blood flow through the anterior descending coronary artery.

the United States. Angioplasty involves inserting a balloon-tipped catheter to widen the inner lumen of the arteries. Health care costs for coronary bypass range between $30,000 and $40,000, and for an angioplasty procedure, $7,500 — or about $11 billion per year for coronary heart disease surgery.

CORONARY HEART DISEASE RISK PROFILE

Although genetic inheritance plays a role in CHD, the most important determinant is personal lifestyle. CHD risk factor analyses are administered to evaluate the impact of a person's lifestyle and genetic endowment as potential factors contributing to the development of coronary disease. The specific objectives of a CHD risk factor analysis are:

■ To screen individuals who may be at high risk for the disease.

■ To educate regarding the leading risk factors for developing CHD.

■ To implement programs aimed at risk reduction.

■ To use the analysis as a starting point from which to compare changes induced by the intervention program.

The leading risk factors contributing to CHD have been identified and are listed in Table 12.1. A

TABLE 12.1
Maximal Number of Risk Points Assigned to the Various Coronary Heart Disease Risk Factors

Risk Factors	Maximal Risk Points
Abnormal cholesterol profile	12
Low HDL-cholesterol	6
High LDL-cholesterol	6
Abnormal stress electrocardiogram	8
Smoking	8
Personal history of heart disease	8
Hypertension	8
Systolic blood pressure	4
Diastolic blood pressure	4
Physical inactivity	8
Diabetes	6
High blood glucose	3
Known diabetes	3
Family history of heart disease	6
Age	4
Excessive body fat	3
Tension and stress	3
Abnormal Resting electrocardiogram	3
Elevated Triglycerides	2

self-assessment CHD risk factor analysis is given in Lab 12A. This CHD risk factor analysis can be done by people with little or no medical information about their cardiovascular health, as well as by those who have had a thorough medical examination. The guidelines for zero risk are outlined for each factor, making this self-assessment analysis a valuable tool in CHD risk factor management.

For example, a person who fills out the form knows that the ideal blood pressure is around 120/80 or lower, that risk is reduced by smoking less or quitting altogether, that HDL-cholesterol should be 45 mg/dl (milligrams per deciliter) or higher for men and 55 mg/dl or higher for women, and that LDL-cholesterol should be less than 170 mg/dl (if unknown, basic nutritional guidelines also are given). The role of HDL- and LDL-cholesterol in protecting against heart disease is discussed later in this chapter.

A risk factor analysis helps to determine the potential effect of lifestyle in the development of coronary heart disease.

To provide a meaningful CHD risk score, a weighing system* was developed to show the impact of each risk factor on developing the disease. This weighing system is based on the latest research and on the work done at leading preventive medicine facilities in the United States. The most significant risk factors are given the heaviest numeric weight.

For example, a poor cholesterol profile seems to be the best predictor for developing CHD. Up to 12 risk points are assigned to individuals with "very high" LDL-cholesterol levels and "very low" HDL-cholesterol levels. On the other hand, the least heavily weighted risk factor is triglycerides. A maximum of only 2 risk points is assigned to this factor. Each risk factor also is assigned a zero risk level, the level at which it does not appear to increase the risk for disease at all.

Based on actual test results, a person receives a score anywhere from zero to the maximum number of points for each factor. When the risk points from all of the risk factors are totaled, the final number is

*The weighing system for the CHD risk factor analysis has been adapted from Hoeger, W. W. K. The Complete Guide for the Development and Implementation of Health Promotion Programs. Englewood, CO: Morton Publishing, 1987.

used to rate an individual in one of five overall risk categories for potential development of CHD (see Lab 12A).

A "very low" CHD risk category designates the group at lowest risk for developing heart disease based on age and gender. "Low" CHD suggests that even though people in this category are taking good care of their cardiovascular health, they can still improve it (unless all of the risk points come from age and family history). "Moderate" CHD risk means the person can definitely improve lifestyle to lower the risk for disease, or medical treatment may be required. A score in the "high" or "very high" CHD risk category points to a strong probability of developing heart disease within the next few years and calls for immediate implementation of a personal risk reduction program, including medical, nutritional, and exercise intervention by professional staff.

With the exception of age, family history of heart disease, and certain electrocardiogram (ECG) abnormalities, the risk factors are preventable and reversible. The leading risk factors for CHD are discussed next, along with the general recommendations for risk reduction.

PHYSICAL INACTIVITY

Physical inactivity is responsible for low levels of cardiovascular endurance, previously defined as the ability of the heart, lungs, and blood vessels to deliver enough oxygen to the cells to meet the demands of prolonged physical activity. The level of cardiovascular endurance (or fitness) is given most commonly by the maximal amount of oxygen (in milliliters) that every kilogram (2.2 pounds) of body weight is able to utilize per minute of physical activity (ml/kg/min). As maximal oxygen uptake increases, so does the efficiency of the cardiovascular system.

Even though physical inactivity has not been assigned the most risk points (8 points for a poor level of fitness, as compared to 12 for a poor cholesterol profile — see Table 12.1), improving cardiovascular endurance through aerobic exercise has a great impact in overall heart disease risk reduction (Figure 12.2).

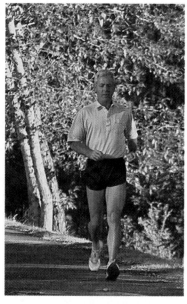

FIGURE 12.2
Lifetime participation in aerobic activities is one of the most important factors in the prevention of cardiovascular disease.

Although specific recommendations can be followed to improve each risk factor, a regular aerobic exercise program helps to control most of the major risk factors that lead to heart disease. Aerobic exercise will:

- Increase cardiovascular endurance.
- Decrease and control blood pressure.
- Reduce body fat.
- Lower blood lipids (cholesterol and triglycerides).
- Improve HDL-cholesterol.
- Help control diabetes.
- Increase and maintain good heart function, sometimes improving certain ECG abnormalities.
- Motivate toward smoking cessation.
- Alleviate tension and stress.
- Counteract a personal history of heart disease.

The significance of physical inactivity in contributing to cardiovascular risk was clearly shown in 1992 when the American Heart Association added physical inactivity as one of the four major risk factors for cardiovascular disease. (The other three factors are smoking, a poor cholesterol profile, and high blood pressure.) In the words of Dr. Kenneth H. Cooper, pioneer of the aerobic movement in the United States, evidence of the benefits of aerobic exercise in reducing heart disease is "far too impressive to be ignored."

Research at the Institute for Aerobics Research in Dallas, Texas, clearly shows the tie between cardiovascular fitness and mortality, regardless of age and other risk factors (see Figure 1.7 in Chapter 1 and Figures 12.8 and 12.11 in this chapter). A higher level of physical fitness benefits even those who have other risk factors such as high blood pressure and serum cholesterol, cigarette smoking, and a family history of heart disease. In most cases, unfit people in the study (group 1) without these risk factors had higher death rates than fit people (groups 4 and 5) with these same risk factors.

Although the findings show that the higher the level of cardiovascular fitness, the longer the life, the largest drop in premature death is seen between the unfit and the moderately fit groups. Even small improvements in cardiovascular endurance, greatly decrease the risk for cardiovascular mortality. Most adults who engage in a moderate exercise program can attain these fitness levels easily.

Subsequent research[34] published in 1993 in the *New England Journal of Medicine* substantiated the importance of exercise in preventing CHD. Dr. Ralph Paffenbarger and colleagues indicated that the benefits of starting a moderate to vigorous physical activity program (by previously inactive adults) were as important as quitting smoking, managing blood pressure, or controlling cholesterol. The increase in physical activity led to the same decrease as giving up cigarette smoking in relative risk for death from CHD.

Even though aerobically fit individuals have a lower incidence of cardiovascular disease, a regular aerobic exercise program by itself does not guarantee a lifetime free of cardiovascular problems. Poor lifestyle habits, such as smoking, eating too many fatty/salty/sweet foods, being overweight, and having high stress levels, increase cardiovascular risk and will not be eliminated completely through aerobic exercise.

Overall risk factor management is the best guideline to lower the risk for cardiovascular disease. Still, aerobic exercise is one of the most important activities in preventing and reducing cardiovascular problems. The basic principles for cardiovascular exercise are given in Chapter 6.

ABNORMAL ELECTROCARDIOGRAM

The electrocardiogram is a valuable measure of the heart's function. The ECG provides a record of the electrical impulses that stimulate the heart to contract (see Figure 12.3). In reading an ECG, five general areas are interpreted: heart rate, heart rhythm, axis of the heart, enlargement or hypertrophy of the heart, and myocardial infarction or heart attack.

On a standard 12-lead ECG, 10 electrodes are placed on the person's chest (see Figure 12.4). From these 10 electrodes, 12 "pictures" or leads of the electrical impulses as they travel through the heart muscle (myocardium) are studied from 12 different positions. By looking at ECG tracings, abnormalities in heart functioning can be identified (see Figure 12.5). Based on the findings, the ECG may be interpreted as normal, equivocal, or abnormal. An

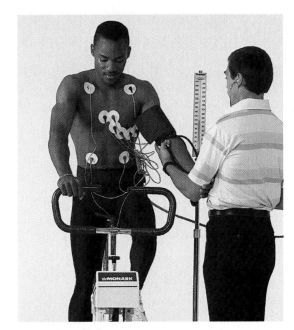

FIGURE 12.4

Exercise tolerance test with 12-lead electrocardiographic monitoring (exercise stress-ECG).

ECG will not always identify problems, so a normal tracing is not an absolute guarantee. On the other hand, an abnormal tracing does not necessarily signal a serious condition.

ECGs are taken at rest, during the stress of exercise (Figure 12.5), and during recovery. An exercise ECG also is known as a graded exercise stress test or a maximal exercise tolerance test. Similar to a high-speed test on a car, a stress ECG reveals the tolerance of the heart to increased physical activity. It is a much better test than a resting ECG to discover CHD.

FIGURE 12.3

Normal electrocardiogram (P wave = atrial depolarization, QRS complex = ventricular depolarization, T wave = ventricular repolarization).

FIGURE 12.5

Abnormal electrocardiogram showing depressed S-T segment. This abnormality is commonly seen during exercise in patients with coronary disease.

Stress ECGs also are used to assess cardiovascular fitness levels, to screen persons for preventive and cardiac rehabilitation programs, to detect abnormal blood pressure response during exercise, and to establish actual or functional maximal heart rate for exercise prescription. The recovery ECG is another important diagnostic tool in monitoring the return of the heart's activity to normal conditions.

An exercise electrocardiogram reveals the tolerance of the heart to increases in physical activity.

Not every adult who wishes to start or continue in an exercise program needs a stress ECG. Some guidelines to determine when this type of test should be administered are:

1. Men over age 40 and women over age 50.
2. A total cholesterol level above 200 mg/dl or an HDL-cholesterol below 35 mg/dl.
3. Hypertensive and diabetic patients.
4. Cigarette smokers.
5. Individuals with a family history of CHD, syncope, or sudden death before age 60.
6. People with an abnormal resting ECG.
7. All individuals with symptoms of chest discomfort, dysrhythmias, syncope, or chronotropic incompetence (heart rate that increases slowly during exercise and never reaches maximum).

At times the stress ECG has been questioned as a reliable predictor of CHD, but it remains the most practical, inexpensive, noninvasive procedure available to diagnose latent (undiagnosed/unknown) CHD. The test is accurate in diagnosing CHD about 65% of the time. Part of the problem with reliability is that many times those who administer stress ECGs do it without clearly understanding the test's indications and limitations. Nevertheless, sensitivity of the test increases along with the severity of the disease. The test also produces more accurate results in people who are at high risk for cardiovascular disease, in particular men over 40 and women over 50 with a poor cholesterol profile, high blood pressure, or a family history of heart disease.

Test protocols, number of leads, electrocardiographic criteria, and the skill of technicians administering the test also affect its sensitivity. In spite of its limitations, it is still a useful tool in identifying people who have high risk for exercise-related sudden death.

ABNORMAL CHOLESTEROL PROFILE

The term "blood lipids" (fats) is used mainly in reference to cholesterol and triglycerides. These lipids are carried in the bloodstream by molecules of protein known as high-density lipoproteins (HDLs), low-density lipoproteins (LDLs), very low-density lipoproteins (VLDLs), and chylomicrons (see Figure 12.6). Although subcategories of these lipoproteins have been identified recently, the discussion here focuses primarily on the four major categories.

Cholesterol has received much attention lately because direct relationships have been established between high total cholesterol, high LDL-cholesterol, low HDL-cholesterol, and the rate of CHD in men and women. *Cholesterol is a waxy substance, technically a steroid alcohol, found only in animal fats and oil.* This fatty substance is used in making cell membranes, as a building block for some hormones, in the fatty sheath around nerve fibers, and in other necessary substances.

An abnormal cholesterol profile contributes to atherosclerotic plaque, the buildup of fatty tissue in the walls of the arteries (see Figure 12.7). As the plaque builds up, it blocks the blood vessels that supply the heart muscle (myocardium) with oxygen and nutrients, and these obstructions can trigger a myocardial infarction or heart attack. Unfortunately, the heart disguises its problems quite well, and typical symptoms of heart disease, such as angina pectoris or chest pain, do not start until the arteries are about 75% blocked. In many cases the first symptom is sudden death. Based on the research conducted at the Institute for Aerobics Research in Dallas, Texas, the relative risk for all causes of mortality by physical fitness and total cholesterol levels is given in Figure 12.8.

The general recommendation by the National Cholesterol Education Program (NCEP) is to keep total cholesterol levels below 200 mg/dl. Other health professionals recommend that total cholesterol in individuals age 30 and younger should not be higher than 180 mg/dl, and for children the level should be below 170 mg/dl. Cholesterol levels

FIGURE 12.6
Approximate content of the four major types of lipo-proteins.

community of Framingham, Massachusetts, not a single individual with a total cholesterol level of 125 mg/dl or lower has had a heart attack. Dr. William Castelli, director of the Framingham Study, recommends a total cholesterol level of less than 150 mg/dl for possible plaque regression in people with atherosclerosis.

Perhaps even more significant is the way in which cholesterol is carried in the bloodstream. Cholesterol is transported primarily in the form of high-density lipoprotein cholesterol (HDL-cholesterol) and low-density lipoprotein cholesterol (LDL-cholesterol). HDL molecules tend to attract cholesterol, which is carried to the liver, changed to bile, and eventually excreted in the stool. HDLs act as "scavengers," removing cholesterol from the body and preventing plaque from forming in the arteries.

LDL-cholesterol, on the other hand, tends to release cholesterol, which then may penetrate the lining of the arteries and speed up the process of atherosclerosis. The NCEP guidelines state that an LDL-cholesterol value below 130 mg/dl is desirable, between 130 and 159 mg/dl is borderline-high, and 160 mg/dl and above is high risk for cardiovascular disease. For people with atherosclerosis, Dr. William Castelli, director of the Framingham Study, recommends an LDL-cholesterol level of 90 mg/dl or lower. A recently discovered subcategory of LDL-cholesterol, a smaller and denser LDL particle, is noteworthy because these particles are a bigger culprit in atherosclerosis than the regular LDL particles.

between 200 and 239 mg/dl are borderline high, and levels of 240 mg/dl and above indicate high risk for disease.

Many preventive medicine practitioners recommend a range between 160 and 180 mg/dl as the ideal level of total cholesterol. In the Framingham Heart Study, a 40-year ongoing project in the

Normal artery

Early stage of atherosclerosis

Progression of the atherosclerotic plaque

Advanced stage of atherosclerosis

FIGURE 12.7
The atherosclerotic process.

MEN

WOMEN

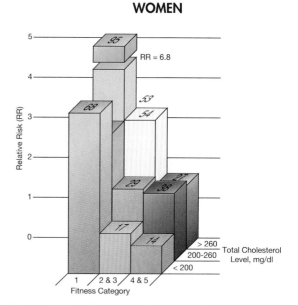

Source: Physical Fitness and All-Cause Mortality: A Prospective Study of Healthy Men and Women, by S. N. Blair, H. W. Kohl III, R. S. Paffenbarger, Jr., D. G. Clark, K. H. Cooper, and L. W. Gibbons, in *Journal of the American Medical Association* 262 (1989): 2395-2401. © American Medical Association. Reproduced by permission.

FIGURE 12.8
Relative risks of all-cause mortality by physical fitness and *serum cholesterol level*. Numbers on top of the bars are all-cause death rates per 10,000 person-years of follow-up for each cell — 1 person-year indicates one person that was followed up one year later. Fitness group 1 is the least fit group, fitness group 5 is the most fit group.

The more HDL-cholesterol (particularly the subcategory HDL_2), the better. HDL-cholesterol, the "good cholesterol" offers some protection against heart disease. In fact, *low levels of HDL-cholesterol could be the best predictor of CHD and may be more significant than the total value*. A low level of HDL-cholesterol has the strongest relationship to CHD at all levels of total cholesterol, including levels below 200 mg/dl.[38]

Researchers at the 1988 annual American Heart Association meeting indicated that people with low total cholesterol (less than 200 mg/dl) and also low HDL-cholesterol (under 40 mg/dl) may have three times greater heart disease risk than those with high cholesterol but with good HDL-cholesterol levels. Other research based on 797 patients whose total cholesterol was less than 200 mg/dl showed that 60% of the patients had heart disease, and almost 75% of this group had HDL-cholesterol levels below 40 mg/dl. The recommended HDL-cholesterol values to minimize the risk for CHD are 45 and 55 mg/dl (or higher) for men and women, respectively.

For the most part, HDL-cholesterol is determined genetically. Generally, women have higher levels than men. The female sex hormone estrogen tends to raise HDL, so premenopausal women have a much lower incidence of heart disease. Black children and adult Black men have higher values than Caucasians. HDL-cholesterol also decreases with age.

Increasing HDL-cholesterol improves the cholesterol profile and lessens the risk for CHD. Habitual aerobic exercise, weight loss, and quitting smoking raise HDL-cholesterol.[16] Beta-carotene,[14] and drug therapy also promote higher HDL-cholesterol levels.

HDL-cholesterol and a regular aerobic exercise program clearly are related, but the exercise program has to be intense to lower LDL and raise HDL. Exercising 20 minutes three times a week may not be enough to alter the lipid profile. Individual responses to aerobic exercise differ, but, generally, the more the exercise, the higher the HDL-cholesterol level. Aerobic exercise five to six times a week and up to 60 minutes a session in the proper heart rate target zone may be needed to see results.

As discussed in Chapter 2, the antioxidant effect of vitamins C and E and beta-carotene also can reduce the risk for CHD.[14] New information suggests that a single unstable free radical (oxygen compounds produced in normal metabolism) can damage LDL particles. Vitamin C seems to inactivate free radicals, and vitamin E protects LDL from oxidation. Beta-carotene not only absorbs free radicals, keeping them from causing damage, but it also seems to increase HDL levels.

Certain cholesterol-lowering drugs also may help raise HDL levels. These agents include colestipol, niacin, cholestyramine, and gemfibrozil.[38] Cholesterol-lowering drugs decrease absorption in the intestines or block cholesterol formation by the cells. Some experts believe HDL levels below 40 mg/dl in combination with triglycerides above 150 mg/dl should be treated with medication.

Many authorities also believe the ratio of LDL-cholesterol to HDL-cholesterol is a strong indicator of potential risk for cardiovascular disease. An LDL-cholesterol to HDL-cholesterol ratio of 3.5 or lower is excellent for men, and 3.0 or lower is best for women. For instance, 50 mg/dl of HDL-cholesterol, as compared to 150 mg/dl of LDL-cholesterol, translates to a ratio of 3.0 (150 ÷ 50 = 3.0).

Although the average American consumes between 400 and 600 mg of cholesterol daily, the body actually manufactures more than that. Saturated fats raise cholesterol levels more than anything else in the diet. Saturated fats produce approximately 1000 mg of cholesterol per day. Because of individual differences, some people can have a higher than normal intake of saturated fats and still maintain normal levels. Others who have a lower intake can have abnormally high levels.

Saturated fats are found mostly in meats and dairy products but seldom in foods of plant origin (see Table 12.2). Poultry and fish contain less saturated fat than beef but should be eaten in moderation (about 3 to 6 ounces per day—see Chapter 2). Unsaturated fats are mainly of plant origin and cannot be converted to cholesterol.

If LDL-cholesterol is higher than ideal, it can be lowered by losing body fat, manipulating the diet, and taking medication. A diet low in fat, saturated fat, and cholesterol (Figure 12.9), and high in fiber is recommended to decrease LDL-cholesterol. The NCEP recommends replacing saturated fat with monounsaturated fat (for example, olive, canola, peanut, and sesame oils), because the latter does not cause a reduction in HDL-cholesterol (also see the discussion on saturated fatty acids in Chapter 2).

Many experts believe that, to have a real effect in lowering LDL-cholesterol, total fat consumption must be much lower than the current 30% of total daily caloric intake guideline. Saturated fat consumption has to be under 10% of the total daily

TABLE 12.2
Cholesterol and Saturated Fat Content of Selected Foods

Food	Serving Size	Cholesterol (mg.)	Sat. Fat (gr.)
Avocado	1/8 med.	—	3.2
Bacon	2 slc.	30	2.7
Beans (all types)	any	—	—
Beef — Lean, fat trimmed off	3 oz.	75	6.0
Beef — Heart (cooked)	3 oz.	150	1.6
Beef — Liver (cooked)	3 oz.	255	1.3
Butter	1 tsp.	12	0.4
Caviar	1 oz.	85	—
Cheese — American	2 oz.	54	11.2
Cheese — Cheddar	2 oz.	60	12.0
Cheese — Cottage (1% fat)	1 cup	10	0.4
Cheese — Cottage (4% fat)	1 cup	31	6.0
Cheese — Cream	2 oz.	62	6.0
Cheese — Muenster	2 oz.	54	10.8
Cheese — Parmesan	2 oz.	38	9.3
Cheese — Swiss	2 oz.	52	10.0
Chicken (no skin)	3 oz.	45	0.4
Chicken — Liver	3 oz.	472	1.1
Chicken — Thigh, Wing	3 oz.	69	3.3
Egg (yolk)	1	250	1.8
Frankfurter	2	90	11.2
Fruits	any	—	—
Grains (all types)	any	—	—
Halibut, Flounder	3 oz.	43	0.7
Ice Cream	1/2 cup	27	4.4
Lamb	3 oz.	60	7.2
Lard	1 tsp.	5	1.9
Lobster	3 oz.	170	0.5
Margarine (all vegetable)	1 tsp.	—	0.7
Mayonnaise	1 tbsp.	10	2.1
Milk — Skim	1 cup	5	0.3
Milk — Low Fat (2%)	1 cup	18	2.9
Milk — Whole	1 cup	34	5.1
Nuts	1 oz.	—	1.0
Oysters	3 oz.	42	—
Salmon	3 oz.	30	0.8
Scallops	3 oz.	29	—
Sherbet	1/2 cup	7	1.2
Shrimp	3 oz.	128	0.1
Trout	3 oz.	45	2.1
Tuna (canned — drained)	3 oz.	55	—
Turkey — Dark Meat	3 oz.	60	0.6
Turkey — Light Meat	3 oz.	50	0.4
Vegetables (except avocado)	any	—	—

FIGURE 12.9
Substituting low-fat for high-fat products in the diet decreases the risk for disease.

caloric intake, and the average cholesterol consumption should be much lower than 300 mg per day.

Research studies on the effects of a 30% fat diet have shown that it has little or no effect in lowering cholesterol, and that CHD actually continues to progress in people who have the disease. The good news comes from a 1991 study published in the *Archives of Internal Medicine*.[3] Men and women in the study lowered their cholesterol by an average of 23% in only 3 weeks following a 10% or less fat-calorie diet combined with a regular aerobic exercise program, primarily walking. In this diet, cholesterol intake was less than 25 mg/day. The author of the study concluded that the exact percent-fat guideline (10% or 15%) is unknown (it also varies from individual to individual), but that 30% total fat calories is definitely too high a level when attempting to lower cholesterol.

A daily 10%-total-fat diet requires the person to limit fat intake to an absolute minimum. Some health care professionals contend that a diet like this is difficult to follow indefinitely. People with high cholesterol levels, however, may not need to follow that diet indefinitely but should adopt the 10%-fat diet while attempting to lower cholesterol. Thereafter, eating a 30%-fat-diet may be adequate to maintain recommended cholesterol levels (1991 national data indicate that current fat consumption in the United States averages 37% of total calories; see Figure 2.7, Chapter 2).

To lower LDL-cholesterol levels, the following general dietary guidelines are recommended:

1. Fewer than three eggs per week.
2. Red meats (3 ounces per serving) fewer than three times per week, and no organ meats (such as liver and kidneys).
3. No commercially baked foods.
4. Low-fat milk (1% or less fat, preferably) and low-fat dairy products.
5. No coconut oil, palm oil, or cocoa butter.
6. Fish, especially fish high in Omega-3 fatty acids (fresh or frozen mackerel, herring, tuna, salmon, and lake trout) twice a week.
7. Baking, broiling, grilling, poaching, or steaming food instead of frying.
8. Removing fat from cooked meat. This can be done by refrigerating it so the fat hardens and can be easily removed.
9. Avoiding fatty sauces made with butter, cream, or cheese.
10. Attaining recommended body weight.

A combination of a healthy diet, sound aerobic exercise program, and weight control is the best prescription for controlling blood lipids. If this does not work, a physician can administer a blood test to break down the lipoproteins into their various subcategories. Most U. S. laboratories, however, do not conduct these tests. Starting in 1991, the American Heart Association established six Lipid Disorder Training Centers that administer comprehensive blood tests. Your local American Heart Association can provide further information.

The NCEP guidelines recommend that people consider drug therapy if, after six months on a low-cholesterol, low-fat diet, cholesterol remains unacceptably high. An unacceptable level is above 190 mg/dl for people with fewer than two risk factors and no signs of heart disease. For people with more than two risk factors and with a history of heart disease, LDL-cholesterol should be below 160 mg/dl.

ELEVATED TRIGLYCERIDES

Triglycerides are also known as *free fatty acids*. In combination with cholesterol, triglycerides speed up the formation of plaque in the arteries. Triglycerides are carried in the bloodstream primarily by very low-density lipoproteins (VLDLs) and chylomicrons.

Although they are found in poultry skin, lunch meats, and shellfish, these fatty acids are manufactured mainly in the liver, from refined sugars, starches, and alcohol. High intake of alcohol and sugars (honey included) significantly raises triglyceride levels. Triglycerides can be lowered by cutting down on these foods along with reducing weight (if overweight) and doing aerobic exercise. An optimal blood triglyceride level is less than 125 mg/dl.

Some people consistently have slightly elevated triglyceride levels (above 140 mg/dl) and HDL-cholesterol levels below 35 mg/dl. About 80% of these people have a genetic condition called LDL phenotype B (approximately 40% of the U. S. population falls in this category). Although the blood lipids may not be notably high, these people are at higher risk for atherosclerosis and CHD.[41]

People who have never had a blood chemistry test should do so, to establish a baseline for future reference. The blood test should include the HDL-cholesterol component. A summary of desirable blood lipid ranges is provided in Figure 12.10.

No definitive guidelines have been set forth, but if the person follows an initial normal baseline test and adheres to the recommended dietary and exercise guidelines, a blood analysis every 3 years prior to age of 35 should suffice. Thereafter, a blood lipid test is recommended every year, in conjunction with a regular preventive medicine physical examination.

A single baseline test is not necessarily a valid measure. Cholesterol levels vary from month to month and sometimes even from day to day. If the initial test reveals cholesterol abnormalities, the test should be repeated within a few weeks to confirm the results.

STANDARDS FOR BLOOD LIPIDS

Total Cholesterol	≤200 mg/dl	Desirable
	201-239 mg/dl	Borderline high
	≥240 mg/dl	High risk
LDL-Cholesterol	≤130 mg/dl	Desirable
	131-159 mg/dl	Borderline high
	≥160 mg/dl	High risk
HDL-Cholesterol	≥45 mg/dl	Desirable
	36-44 mg/dl	Borderline high
	≤35 mg/dl	High risk
Triglycerides	≤125 mg/dl	Desirable
	126-499 mg/dl	Borderline high
	≥500 mg/dl	High risk

FIGURE 12.10
Standards for blood lipids.

DIABETES

Diabetes mellitus is a condition in which the blood glucose is unable to enter the cells because the pancreas either totally stops producing insulin or does not produce enough to meet the body's needs. As a result, glucose absorption by the cells and the liver is low, leading to high glucose levels in the blood.

The incidence of cardiovascular disease and death in the diabetic population is quite high. People with chronically high blood glucose levels also may have problems metabolizing fats, making them more susceptible to atherosclerosis, increasing the risk for coronary disease, and contributing to other conditions such as vision loss and kidney damage.

Fasting blood glucose levels above 120 mg/dl may be an early sign of diabetes and should be brought to the attention of a physician. Many health care practitioners consider blood glucose levels around 150 to 160 mg/dl as borderline diabetes.

A single cholesterol test may not be a true indicator of a person's regular cholesteral values.

Diabetes is of two types: Type I, or insulin-dependent diabetes, and Type II, or non-insulin-dependent diabetes. **Type I** also is called juvenile diabetes because it is found mainly in young people. In insulin-dependent diabetes, the pancreas produces little or no insulin. In **Type II**, often referred to as adult-onset diabetes, the insulin-producing cells function adequately but the body is unable to use insulin correctly.

Although there is a genetic predisposition to diabetes, adult-onset diabetes is related closely to overeating, obesity, and lack of physical activity. In most cases, this condition can be corrected through a special diet, a weight-loss program, and a regular exercise program.

A diet high in water-soluble fibers (found in fruits, vegetables, oats, and beans) is helpful in treating diabetes. A simple aerobic exercise program (walking, cycling, or swimming four to five times a week) often is prescribed because it increases the body's sensitivity to insulin. Individuals who have high blood glucose levels should consult a physician to decide on the best treatment.

According to research published in 1991 in the *New England Journal of Medicine*,[19] aerobic exercise helps prevent diabetes in middle-aged men. The protective effect is even greater in those with risk factors such as obesity, high blood pressure, and family propensity.

The preventive effect is attributed to less body fat and better sugar and fat metabolism resulting from regular exercise program. At 3,500 calories per week, the risk was cut in half, as compared to sedentary men. This preventive effect, according to one of the authors of the study, should hold for women, too.

HYPERTENSION

Some 60,000 miles of blood vessels run through the human body. As the heart forces the blood through these vessels, the fluid is under pressure. Blood pressure is a measure of the force exerted against the walls of the vessels by the blood flowing through them. Blood pressure is measured in milliliters of mercury (mmHg), usually expressed in two numbers. The higher number reflects the pressure exerted during the forceful contraction of the heart or systole (therefore, the term systolic pressure), and the lower pressure is taken during the heart's relaxation, or diastolic phase, when no blood is being ejected. Ideal blood pressure is 120/80 or below.

STANDARDS

A few years ago, a systolic pressure of 100 plus your age was the acceptable standard. Hypertension was viewed as the point at which the pressure doubled the mortality risk, about 160/96. Readings between 140/90 and 160/96 (either number being in that range) were classified as mild hypertension.

This is no longer the case. Statistical evidence now indicates that blood pressure readings above 140/90 increase the risk for disease and premature death. Consequently, the American Heart Association revised its standards in 1986 and now considers all blood pressures above 140/90 as hypertension.

Even though the threshold for hypertension has been set at 140/90, many experts believe that the lower the blood pressure, the better. Even if the

pressure is around 90/50, as long as that person does not have any symptoms of low blood pressure, or hypotension, he or she need not be concerned. Typical hypotension symptoms are dizziness, lightheadedness, and fainting.

Hypertensive people who are physically active have a lower relative risk of all cause mortality than inactive individuals with normal blood pressure.

Blood pressure also may fluctuate during a regular day. Many factors affect blood pressure, and one single reading may not be a true indicator of your real pressure. For example, physical activity and stress increase blood pressure, and rest and relaxation decrease it. Consequently, several measurements should be taken before diagnosing high pressure.

Based on 1993 estimates by the American Heart Association, nearly 61 million adults and 2.8 million children (6 to 17 years old) in the United States are hypertensive. As a disease, hypertension has been referred to as the silent killer. It does not hurt, it does not make you feel sick, and, unless you check it, years may go by before you even realize you have a problem. High blood pressure is a risk factor not only for CHD, but also for congestive heart failure, strokes, and kidney failure. The relative risk for all-cause mortality by systolic blood pressure and various fitness levels is shown in Figure 12.11.

WHAT MAKES HYPERTENSION A KILLER

All inner walls of arteries are lined by a layer of smooth endothelial cells. Blood lipids cannot penetrate the lining and build up unless damage is done to the cells. High blood pressure is thought to be a leading contributor to destruction of this lining. As blood pressure rises, so does the risk for atherosclerosis. The higher the pressure, the greater is the damage to the arterial wall, making the vessels susceptible to fat deposits, especially if serum cholesterol also is high. Blockage of the coronary vessels decreases blood supply to the heart muscle and can lead to heart attacks. When brain arteries are involved, strokes may follow.

A clear example of the connection between high blood pressure and atherosclerosis can be seen by

Source: Physical Fitness and All-Cause Mortality: A Prospective Study of Healthy Men and Women, by S. N. Blair, H. W. Kohl III, R. S. Paffenbarger, Jr., D. G. Clark, K. H. Cooper, and L. W. Gibbons, in *Journal of the American Medical Association* 262 (1989): 2395-2401. © American Medical Association. Reproduced by permission.

FIGURE 12.11
Relative risks of all-cause mortality by physical fitness and systolic blood pressure. All-cause death rates per 10,000 person-years of follow-up for each cell; 1 person-year indicates one person that was followed up 1 year later. Fitness group 1 is the least fit group; fitness group 5 is the most fit group.

comparing blood vessels in the human body. Even when atherosclerosis is present throughout major arteries, fatty plaques rarely are seen in the pulmonary artery, which goes from the right part of the heart to the lungs. The pressure in this artery normally is below 40 mmHg, and at such low pressure significant deposits do not occur. This is one of the reasons people with low blood pressure have a lower incidence of cardiovascular disease.

Constantly elevated blood pressure also causes the heart to work much harder. At first the heart does well, but in time this continual strain produces an enlarged heart, followed by congestive heart failure. Furthermore, high blood pressure damages blood vessels to the kidneys and eyes, which may result in kidney failure and loss of vision.

TREATMENT

Of all hypertension, 90% has no definite cause. Referred to as *essential hypertension*, this type is treatable. Aerobic exercise, weight reduction, a low-sodium/high-potassium diet, stress reduction, no smoking, a diet designed to lower blood lipids, lower caffeine and alcohol intake, and antihypertensive

medication have all been used effectively to treat essential hypertension.

The remaining 10% of hypertensive cases is caused by pathological conditions such as narrowing of the kidney arteries, glomerulonephritis (a kidney disease), tumors of the adrenal glands, and narrowing of the aortic artery. With this type of hypertension, the pathological cause has to be treated first to correct the blood pressure problem.

Antihypertensive medicines often are the first choice of treatment, but they produce many side effects, such as lethargy, sleepiness, sexual difficulties, higher blood cholesterol and glucose levels, lower potassium levels, and elevated uric acid levels. A physician may end up treating these side effects as much as the hypertension itself. Because of the multiple side effects, about half of the patients stop taking the medication within the first year of treatment.

Another factor contributing to elevated blood pressure is too much sodium in the diet (salt, or sodium chloride, contains approximately 40% sodium). With high sodium intake the body retains more water, which increases the blood volume and, in turn, drives up the pressure. On the other hand, high intake of potassium seems to regulate water retention and lower the pressure slightly.

Although sodium is essential for normal body functions, the body can function with as little as 200 mg, or a tenth of a teaspoon daily. Even under strenuous conditions of job and sports participation that incite heavy perspiration, the amount of sodium required is seldom more than 3,000 mg per day. Yet, sodium intake in the typical American diet ranges between 6,000 and 20,000 mg per day!

Hypertension is practically unknown in populations where daily sodium intake rarely exceeds 2,000 mg.

In underdeveloped countries and American Indian tribes where no salt is used in cooking or added at the table, and the only sodium comes from food in its natural form, daily intake rarely is more than 2,000 mg. Blood pressure in these people does not get higher with age, and hypertension is practically unknown. These findings suggest that the human body may be able to handle 2,000 mg per day, but intakes higher than that over the years may cause a gradual rise in blood pressure.

Where does all the sodium come from? The answer is found in Table 12.3. Most people do not realize the amount of sodium in various foods (the list in Table 12.3 does not include salt added at the table).

A recent national dietary survey has linked calcium deficiency to high blood pressure. Magnesium supplementation also has been used to lower blood pressure in patients with hypertensive encephalopathy (brain dysfunction) and in those affected by diuretic-induced low magnesium levels. No evidence at this point shows lower blood pressure in people with normal magnesium levels.

When treating high blood pressure (unless it is extremely high), before recommending medication many sports medicine physicians recommend a combination of aerobic exercise, weight loss, and less sodium in the diet. In most instances, this treatment brings blood pressure under control.

The link between hypertension and obesity has been well-established. Not only does blood volume increase with excess body fat, but every additional pound of fat requires an estimated extra mile of blood vessels to feed this tissue. Furthermore, blood capillaries are constricted by the adipose tissues as these vessels run through them. As a result, the heart muscle must work harder to pump the blood through a longer, constricted network of blood vessels.

The role of aerobic exercise in managing blood pressure is becoming more important each day. On the average, cardiovascularly fit individuals have lower blood pressures than unfit people do. An 18-year follow-up study on exercising and nonexercising subjects showed much lower blood pressures in the active group. The exercise group had an average resting blood pressure of 120/79 as compared to 150/90 for the nonexercise group (see Table 12.4).

Aerobic exercise often is prescribed for hypertensive patients. Several well-documented studies have shown that nearly 90% of hypertensive patients who begin a moderate aerobic exercise program can expect a notable decrease in blood pressure after only a few weeks of training. The research data also show that exercise, not weight loss, is the major contributor to the lowered blood pressure of exercisers. If aerobic exercise is discontinued, these changes are not maintained.

A moderate exercise program appears to have the best effect in lowering blood pressure.

Research presented by Dr. Larry Gibbons (Institute for Aerobics Research, Dallas, Texas) at the 1990 American College of Sports Medicine meeting also indicates that exercise programs for hypertensive patients should be of moderate intensity. Training at about 50% of heart rate reserve seems to have the same effect in lowering blood pressure as training at a 70% heart rate reserve. High-intensity training in hypertensive patients actually may cause the blood pressure to rise slightly. Even so, a person may be better off to be highly fit and have high blood pressure than to be unfit and have low blood pressure. As illustrated in Figure 12.11, the death rates for unfit individuals with low systolic blood pressure are much higher than in highly fit people with high systolic blood pressure.

The best tip, though, is to take a preventive approach. Keeping blood pressure under control is easier than trying to bring it down once it is high. Regardless of your past blood pressure history, high or low, you should check it routinely. Regular

TABLE 12.3
Sodium, Potassium, Calcium, and Magnesium Levels of Selected Foods

Food	Serving Size	Sodium (mg)	Potassium (mg)	Calcium (mg)	Magnesium (mg)
Apple	1 med.	1	182	10	6
Asparagus	1 cup	2	330	26	24
Avocado	1/2	4	680	11	39
Banana	1 med.	1	440	8	33
Bologna	3 oz.	1,107	133	6	12
Bouillon Cube	1	960	4	0	0
Cantaloupe	1/4	17	341	20	22
Carrot (raw)	1	34	225	27	12
Cheese					
American	2 oz.	614	93	376	16
Cheddar	2 oz.	342	56	408	16
Muenster	2 oz.	356	77	406	16
Parmesan	2 oz.	1,056	53	672	24
Swiss	2 oz.	148	64	410	16
Chicken (light meat)	6 oz.	108	700	20	20
Corn (canned)	1/2 cup	195	80	4	15
Corn (natural)	1/2 cup	3	136	2	29
Frankfurter	1	627	136	4	5
Haddock	6 oz.	300	594	66	41
Hamburger (reg)	1	500	321	63	25
Lamb (leg)	6 oz.	108	700	18	22
Milk (whole)	1 cup	120	351	288	33
Milk (skim)	1 cup	126	406	296	28
Orange	1 med.	1	263	54	13
Orange Juice	1 cup	1	200	26	27
Peach	1 med.	2	308	14	9
Pear	1 med.	2	130	13	9
Peas (canned)	1/2 cup	200	82	22	20
Peas (boiled-natural)	1/2 cup	2	178	18	24
Pizza (cheese - 14" diam.)	1/8	456	85	110	25
Potato	1 med.	6	763	14	75
Potato Chips	10	150	226	8	25
Potato (french fries)	10	5	427	12	40
Pork	6 oz.	96	438	17	25
Roast Beef	6 oz.	98	448	15	27
Salami	3 oz.	1,047	170	12	5
Salmon (canned)	6 oz.	198	756	262	50
Salt	1 tsp.	2,132	0	14	7
Soups					
Chicken Noodle	1 cup	979	55	17	5
Clam Chowder					
(New England)	1 cup	914	146	43	7
Cream of Mushroom	1 cup	955	98	191	5
Vegetable Beef	1 cup	1,046	162	12	6
Soy Sauce	1 tsp.	1,123	22	13	2
Spaghetti (tomato sauce and cheese)	6 oz.	648	276	54	20
Strawberries	1 cup	1	244	31	16
Tomato (raw)	1 med.	3	444	12	11
Tuna (drained)	3 oz.	38	255	7	0

TABLE 12.4
Effects of a Regular Aerobic Exercise Program*
on Resting Blood Pressure: An 18-Year Follow-
up Study**

	Initial	Final
Exercise Group		
Age	44.6	68.0
Blood Pressure	120/79	120/78
Nonexercise Group		
Age	51.6	69.7
Blood Pressure	135/85	150/90

*The aerobic exercise program consisted of an average four
training sessions per week, each 66 minutes long, at about 76
percent of heart rate reserve.

**Based on data from Kash, F. W., J. L. Boyer, S. P. Van Camp,
L. S. Verity, and J. P. Wallace. "The Effect of Physical Activity
on Aerobic Power in Older Men (A Longitudinal Study)." *The
Physician and Sports Medicine* 18(4):73–83, 1990.

physical exercise, weight control, a low-salt diet, no smoking, and stress management are the keys to controlling blood pressure.

Those who are taking medication for hypertension should not stop unless the prescribing physician gives the go-ahead. If it is not treated properly, high blood pressure can kill. By combining medication with the other treatments, drug therapy eventually may be reduced or completely eliminated.

EXCESSIVE BODY FAT

Body composition refers to the ratio of lean body weight to fat weight. If the body contains too much fat, the person is considered obese (see guidelines in Chapter 3, Table 3.7).

Obesity has long been recognized as a risk factor for CHD. Until a few years ago, experts believed that CHD actually was brought on by some of the other risk factors that usually accompany obesity (higher cholesterol and triglycerides, hypertension, diabetes, lower level of cardiovascular fitness). More recent evidence, however, suggests that too much body fat is a serious coronary risk factor in and of itself. Even when all of the other risk factors are in good range, people with body fat percentages higher than the recommended standard have a higher incidence of coronary disease.

Attaining recommended body composition is important not only in lowering the risk for cardiovascular disease but also in reaching a better state of health and wellness. The only positive thing that can be said about too much body fat is that it can be lost through a combination of diet and exercise. Dieting by itself seldom works.

If you have a weight problem and want to get down to your recommended weight, you must: (a) increase your physical activity; (b) follow a diet low in fat and refined sugars and high in complex carbohydrates and fiber; and (c) moderately reduce your total caloric intake while still getting the necessary nutrients to sustain normal body functions. Additional recommendations for weight reduction and weight control are discussed in Chapter 4.

SMOKING

More than 48 million adults and 3.5 million adolescents in the United States smoke. Cigarette smoking is the single largest preventable cause of illness and premature death in the United States. Smoking has been linked to cardiovascular disease, cancer, bronchitis, emphysema, and peptic ulcers. In relation to coronary disease, not only does smoking speed up the process of atherosclerosis, but it also carries a threefold increase in the risk of sudden death following a myocardial infarction.

> *Smoking presents a much greater risk of death from heart disease than from lung disease.*

Smoking prompts the release of nicotine and some other 1,200 toxic compounds into the bloodstream. Similar to hypertension, many of these substances are destructive to the inner membrane that protects the walls of the arteries. As mentioned, once the lining is damaged, cholesterol and triglycerides can be deposited readily in the arterial wall. As the plaque builds up, it obstructs blood flow through the arteries.

Furthermore, smoking encourages the formation of blood clots, which can completely block an artery already narrowed by atherosclerosis. In addition, carbon monoxide, a by-product of cigarette smoke, decreases the blood's oxygen-carrying capacity. A combination of obstructed arteries, less oxygen, and nicotine in the heart muscle heightens the risk for a serious heart problem.

Smoking also increases heart rate, raises blood pressure, and irritates the heart, which can trigger fatal cardiac arrhythmias (irregular heart rhythms). Another harmful effect is a decrease in HDL-cholesterol, the "good" type that helps control blood lipids. Smoking actually presents a much greater risk of death from heart disease than from lung disease.

Pipe and cigar smoking and chewing tobacco also increase the risk for heart disease. Even if the smoker inhales no smoke, he or she absorbs toxic substances through the membranes of the mouth, and these end up in the bloodstream. Individuals who use tobacco in any of these three forms also have a much greater risk for cancer of the oral cavity.

The risk for both cardiovascular disease and cancer starts to decrease the moment you quit smoking. The risk approaches that of a lifetime non-smoker 10 and 15 years, respectively, after quitting. A more thorough discussion of the harmful effects of cigarette smoking, the benefits of quitting, and a complete program for quitting are detailed in Chapter 15.

TENSION AND STRESS

Tension and stress have become a part of life. Everyone has to deal daily with goals, deadlines, responsibilities, pressures. Almost everything in life (whether positive or negative) is a source of stress. The stressor itself is not what creates the health hazard but, rather, the individual's response to it.

The human body responds to stress by producing more catecholamines (hormones) to prepare the body for "fight or flight." These hormones increase heart rate, blood pressure, and blood glucose levels, enabling the person to take action. If the person fights or flees, the higher levels of catecholamines are metabolized and the body is able to return to a normal state. If, however, a person is under constant stress and unable to take action (as in the death of a

close relative or friend, loss of a job, trouble at work, financial insecurity), the catecholamines remain elevated in the bloodstream.

People who are not able to relax will experience a constant low-level strain on the cardiovascular system that could manifest itself in heart disease. In addition, when a person is in a stressful situation, the coronary arteries that feed the heart muscle constrict, reducing the oxygen supply to the heart. If the blood vessels are largely blocked by atherosclerosis, abnormal heart rhythms or even a heart attack may follow.

Individuals who are under a lot of stress and do not cope well with it need to take measures to counteract the effects of stress in their lives. One way is to identify the sources of stress and learn how to cope with them. People need to take control of themselves, examine and act upon the things that are most important in their lives, and ignore less meaningful details.

Physical activity is one of the best ways to relieve stress (Figure 12.12). When a person takes part in physical activity, the body metabolizes excess catecholamines and is able to return to a normal state. Exercise also steps up muscular activity, which contributes to muscular relaxation after completing the physical activity.

Many executives in large cities are choosing the evening hours for their physical activity programs, stopping after work at the health or fitness club. In doing this, they are able to "burn up" the excess tension accumulated during the day and enjoy the evening hours. This has proven to be one of the best

FIGURE 12.12
Physical activity is one of the best ways to relieve stress.

stress management techniques. More information on stress management techniques is presented in Chapter 14.

PERSONAL AND FAMILY HISTORY

Individuals who have had cardiovascular problems are at higher risk than those who have never had a problem. People with this history should control the other risk factors as much as they can. Most risk factors are reversible, so this will greatly decrease the risk for future problems. The more time that has passed since the cardiovascular problem occurred, the lower is the risk for recurrence.

Genetic predisposition toward heart disease has been demonstrated clearly and seems to be gaining in importance. All other factors being equal, a person with blood relatives who now have or did have heart disease before age 60 runs a greater risk than someone with no such history. The younger the age at which the cardiovascular incident happened to the relative, the greater is the risk for the disease.

In many cases there is no way of knowing whether a person's true genetic predisposition or simply poor lifestyle habits led to a heart problem. A person may have been physically inactive, overweight, have smoked, and had bad dietary habits, leading to heart attack. Regardless, blood relatives would fall in the family history category. Because we have no reliable way to differentiate all the factors contributing to cardiovascular disease, a person with a family history should watch all other factors closely and maintain as low a risk level as possible. In addition, the person should have a blood chemistry analysis annually to make sure the body is handling blood lipids properly.

AGE

Age is a risk factor because of the higher incidence of heart disease in older people. This tendency may be induced partly by other factors stemming from changes in lifestyle as we get older — less physical activity, poor nutrition, obesity, and so on.

Young people should not think they are exempt from heart disease. The process begins early in life. Autopsies conducted on soldiers killed at age 22 and younger revealed that approximately 70% had early stages of atherosclerosis. Other studies found elevated blood cholesterol levels in children as young as 10 years old.

Although the aging process cannot be stopped, it certainly can be slowed down. Physiological versus chronological age is important in preventing disease. Some individuals in their sixties or older have the body of a twenty-year-old. And twenty-year-olds often are in such poor condition and health that they almost seem to have the body of a sixty-year-old. Risk factor management and positive lifestyle habits are the best ways to slow down the natural aging process.

A FINAL WORD ON CORONARY RISK REDUCTION

Most of the risk factors for CHD are reversible and preventable. The fact that a person has a family history of heart disease and possibly some of the other risk factors because of neglect in lifestyle does not mean this person is doomed. A healthier lifestyle — free of cardiovascular problems — is something over which you have much control. You are encouraged to be persistent. Willpower and commitment are required to develop patterns that will eventually turn into healthy habits contributing to total well-being.

LABORATORY EXPERIENCE

LAB 12A
Self-Evaluation of Cardiovascular Risk

Lab Preparation
If time allows, reassess cardiovascular endurance, body composition, and blood pressure during this lab. Wear appropriate exercise clothing for this reassessment (see Labs 1B, 4A, and 6A). Also, if you have had a blood chemistry analysis that included total cholesterol, HDL-cholesterol, triglycerides, and glucose levels, you may use the results for this laboratory experience.

REFERENCES

1. American Heart Association. *Heart and Stroke Facts*. Dallas, TX: AHA, 1992.

2. American Heart Association. *Heart and Stroke Facts Statistics*. Dallas, TX: AHA, 1992.

3. Barnard, R. J. "Effects of Lifestyle Modification on Serum Lipids." *Archives of Internal Medicine* 151:1389-1394, 1991.

4. Blair, S. N., K. H. Cooper, L. W. Gibbons, L. R. Gettman, S. Lewis, and N. N. Goodyear. "Changes in Coronary Heart Disease Risk Factors Associated with Increased Treadmill Time in 753 Men." *American Journal of Epidemiology* 3:352-359, 1983.

5. Blair, S. N., N. N. Goodyear, L. W. Gibbons, and K. H. Cooper. "Physical Fitness and Incidence of Hypertension in Healthy Normotensive Men and Women." *Journal of the American Medical Association* 252:487-490, 1984.

6. Blair, S. N., H. W. Kohl III, R. S. Paffenbarger, Jr, D. G. Clark, K. H. Cooper, and L. W. Gibbons. "Physical Fitness and All-Cause Mortality: A Prospective Study of Healthy Men and Women." *Journal of the American Medical Association* 262:2395-2401, 1989.

7. Blankenhorn, D. H ., et al. "Beneficial Effects of Combined Colestipol-Niacin Therapy on Coronary Atherosclerosis and Coronary Venous Bypass Grafts." *Journal of the American Medical Association* 257:3233-3240, 1987.

8. Blankenhorn, D. H. and H. N. Hodis. "Status Report on Coronary Atherosclerosis Regression: Clinical Implications." *Practical Cardiology* 16(11):41-56, 1990.

9. Cristian, J. L., and J. L. Greger. *Nutrition for Living*. Menlo Park, CA: The Benjamin/Cummings Publishing Co., 1991.

10. Cooper, K. H. *Running Without Fear*. New York: Mount Evans and Co., 1985.

11. Cooper, K. H. *The Aerobics Program for Total Well-Being*. New York: Mount Evans and Co., 1982.

12. Diethrich, E. B. *The Arizona Heart Institute's Heart Test*. New York, NY: International Heart Foundation, 1981.

13. Frick, M. H., et al. "Helsinki Heart Study: Primary-Prevention Trial with Gemfibrozil in Middle-Aged Men with Dyslipidemia." *The New England Journal of Medicine* 317:1237-1245, 1987.

14. Gaziano, J. M. and C. H. Hennekens. "A New Look at What Can Unclog Your Arteries." *Executive Health Report* 27(8):16, 1991.

15. Gibbons, L. W., S. Blair, K. H. Cooper, and M. Smith. "Association Between Coronary Heart Disease Risk Factors and Physical Fitness in Healthy Adult Women." *Circulation* 5:977-983, 1983.

16. Gluek, C. J. "Nonpharmacologic and Pharmacologic Alteration of High Density Lipoprotein Cholesterol: Therapeutic Approaches to Prevention of Atherosclerosis." *American Heart Journal* 110:1107-1115, 1985.

17. Gordon, D. J., et al. "High-Density Lipoprotein Cholesterol and Coronary Heart Disease in Hypercholesterolemic Men: The Lipid Research Clinics Coronary Primary Prevention Trial." *Circulation* 74:1217-1225, 1986.

18. Guss, S. B. "Heart Attack Risk Score." *Cardiac Alert*, 1983.

19. Helmrich, S. P., D. R. Ragland, R. W. Leung, and R. S. Paffenbarger. "Physical Activity and Reduced Occurrences of Non-Insulin-Dependent Diabetes Mellitus." *The New England Journal of Medicine* 325:147-152, 1991.

20. Hoeger, W. W. K. *Ejercicio, Salud y Vida [Exercise, Health and Life]*. Caracas, Venezuela: Editorial Arte, 1980.

21. Hoeger, W. W. K. *The Complete Guide for the Development & Implementation of Health Promotion Programs*. Englewood, CO: Morton Publishing Company, 1987.

22. Hoeger, W. W. K. "Self-Assessment of Cardiovascular Risk." *Corporate Fitness & Recreation* 5(6):1316, 1986.

23. "How Good is 'Good' Cholesterol?" *The Health Letter*. April 9, 1982.

24. Hubert, H. B., M. Feinleib, P. M. MacNamara, and W. P. Castelli. "Obesity as an Independent Risk Factor for Cardiovascular Disease: A 26-year Follow-up of Participants in the Framingham Heart Study." *Circulation* 5:968-977, 1983.

25. Johnson, L.C. *Interpreting Your Test Results*. Chattanooga, TN: Blue Cross Blue Shield of Tennessee, 1990.

26. Kannel, W. B., D. McGee, and T. Gordon. "A General Cardiovascular Risk Profile: The Framingham Study." *The American Journal of Cardiology* 7:46-51, 1976.

27. Kash, F. W., J. L. Boyer, S. P. Van Camp, L. S. Verity, and J. P. Wallace. "The Effect of Physical Activity on Aerobic Power in Older Men (A Longitudinal Study)." *The Physician and Sports Medicine* 18(4):73-83, 1990.

28. Kostas, G. "Three Nutrients May Help Control Blood Pressure." *The Aerobics News* 1(7):6, 1986.

29. Leon, A., J. Connett, D. R. Jacobs, and R. Rauramaa. "Leisure-time Physical Activity Levels and Risk of Coronary Heart Disease and Death: The Multiple Risk Factor Intervention Trial." *Journal of the American Medical Association* 258:2388-2395, 1987.

30. Manninen, V., et al. "Lipid Alterations and Decline in the Incidence of Coronary Heart Disease in the Helsinki Heart Study." *Journal of the American Medical Association* 260:641651, 1988.

31. Multiple Risk Factor Intervention Trial. "Risk Factor Changes and Mortality Results." Multiple risk factor intervention trial research group. *Journal of the American Medical Association* 248:1465-1477, 1982.

32. Neufeld, H. N., and U. Gouldbourt. "Coronary Heart Disease: Genetic Aspects." *Circulation.* 5:943-954, 1983.

33. Ornish, D. S. E. Brown, L. W. Scherwitz, et al., "Can Lifestyle Changes Reverse Coronary Heart Disease? The Lifestyle Heart Trial." *Lancet.* 336:129-133.

34. Paffenbarger, R. S., Jr, R. T. Hyde, A. L. Wing, I. Lee, D. L. Jung, and J. B. Kampert. "The Association of Changes in Physical-Activity Level and Other Lifestyle Characteristics with Mortality Among Men." *The New England Journal of Medicine*, 328:538-545, 1993.

35. Page, L. B. "On Making Sense of Salt and Your Blood Pressure." *Executive Health*. August 1982.

36. Peters, R. K., L. D. Cady, Jr, D. P. Bischoff, L. Bernstein, and M. C. Pike. "Physical Fitness and Subsequent Myocardial Infarction in Healthy Workers." *Journal of the American Medical Association* 249:3052-3056, 1983.

37. Powell, K. E., P. D. Thompson, C. J. Caspersen, and J. S. Kendrick. "Physical Activity and the Evidence of Coronary Heart Disease." *Public Health Reviews* 8:253-287, 1987.

38. Romm, P. A., M. K. Hong, and C. E. Rackley. "High-Density-Lipoprotein Cholesterol and Risk of Coronary Heart Disease." *Practical Cardiology* 16:28-40, 1990.

39. Sandvik, L., J. Erikssen, E. Thaulow, G. Erikssen, R. Mundal, and K. Rodahl. "Physical Fitness as a Predictor of Mortality Among Healthy, Middle-Aged Norwegian Men." *The New England Journal of Medicine*, 328:533-537, 1993.

40. Sobolski, J., et al. "Protection Against Ischemic Heart Disease in the Belgian Physical Fitness Study: Physical Fitness Rather than Physical Activity." *American Journal of Epidemiology* 125:601-610, 1987.

41. Superko, R. "Platelets and Lipid Interaction with a Vessel Wall." Symposium presented at the American College of Sports Medicine Annual Meeting, 1991.

42. Van Camp, S. P. "The Fixx Tragedy: A Cardiologist's Perspective." *Physician and Sportsmedicine* 12:153-155, 1984.

43. Wiley, J. A., and T. C. Camacho. "Lifestyle and Future Health: Evidence from the Alameda County Study." *Preventive Medicine* 9:121, 1980.

CANCER RISK MANAGEMENT

13

OBJECTIVES

Define cancer and how it starts and spreads.

Recognize the importance of health education in a cancer prevention program.

Become acquainted with the American Cancer Society's guidelines for cancer prevention.

Learn to recognize early warning signs of possible serious illness.

Become familiar with major risk factors that lead to specific types of cancer.

Assess the risk for developing certain types of cancer.

The human body has approximately 100 trillion cells, and under normal conditions these cells reproduce themselves in an orderly way. The cell growth has to take place so old, worn-out tissue can be replaced and injuries can be repaired.

Cell growth is controlled by deoxyribonucleic acid (DNA) and ribonucleic acid (RNA), found in the nucleus of each cell. When nuclei lose their ability to regulate and control cell growth, cell division is disrupted and mutant cells may develop. Some of these cells may grow uncontrollably and abnormally, forming a mass of tissue called a tumor, which can be either benign or malignant. *A malignant tumor is a cancer.*

Cancer can be caused by external factors such as radiation, chemicals, and viruses; as well as internal factors such as immune conditions, hormones, and genetic mutations.[2] Often a decade or more can pass between carcinogenic exposure or mutations and the time cancer is diagnosed.

Cancer cells grow and multiply uncontrollably, destroying normal tissue (see Figure 13.1). The rate at which cancer cells grow varies from one type to another. Some types grow fast; others take years.

More than 100 types of cancer can develop in any tissue or organ of the body. Cancer probably starts with the abnormal growth of one cell, which then can multiply into billions of cancerous cells. The accumulation of approximately one billion cells, the equivalent of a one-centimeter tumor, is required to detect cancer.

Through metastasis (the movement of bacteria or body cells from one part of the body to another), cells break away from a malignant tumor and migrate to other parts of the body, where they can cause new cancer. Although the immune system destroys most cancer cells, only one abnormal cell lodging elsewhere can start a new cancer. In contrast, benign tumors do not invade other tissue. They can interfere with normal bodily functions, but they rarely cause death.

L A B S

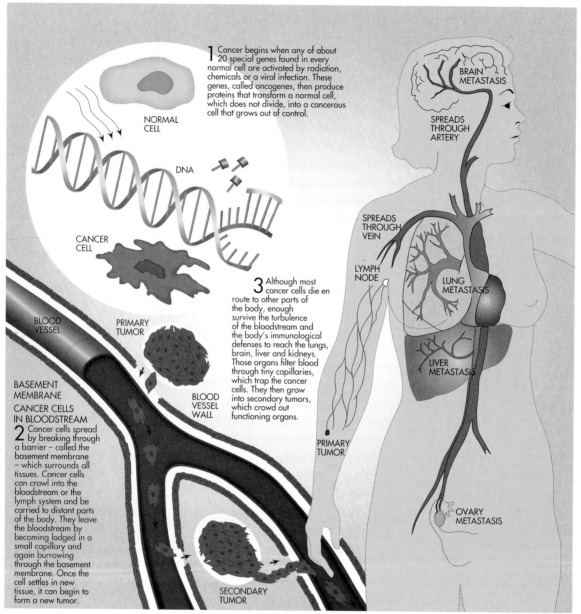

FIGURE 13.1
How cancer starts and spreads.

Illustration by John Stone Quinan and Jo Ellen Murphy of the *Washington Post* (edited by *Cancer News*, American Cancer Society, Texas Division, Winter 1986). Reprinted by permission of the *Washington Post*, © 1985.

INCIDENCE OF CANCER

According to a 1990 report by the National Center for Health Statistics, cancer was the cause of 23.5% of all deaths in the United States. It is the second leading cause of death in the country and the leading cause in children between ages 1 and 14.

The American Hospital Association estimates that the number of people with cancer will double in this decade as the population ages. This means that 85 million Americans, based on the total 1993 population, will develop cancer in their lifetime, striking approximately three of every four families. By the year 2000, cancer is expected to replace heart disease as the number-one killer in the United States. About 526,000 people died from the disease in 1993, and approximately 1,170,000 new cases were diagnosed that same year.

The 1993 statistical estimates of cancer incidence and deaths by gender and site are given in

Figure 13.2. These estimates exclude nonmelanoma skin cancer (cancer that spreads or grows directly from the original site but does not metastasize to other regions of the body) and carcinoma in situ (encapsulated tumor that is found at an early stage and has not spread).

As with coronary heart disease, cancer is largely preventable. As much as 80% of all human cancer is related to lifestyle or environmental factors (including diet, tobacco use, excessive use of alcohol, sexual and reproductive history, and exposure to occupational hazards — see Figure 13.3). Most of these cancers could be prevented through positive lifestyle habits.

Research sponsored by the American Cancer Society and the National Cancer Institute[7] showed that individuals who have a healthy lifestyle have some of the lowest cancer mortality rates ever reported in scientific studies (also see the discussion on wellness, fitness, and longevity in Chapter 1). A group of about 10,000 members of the Church of Jesus Christ of Latter Day Saints (commonly referred to as the Mormon church) in California was reported to have only about one third (men) to one half (women) the rate of cancer mortality as the general White population (Figure 13.4). In this study the investigators looked at three general health habits in the participants: lifetime abstinence from smoking, regular physical activity, and sleep. In addition, healthy lifestyle guidelines instituted by the church since 1833 include abstention from tobacco, alcohol, caffeine, and drugs, and adhering to a well-balanced diet. Nutrition recommendations include a diet based on grains, fruits, and vegetables, and moderate use of poultry and red meat.

Equally important is the fact that more than 8

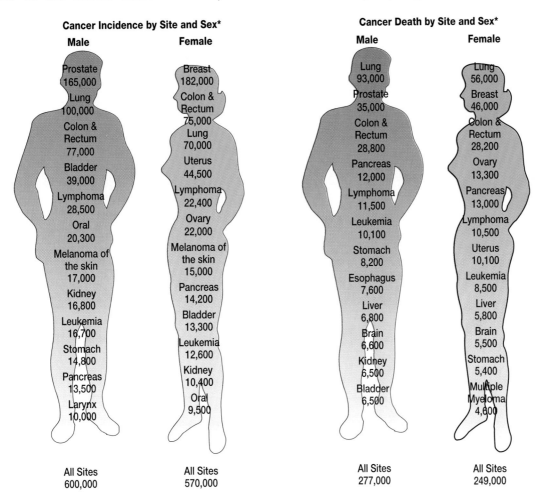

*Excluding basal and squamous cell skin cancer and carcinoma in situ.

FIGURE 13.2

Cancer incidence and deaths by site and gender.

Estimated 1993. From *Cancer Facts & Figures — 1993*. New York: American Cancer Society.

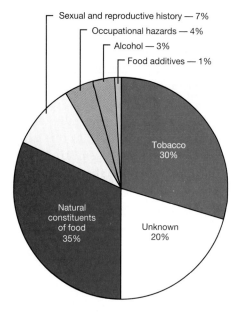

FIGURE 13.3
Estimate of relative roles of major cancer-causing factors.

million Americans with a history of cancer were alive in 1993, nearly 5 million of whom were considered cured. For most patients, "cured" means 5 years without symptoms after treatments stop. Life expectancy for these individuals is the same as for those who have never had cancer.[2]

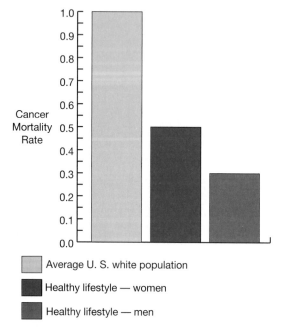

FIGURE 13.4
Effects of healthy Lifestyle* on cancer mortality rate.[7]

*Healthy lifestyle factors include proper nutrition, abstinence from cigarette smoking, regular sleep (7–8 hours per night), and regular physical activity.

GUIDELINES FOR CANCER PREVENTION

The biggest factor in fighting cancer today is health education. People need to be informed about the risk factors for cancer and the guidelines for early detection. The most effective way to protect against cancer is to change negative lifestyle habits and behaviors. Following are guidelines for cancer prevention, from the American Cancer Society:

1. **Make dietary changes.** The diet should be low in fat and high in fiber, and contain vitamins A and C from natural sources (Figure 13.5). Protein intake should be within the RDA guidelines. Cruciferous vegetables (plants that produce cross-shaped leaves) are encouraged. Alcohol should be consumed in moderation, and obesity should be avoided.

   High fat intake has been linked primarily to breast, colon, and prostate cancers. Low intake of fiber seems to increase the risk for colon cancer. Foods high in vitamins A and C may deter larynx, esophagus, and lung cancers. Salt-cured, smoked, and nitrite-cured foods have been associated with cancer of the esophagus and stomach. Vitamin C seems to discourage the formation of nitrosamines (cancer-causing substances formed from eating cured meats).

   Carrots, squash, sweet potatoes, and cruciferous vegetables (cauliflower, broccoli, cabbage, Brussels sprouts, and kohlrabi) seem to protect against cancer (Figure 13.6). These vegetables contain a lot of beta-carotene (a precursor to vitamin A) and vitamin C. Although the cancer-protecting mechanism of these vegetables is not known, researchers believe the antioxidant effect of these vitamins protects the body from oxygen free radicals.

   As discussed in Chapter 2, during normal metabolism most of the oxygen in the human body is converted into stable forms of carbon dioxide and water. A small amount, however, ends up in an unstable form known as oxygen free radicals, which are thought to attack and damage the cell membrane and DNA, leading to the formation of cancers. Antioxidants absorb free radicals before they can cause damage, and they also interrupt the sequence of reactions once damage has begun.[8]

FIGURE 13.5
Nutrition guidelines for a cancer prevention program include a diet low in fat and high in fiber, with ample amounts of vitamins A and C from natural sources.

Daily protein intake for some Americans is almost twice the amount the human body needs. Too much animal protein seems to decrease blood enzymes that prevent precancerous cells from developing into tumors.

Some research suggests that grilling protein (fat or lean) at high temperatures for a long time increases the formation of carcinogenic substances on the skin or surface of the meat. Microwaving the meat for a couple of minutes before barbecuing decrease the risk, as long as the fluid released by the meat is discarded. Most potential carcinogens collect in this solution. Removing the skin before serving and cooking at lower heat to a medium stage rather than well done also seems to lower the risk.

Alcohol should be consumed in moderation, as too much alcohol raises the risk for developing certain cancers, especially when it is combined with tobacco smoking or smokeless tobacco. In combination, these substances significantly increase the risk for mouth, larynx, throat, esophagus, and liver cancers. Approximately 17,000 cancer deaths yearly are attributed to excessive use of alcohol, often in combination with smoking. According to some research, the combined action of heavy use of alcohol and tobacco increases cancer of the oral cavity fifteenfold.

Maintaining recommended body weight also is encouraged. Obesity has been associated with cancers of the colon, rectum, breast, prostate, gallbladder, ovary, and uterus.

2. **Abstain from tobacco.** Smoking is the culprit in 83% of lung cancers and 30% of all cancers. Smokeless tobacco also increases the risk for mouth, larynx, throat, and esophagus cancers. About 138,600 cancer deaths annually stem from tobacco use.

Cigarette smoking by itself is a major health hazard. When considering all related deaths, cigarette smoking is responsible for more than 450,000 unnecessary deaths each year. The average life expectancy for a chronic smoker is up to 18 years less than for a nonsmoker.

3. **Avoid too much sun.** Excessive exposure to sunlight (or any ultraviolet source, including tanning booths) is a major contributor to the development of skin cancer. The most common sites of skin cancer are those most often exposed to the sun (face, neck, and back of the hands).

The three types of skin cancer are: (a) basal cell carcinoma, (b) squamous cell carcinoma, and (c) malignant melanoma. The latter is the most deadly, causing approximately 6,800 deaths in 1993.

Nearly 90% of the 700,000 cases of skin cancer reported yearly in the United States could

FIGURE 13.6
Cruciferous vegetables are recommended in a cancer-prevention diet.

have been prevented by protecting the skin from the sun's rays. One in every six Americans eventually will develop some type of skin cancer.

There is nothing healthy about a "healthy tan." Tanning of the skin is the body's natural reaction to permanent and irreversible damage from too much exposure to the sun. Even small doses of sunlight add up to a greater risk for skin cancer and premature aging. The tan fades at the end of the summer season, but the underlying skin damage does not disappear. People with sensitive skin should avoid sun exposure between 10:00 a.m. and 3:00 p.m.

The stinging sunburn comes from ultraviolet B rays (UVB), which also are thought to be the main cause of premature wrinkling and skin aging, roughened/leathery/sagging skin, and skin cancer. Unfortunately, the damage may not become evident until up to 20 years later. In comparison, skin that has not been overexposed to the sun remains smooth and unblemished, and, over time, shows less evidence of aging.

Sunscreen lotion should be applied about 30 minutes before lengthy exposure to the sun because the skin takes that long to absorb the protective ingredients. A sun protection factor (SPF) of at least 15 is recommended. SPF 15 means it takes 15 times longer to burn than with no lotion. If you ordinarily get a mild sunburn after 20 minutes of noonday sun, an SPF 15 allows you to remain in the sun about 300

minutes before burning. The higher the number, the more the protection. When swimming or sweating, waterproof sunscreens should be reapplied more often because all sunscreens lose strength when they are diluted.

4. **Carefully consider estrogen use, radiation exposure, and potential occupational hazards.** Estrogen intake has been linked to endometrial cancer but can be taken safely under careful supervision by a physician. Although radiation exposure increases the risk for cancer, the benefits of x-rays may outweigh the risk involved, and most medical facilities use the lowest dose possible to lower the risk to a minimum. Occupational hazards, such as asbestos fibers, nickel and uranium dusts, chromium compounds, vinyl chloride, and bischlormethyl ether, increase the risk for cancer. Cigarette smoking magnifies the risk from occupational hazards.

A more active lifestyle and lower stress levels also seem to offer a protective effect against cancer. Although the mechanism is not clear, physical fitness and cancer mortality in men and women may have a graded and consistent inverse relationship (see Figure 13.7).

A moderately intense lifetime exercise program has been shown to lower the risk for cancers of the breast, colon, and reproductive system. In addition, growing evidence suggests that the body's autoimmune system may play a role in preventing cancer.

*Age-adjusted cancer death rates per 10,000 person-years of follow-up (1970-1985).

**Least fit group = 1. Most fit group = 5.

FIGURE 13.7

Association between physical activity and health.

Studies have indicated that exercise improves the autoimmune system. In contrast, high levels of tension and stress and poor coping may affect this system negatively and render the body less effective in dealing with the various cancers.

The contribution of many of the other much-publicized factors is not as significant as those just pointed out. Intentional food additives, saccharin, processing agents, pesticides, and packaging materials currently used in the United States and other developed countries appear to have minimal consequences.

Genetics plays a role in susceptibility in only 2% of all cancers. Most of the effect is seen in the early childhood years. Some cancers are a combination of genetic and environmental liability. Genetics may add to the environmental risk of certain types of cancers. The biggest carcinogenic exposure in the workplace is cigarette smoke. Environment, however, means more than pollution and smoke. It incorporates diet, lifestyle-related events, viruses, and physical agents such as x-rays and exposure to the sun.

Fortunately, through early detection, many cancers can be controlled or cured. The real problem comes when cancerous cells spread. Once they spread, the cancer is difficult to wipe out. Therefore, effective prevention, or at least early detection, is crucial. Herein lies the importance of periodic screening.

Everyone should become familiar with the following seven warning signals for cancer and bring them to a physician's attention if any are present:

1. Change in bowel or bladder habits.
2. Sore that does not heal.
3. Unusual bleeding or discharge.
4. Thickening or lump in breast or elsewhere.
5. Indigestion or difficulty in swallowing.
6. Obvious change in wart or mole.
7. Nagging cough or hoarseness.

Furthermore, the American Medical Association has developed a questionnaire to alert people to symptoms that may indicate a serious health problem. The questionnaire is given in Lab 13B. Although in most cases nothing serious will be found, any of the symptoms calls for a physician's attention as soon as possible. Finally, the Guidelines for Screening Recommendations by the American Cancer Society, outlined in Table 13.1, should be included in regular physical examinations as part of a cancer prevention program.

Scientific evidence and testing procedures for prevention and early detection of cancer do change. Studies continue to provide new information about cancer prevention and detection. The intent of cancer prevention programs is to educate and guide individuals toward a lifestyle that will help prevent cancer and enable early detection of malignancy.

Treatment of cancer always should be left to specialized physicians and cancer clinics. Current treatment modalities include surgery, radiation, radioactive substances, chemotherapy, hormones, and immunotherapy.

CANCER HEALTH PROTECTION PLAN

The Health Protection Plan for Cancer at the end of this chapter (Figure 13.8) was designed by the Preventive Medicine Institute/Strang Clinic in New York to help people assess their risk for certain common types of cancer. People who may have more than the average risk for developing certain cancers can be identified by some of the risk factors for these cancer sites. The questions to be answered for each cancer site make reference to the major risk factors and by no means represent the only factors that might be involved. The questions are grouped into four categories: (a) symptoms that may indicate something is wrong, (b) family history, (c) personal history, and (d) preventive measures that can help to protect you from certain health hazards. In Lab 13C you are asked to complete this questionnaire. Nevertheless, the questionnaire is included at the end of this chapter so it can be retained for future reference.

OTHER CANCER SITES

Risk factors and prevention techniques for types of cancer not contained in the cancer questionnaire also have been outlined in the Cancer Book published by the American Cancer Society, as well as in a series of pamphlets on Facts on Cancer (one each for selected cancer sites). Some of these types of cancer are discussed next, along with the risk factors associated with each type and preventive techniques to help lower the risk.

TABLE 13.1
Guidelines for Cancer Screening

Test	Patient age	Frequency
Breast physical examination	20-40 Over 40	Every 3 yrs Annually
Breast self-examination	Over 20	Monthly
Chest X-ray	No specific recommendation	No specific recommendation
Digital rectal examination	Over 40	Annually
Endometrial tissue examination	At menopause[a]	At menopause
Mammography	35-40 40-49 Over 50	One baseline Every 1-2 yrs Annually
Pap smear	20-65 and sexually active teenagers	2 consecutive yrs, then every 3 yrs
Pelvic examination	20-40 Over 40 At menopause	Every 3 yrs Annually
Sigmoidoscopy	Over 50	2 consecutive yrs, then every 3-5 yrs
Sputum cytology	No specific recommendation	No specific recommendation
Stool guaiac	Over 50	Annually
Health counseling and cancer check-up[b]	Over 20 Over 40	Every 3 yrs Every yr

From *Guidelines for the Cancer-Related Checkup: Recommendations and Rationale.* New York: American Cancer Society, July/August 1980. Reproduced with permission.

[a] Recommended for obese women with a history of involuntary infertility, failure of ovulation, abnormal uterine bleeding, or estrogen therapy.

[b] To include examinations for cancers of the thyroid, testicles, prostate, ovaries, lymph nodes, oral region, and skin.

PANCREATIC CANCER

The pancreas is a thin gland that lies behind the stomach. This gland releases insulin and pancreatic juice. Insulin regulates blood sugar, and pancreatic juice contains enzymes that aid in food digestion.

Possible Risk Factors

1. Age. The incidence increases between ages of 35 and 70 and is significantly higher around age 55.
2. Cigarette smoking.
3. High cholesterol diet.
4. Exposure to unspecified environmental agents.

Prevention and Warning Signals

Detecting pancreatic cancer is difficult because (a) no symptoms are evoked early in the disease process, and (b) advanced disease symptoms are similar to those of other diseases. Warning signals that may be related to pancreatic cancer include pain in the abdomen or lower back, jaundice, loss of weight and appetite, nausea, weakness, agitated depression, loss of energy and feeling weary, dizziness, chills, muscle spasms, double vision, and coma.

ORAL CANCER

Oral cancer includes cancer of the mouth, lips, tongue, salivary glands, pharynx, larynx, and floor of the mouth. Most of these cancers seem to be related to cigarette smoking and excessive alcohol consumption.

Risk Factors

1. Heavy smoking/drinking.
2. Broken or ill-fitting dentures.
3. A broken tooth that irritates the inside of the mouth.
4. Chewing and dipping tobacco.
5. Excessive exposure to sun (lip cancer).

Prevention and Warning Signals

Regular examinations and good dental hygiene help in the prevention and early detection of oral cancer. Warning signals include: a nonhealing sore or white patch in the mouth, a lump, problems with chewing and swallowing, and a constant feeling of having "something" in the throat. A person with any of these conditions should be evaluated by a physician or a dentist. A tissue biopsy normally is conducted to diagnose the presence of cancer.

THYROID CANCER

The thyroid gland is located in the lower portion of the front of the neck and helps to regulate growth and metabolism. Thyroid cancer among women occurs almost twice as often as in men, and the incidence also is higher in Whites than in Blacks.

Risk Factors

1. Age. Risk increases with age.
2. Radiation therapy of the head and neck region in childhood or adolescence.
3. A family history of thyroid cancer.

Prevention and Warning Signals

Regular inspection for thyroid tumors is done by palpating of the gland and surrounding areas during a physical examination. Thyroid cancer is slow growing. Therefore, this malignancy is highly treatable. Even so, any unusual lumps in front of the neck should be reported promptly to a physician. Although thyroid cancer has few symptoms, warning signals (besides a lump) may be: difficulty in swallowing or choking, labored breathing, and persistent hoarseness.

Adherence to a healthy lifestyle and following cancer screening guidelines can prevent 60% to 80% of all cancers.

LIVER CANCER

The incidence of liver cancer in the United States is low. Men are more prone to liver cancer, and the disease is more common after age 60.

Risk Factors

1. A history of cirrhosis of the liver.
2. A history of hepatitis B virus.
3. Exposure to vinyl chloride (industrial gas used in manufacturing plastics) and aflotoxin (natural food contaminant).
4. Heavy alcohol consumption.

Prevention and Warning Signals

Prevention is accomplished primarily by avoiding the risk factors and being aware of warning signals. Possible signs and symptoms are a lump or pain in the upper right abdomen (which may radiate into the back and the shoulder), fever, nausea, rapidly deteriorating health, jaundice, and tenderness in the area of the liver.

LEUKEMIA

Leukemia is a type of cancer that interferes with blood-forming tissues (bone marrow, lymph nodes, and spleen), bringing about the production of too many immature white blood cells. Consequently, people afflicted by leukemia cannot fight infection effectively. For the most part, the causes of leukemia are unknown, although suspected risk factors have been identified.

Risk Factors

1. Inherited susceptibility, but not transmitted directly from parent to child.
2. Higher incidence in children with Down syndrome (mongolism) and a few other genetic abnormalities.
3. Excessive exposure to ionizing radiation.
4. Environmental exposure to chemicals such as benzene.

Prevention and Warning Signals

Detection is not easy, because early symptoms may be attributed to less serious ailments. Early warning signals include fatigue, pallor, weight loss, easy bruising, nosebleeds, paleness, loss of appetite, recurring infections, hemorrhages, night sweats, bone and joint pain, and fever. At a more advanced stage, fatigue increases, hemorrhages become more severe, pain and high fever continue, and swelling of the gums and various skin disorders occur.

A FINAL WORD ON CANCER RISK MANAGEMENT

If you are at high risk for any of the cancer sites, you are advised to discuss this with your physician. An ounce of prevention is worth a pound of cure. Although cardiovascular disease is the number-one killer in the country, cancer is the number-one fear. Of all cancers, 60% to 80% are preventable, and about 50% are curable. Most cancers are lifestyle-related, so being aware of the risk factors and following the screening guidelines (Table 13.1) and basic recommendations for cancer prevention will greatly decrease the risk for developing cancer.

LABORATORY EXPERIENCE

LAB 13A
Cancer Prevention: Are You Taking Control?

Lab Preparation
None required.

LAB 13B
Early Warning Signs of Possible Serious Illness

Lab Preparation
None required.

LAB 13C
Health Protection Plan for Cancer

Lab Preparation
None required.

REFERENCES

1. American Cancer Society, Texas Division. *Cancer: Assessing Your Risk*. Dallas, TX: ACS, 1982.
2. American Cancer Society. *Cancer Facts & Figures - 1993*. New York: ACS, 1993.
3. American Cancer Society. *Cancer Book*. New York: ACS, 1986.
4. American Cancer Society. *Guidelines for the Cancer-Related Checkup: Recommendations and Rationale*. New York: ACS, 1980.
5. American Cancer Society. Pamphlets on Facts on "Selected" Cancer Sites. New York: ACS, pamphlets published between 1978 and 1983.
6. Blair, S. N., H. W. Kohl III, R. S. Paffenbarger, Jr, D. G. Clark, K. H. Cooper, and L. W. Gibbons. "Physical Fitness and All-Cause Mortality: A Prospective Study of Healthy Men and Women." *Journal of the American Medical Association* 262:2395-2401, 1989.
7. Enstrom, J. E. "Health Practices and Cancer Mortality Among Active California Mormons." *Journal of the National Cancer Institute* 81:1807-1814, 1989.
8. Gaziano, J. M. and C. H. Hennekens. "A New Look at What Can Unclog Your Arteries." *Executive Health Report* 27(8):16, 1991.
9. Greenwald, P. "Assessment of Risk Factors for Cancer." *Preventive Medicine* 9:260-263, 1980.
10. Hammond, E. C., and H. Seidman. "Smoking and Cancer in the United States." *Preventive Medicine* 9:169-173, 1980.
11. Higginson, J. "Proportion of Cancers Due to Occupation." *Preventive Medicine* 9:180-188, 1980.
12. Paffenbarger, R. S., R. T. Hyde, A. L. Wing, and C. H. Steinmetz. "A Natural History of Athleticism and Cardiovascular Health." *Journal of the American Medical Association* 252:491-495, 1984.
13. Rothman, K. J. "The Proportion of Cancer Attributable to Alcohol Consumption." *Preventive Medicine* 9:174-179, 1980.
14. Weisburger, J. H., D. M. Hegsted, G. B. Gori, and B. Lewis. "Extending the Prudent Diet to Cancer Prevention." *Preventive Medicine* 9:297-304, 1980.
15. Williams, C. L. "Primary Prevention of Cancer Beginning in Childhood." *Preventive Medicine* 9:275-280, 1980.
16. Williams, P. A. "A Productive History and Physical Examination in the Prevention and Early Detection of Cancer." *Cancer* 47:1146-1150, 1981.

Skin and Lymph Nodes

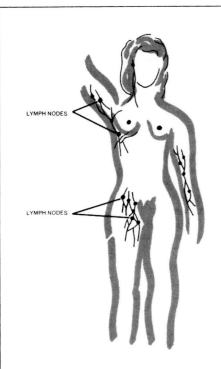

LYMPH NODES

LYMPH NODES

Both skin and lymph nodes cover the entire body. Lymph nodes are located at strategic points in the body to fight infection.

An enlarged lymph node will appear as a single firm swelling under the skin. It is often confused with a hernia, infection or cyst.

		YES	NO
A.	**Do you now have . . . ?**		
	. . . Any unexplained itching	○	○
	. . . Unexplained sweating or fever during the night which has lasted for more than two weeks	○	○
	. . . Swelling or enlargement (painful or not) of lymph glands	○	○
	. . . Non-healing ulcers, sores, or growths which have lasted for more than a month	○	○
	. . . Red scaling patches of skin which do not heal	○	○
	. . . Any moles which have changed color, changed size, become ulcerated (sore) or bleed	○	○
B.	**Has a member of your family ever had . . . ?**		
	. . . Cancer of the skin	○	○
	. . . Leukemia	○	○
	. . . Lymphosarcoma	○	○
	. . . Hodgkin's disease	○	○
C.	**Have you ever had . . . ?**		
	. . . Cancer of the skin	○	○
	. . . A mole removed	○	○
	. . . A skin growth removed	○	○
	. . . Treatment with X-rays (radiation therapy)	○	○
	. . . A burn with scarring	○	○
D.	**Do you . . . ?**		
	. . . Have frequent boils or other skin infections	○	○
	. . . Have skin that sunburns more easily than others	○	○
	. . . Have an outdoor occupation (example: farmer, fisherman, etc.)	○	○

CANCER OF THE SKIN

RISK FACTORS:
- Extremely fair skin
- Prolonged exposure to the sun (more than 4 hours a day for 4 months out of the year)
- A history of skin cancer or malignant moles
- Moles on the soles of your feet or in areas irritated by tight clothing or shaving
- Scars from severe burns
- A non-healing scaling sore on your skin

AWARENESS COUNTS:

You can reduce your risks for skin cancer by wearing protective clothing, such as sun hats, or by lightly covering the over-exposed parts of your body when out in the sun for long periods.

Avoid excess sun-bathing if you are fair-skinned; apply *sun-screening ointment* (different from regular suntan lotion) to filter out harmful rays.

Avoid contact with arsenic (found in some insecticides) and coal tar derivatives since these agents play a role in the development of skin cancer.

FIGURE 13.8
Health Protection Plan for Cancer.*

*Questionnaire published by the Preventive Medicine Institute/Strang Clinic. New York, 1982. Reproduced with permission.

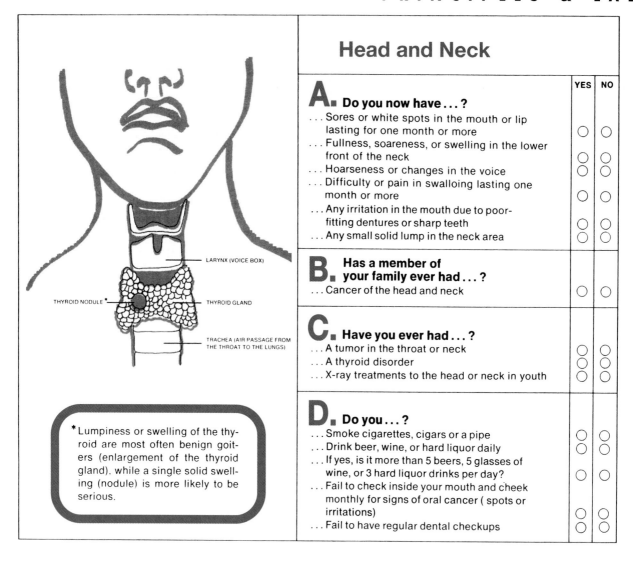

Head and Neck

	YES	NO
A. **Do you now have . . . ?**		
. . . Sores or white spots in the mouth or lip lasting for one month or more	○	○
. . . Fullness, soareness, or swelling in the lower front of the neck	○	○
. . . Hoarseness or changes in the voice	○	○
. . . Difficulty or pain in swalloing lasting one month or more	○	○
. . . Any irritation in the mouth due to poor-fitting dentures or sharp teeth	○	○
. . . Any small solid lump in the neck area	○	○
B. **Has a member of your family ever had . . . ?**		
. . . Cancer of the head and neck	○	○
C. **Have you ever had . . . ?**		
. . . A tumor in the throat or neck	○	○
. . . A thyroid disorder	○	○
. . . X-ray treatments to the head or neck in youth	○	○
D. **Do you . . . ?**		
. . . Smoke cigarettes, cigars or a pipe	○	○
. . . Drink beer, wine, or hard liquor daily	○	○
. . . If yes, is it more than 5 beers, 5 glasses of wine, or 3 hard liquor drinks per day?	○	○
. . . Fail to check inside your mouth and cheek monthly for signs of oral cancer (spots or irritations)	○	○
. . . Fail to have regular dental checkups	○	○

LARYNX (VOICE BOX)

THYROID NODULE *

THYROID GLAND

TRACHEA (AIR PASSAGE FROM THE THROAT TO THE LUNGS)

*Lumpiness or swelling of the thyroid are most often benign goiters (enlargement of the thyroid gland), while a single solid swelling (nodule) is more likely to be serious.

CANCER OF THE LARYNX

RISK FACTORS:
• Heavy smoking
• Heavy drinking
• Cancer of the oral cavity or lung

AWARENESS COUNTS:
WHEN DETECTED EARLY, CANCER OF THE LARYNX CAN BE CURED. The preventive measure you can take is to cut down on your drinking and smoking. Alcohol and smoke are irritants to the lining of your mouth and throat. Any reduction of this kind of irritation to your mouth and throat decreases your risk.

CANCER OF THE MOUTH AND THROAT

RISK FACTORS:
• A broken tooth which irritates the inside of your mouth
• Broken or ill-fitting dentures
• Heavy smoking or drinking
• A non-healing sore or white patch in your mouth

AWARENESS COUNTS:
Any sores of the mouth, throat or gums which do not heal properly should be brought to the attention of a physician or dentist.

Cutting down on alcohol consumption and smoking is an important preventive measure and can reduce your risks.

FIGURE 13.8 *(Continued)*
Health Protection Plan for Cancer.

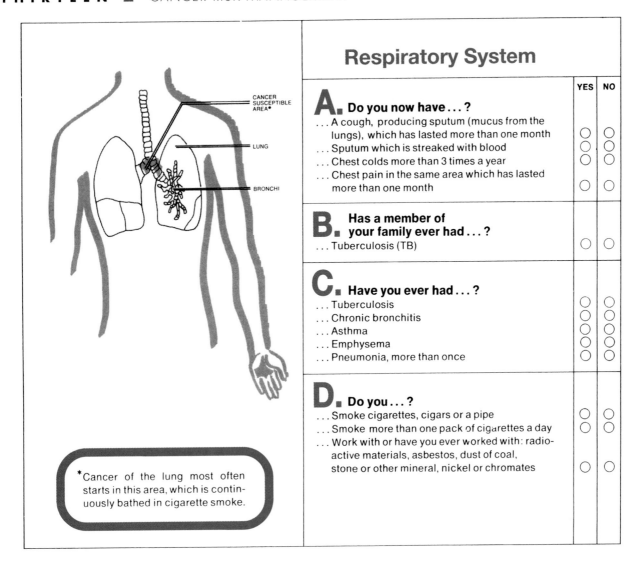

Respiratory System

CANCER
SUSCEPTIBLE
AREA*

LUNG

BRONCHI

*Cancer of the lung most often starts in this area, which is continuously bathed in cigarette smoke.

	YES	NO
A. Do you now have...?		
...A cough, producing sputum (mucus from the lungs), which has lasted more than one month	○	○
...Sputum which is streaked with blood	○	○
...Chest colds more than 3 times a year	○	○
...Chest pain in the same area which has lasted more than one month	○	○
B. Has a member of your family ever had...?		
...Tuberculosis (TB)	○	○
C. Have you ever had...?		
...Tuberculosis	○	○
...Chronic bronchitis	○	○
...Asthma	○	○
...Emphysema	○	○
...Pneumonia, more than once	○	○
D. Do you...?		
...Smoke cigarettes, cigars or a pipe	○	○
...Smoke more than one pack of cigarettes a day	○	○
...Work with or have you ever worked with: radioactive materials, asbestos, dust of coal, stone or other mineral, nickel or chromates	○	○

CANCER OF THE LUNG

RISK FACTORS:

- Cigarette smoking — the smoker's risk of developing lung cancer is proportional to the number of cigarettes smoked, number of years smoking, age at which smoking started, and how deeply smoke is inhaled.
- Working in an occupation which brings you into contact with asbestos, nickel, chromates or radioactive material
- A history of tuberculosis
- A chronic cough

AWARENESS COUNTS:

Your risk for lung cancer can be reduced if you avoid cigarette smoking. This is an effective preventive measure. Cigarette smoking can not only lead to death from lung cancer, but can also increase the chances of dying from other lung diseases (asthma, emphysema, pneumonia) or heart disease.

Occupational exposure to the cancer causing agents mentioned should be avoided or carefully controlled. Be aware of the materials you work with.

FIGURE 13.8 *(Continued)*
Health Protection Plan for Cancer.

Urinary Tract

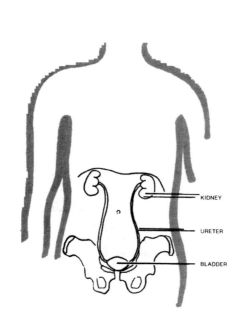

	YES	NO
A. Do you now have...?		
...An urge to urinate more frequently than usual	○	○
...Pain or burning upon urination	○	○
...Narrowing stream of urine	○	○
...Blood in the urine	○	○
B. Has a member of your family ever had...?		
...Cancer of the kidney or bladder	○	○
...Any congenital (present from birth) urinary tract disease	○	○
C. Have you ever had...?		
...A urinary tract infection	○	○
...Blood in the urine	○	○
...Kidney stones	○	○
...Any chronic (long-lasting) kidney disease	○	○
D. Do you...?		
..Work daily with cleaning fluids, paints, dyes or in factories which manufacture these substances	○	○
...Smoke cigarettes	○	○

Kidney stones or urinary infections will cause bleeding and pain, but tumors in the kidney or bladder usually cause painless bleeding.

CANCER OF THE KIDNEY AND BLADDER

RISK FACTORS:
- Congenital abnormalities of the kidney or bladder (your physician should have informed you if these conditions exist)
- Exposure to certain chemicals such as naphthalines, aniline dyes, or benzidine (be sure to read labels)
- Blood in the urine
- Frequent urinary tract infections, especially after age 50
- A history of schistosomiasis (a tropical disease)
- Heavy cigarette smoking — smoking leads to the presence of chemicals in the urine which may contribute to the development of cancer of the urinary tract

AWARENESS COUNTS:
You can prevent urinary tract cancer by avoiding occupational exposure to cancer-causing chemicals and by seeking medical attention when any symptoms exist.

Blood in the urine is always an important sign and requires *immediate* medical evaluation.

These symptoms are not specific for cancer; more commonly, they are found with bladder infection. However, a physician should be consulted. Frequent urinary tract infections may be due to underlying cancer.

FIGURE 13.8 *(Continued)*
Health Protection Plan for Cancer.

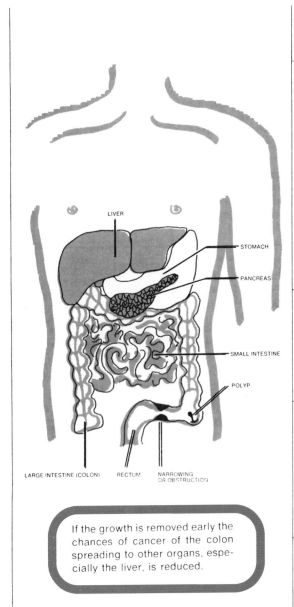

If the growth is removed early the chances of cancer of the colon spreading to other organs, especially the liver, is reduced.

Gastrointestinal Tract

	YES	NO
A. **Do you now have ... ?**		
... Heartburn, indigestion or abdominal pain which has lasted for more than one month	○	○
... Nausea or vomiting which has lasted more than one week	○	○
... Fullness after eating small amounts	○	○
... Unexplained weight loss, more than 10 lbs. in three months or less	○	○
... Any vomiting of blood	○	○
... Bowel movements more frequently or less frequently than usual	○	○
... Increasing narrowness of stool (ribbon-like)	○	○
... Pain in rectum with bowel movements	○	○
... Blood in stool, or tarry-black stool	○	○
... Passage of mucus alone or with stool	○	○
B. **Has a member of your family ever had ... ?**		
... Cancer of the stomach	○	○
... Stomach or duodenal ulcer	○	○
... Pernicious anemia	○	○
... Polyps of the colon	○	○
... Cancer of the colon or rectum	○	○
C. **Have you ever had ... ?**		
... Gall bladder disorder	○	○
... Stomach or duodenal ulcer	○	○
... Pernicious anemia	○	○
... Jaundice, hepatitis, cirrhosis of the liver	○	○
... Polyps of the stomach or colon	○	○
... Ulcerative colitis or other chronic bowel problems	○	○
D. **Do you ... ?**		
... Have more than 5 beers, 5 glasses of wine, or 3 hard liquor drinks a day	○	○

CANCER OF THE STOMACH

RISK FACTORS:
- A lack of normal stomach acid
- Pernicious anemia (a special kind of anemia treated by vitamin B₁₂ injections)
- Chronic gastritis or stomach polyps

AWARENESS COUNTS:
Ulcers and ulcer symptoms may be mistaken for stomach cancer and vice versa. If any symptoms listed above last for more than one month, consult a physician.

CANCER OF THE COLON

RISK FACTORS:
- Polyps in the colon
- A family history of cancer of the colon or rectum

AWARENESS COUNTS:
Any changes in your regular bowel habits should be reported to your physician promptly.

Cancer of the colon is infrequent in countries where the diet is high in fruits, vegetables and fish and low in meat.

FIGURE 13.8 *(Continued)*
Health Protection Plan for Cancer.

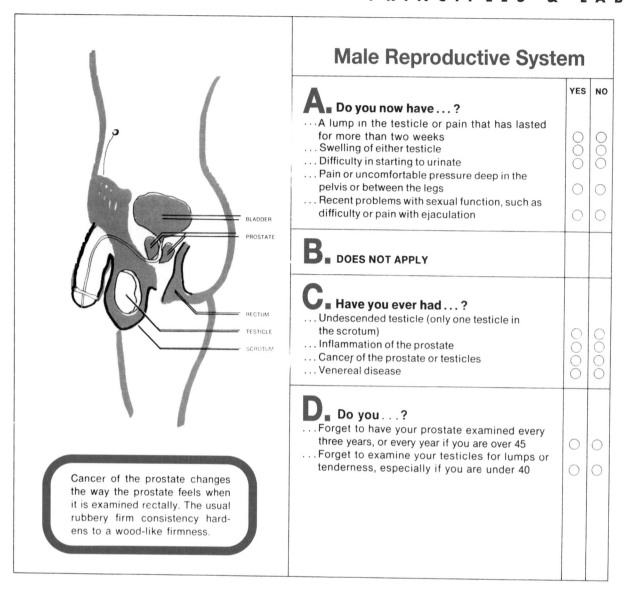

Male Reproductive System

	YES	NO
A. **Do you now have . . . ?**		
. . . A lump in the testicle or pain that has lasted for more than two weeks	○	○
. . . Swelling of either testicle	○	○
. . . Difficulty in starting to urinate	○	○
. . . Pain or uncomfortable pressure deep in the pelvis or between the legs	○	○
. . . Recent problems with sexual function, such as difficulty or pain with ejaculation	○	○
B. **DOES NOT APPLY**		
C. **Have you ever had . . . ?**		
. . . Undescended testicle (only one testicle in the scrotum)	○	○
. . . Inflammation of the prostate	○	○
. . . Cancer of the prostate or testicles	○	○
. . . Venereal disease	○	○
D. **Do you . . . ?**		
. . . Forget to have your prostate examined every three years, or every year if you are over 45	○	○
. . . Forget to examine your testicles for lumps or tenderness, especially if you are under 40	○	○

BLADDER

PROSTATE

RECTUM

TESTICLE

SCROTUM

Cancer of the prostate changes the way the prostate feels when it is examined rectally. The usual rubbery firm consistency hardens to a wood-like firmness.

CANCER OF THE PROSTATE

RISK FACTORS:
- A history of venereal disease
- A history of prostate infections (more than 2)
- Risk increases after the age of 50

AWARENESS COUNTS:
The occurrence of cancer of the prostate cannot be controlled since the causes are not known. However, the death rate can be greatly lowered if men, especially those over age 50, are familiar with the above symptoms of the disease and if the prostate is examined regularly. Ask your physician to examine the prostate.

CANCER OF THE TESTES

RISK FACTOR:
- Undescended testicle not corrected before age 6

AWARENESS COUNTS:
There is a high incidence of cancer of the testicle in persons born with an undescended testicle, so this condition should be corrected early. Cancer of the testicle is most common in men under 40. Perform testicular self-exam once a month after a warm bath or shower, when the scrotal skin is most relaxed. Examine each testicle gently by rolling it between the thumb and fingers. Feel for a firm lump about the size of a pea. Most lumps are non-cancerous.

FIGURE 13.8 *(Continued)*
Health Protection Plan for Cancer.

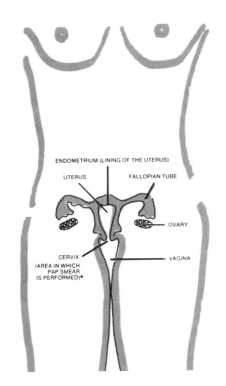

*A Pap smear is done by placing a cotton swab in the vagina and wiping cells off the surface of the cervix. The cells are then examined under a microscope for evidence of cancer. Having a Pap smear is a painless procedure.

Female Reproductive System

	YES	NO
A. Do you now have . . . ?		
. . . Bleeding between menstrual periods	○	○
. . . Bloody discharge unrelated to menstrual periods	○	○
. . . Bleeding after sexual intercourse	○	○
. . . Having completed the menopause, any bleeding or spotting	○	○
B. Has a member of your mother's side of the family ever had . . . ?		
. . . Cancer of the cervix, vagina, uterus (womb), or ovary	○	○
Did your mother take female hormones when she was pregnant with you?	○	○
C. Have you ever had . . . ?		
. . . Abnormal cervical (Pap) smear	○	○
. . . Ovarian cyst or tumor	○	○
. . . Fibroid tumor of the uterus	○	○
. . . A Dilatation and Curettage operation ("D & C" or scraping)	○	○
. . . Cauterization of the cervix	○	○
. . . Other surgery of female organs	○	○
Do you use birth control pills?	○	○
Do you use female hormones (estrogens)?	○	○
D. Do you . . . ?		
. . . Forget to have a Pap smear . . .		
. . . Every 3 years (if between 25-35 years of age)	○	○
. . . Every 2 years (if between 35-45 years of age)	○	○
. . . Every year (if over age 45)	○	○

CANCER OF THE CERVIX

RISK FACTORS:
• Completed pregnancies (more than 5)
• Marriage at an early age (intercourse before age 18)
• A history of syphilis or gonorrhea
• Any of the symptoms listed under A

AWARENESS COUNTS:
Cancer of the cervix is usually slow-growing and can be detected early by the Pap smear and cured. Examination of any adult female should include a Pap smear and pelvic examination as well as an examination of the breasts.

CANCER OF THE ENDO-METRIUM

RISK FACTORS:
• Having completed the menopause
• Never having been pregnant
• A family history of cancer of the endometrium (lining of the uterus)
• Being a diabetic
• Having hypertension
• Being obese
• Any of the symptoms listed under A

CANCER OF THE OVARY

AWARENESS COUNTS:
In most cases, a woman is unaware of the presence of tumors in the ovaries. There are seldom early symptoms. The ovaries are examined at the time of a Pap and pelvic examination. These examinations should be done on a regular basis (see **D.** above).

FIGURE 13.8 *(Continued)*
Health Protection Plan for Cancer.

Look for any changes in size, shape, or contour of the breasts. Look for skin changes such as puckering or dimpling. Squeeze nipples gently for discharge. *(Remember it is perfectly normal to have one breast which is larger than the other.)*

Lying down, examine the breasts one at a time with one hand behind your head and the other hand crossed over to examine the opposite breast.

Still lying down, hold your fingers closely together; use gentle pressure and small circular motions. Start at the outer margins, proceed in the same way in smaller circles until you have covered the entire breast.

Cancer of the Breast (For Women)

	YES	NO
A. **Do you now have...?**		
...Breast pain not related to menstrual periods	○	○
...A lump in either breast	○	○
...Any discharge from the nipples	○	○
...Ulceration (sores), puckering or scaling of breast or any unusual color change of skin or scaling or peeling of nipples	○	○
B. **Has a member of your mother's side of the family ever had...?**		
...Cancer of the breast	○	○
...Cysts or tumors of the breast (which were not cancer)	○	○
...Any surgery of the breast	○	○
C. **Have you ever had...?**		
...Cancer of the breast	○	○
D. **Do you...?**		
...Forget to examine your breasts each month after your period?	○	○

CANCER OF THE BREAST

RISK FACTORS:

- A family or personal history of breast cancer
- Never having had a baby, if you are over age 45
- Having a first pregnancy after age 35
- Any of the symptoms under **A.**

If you have any of the above risks and are over 45, X-ray examination of the breasts (a mammography) is recommended.

AWARENESS COUNTS:

Breast cancer is curable if detected early. Breast examinations should be performed regularly and each time a Pap smear is done. Ask the doctor or nurse to teach you to do breast self-examination. Practice this yourself once a month 2 or 3 days after your menstrual period is over. Many women have cystic breasts. When cysts are present it is advisable to have breast examinations more frequently. This is not a premalignant condition, it just makes the breasts more difficult to examine. Most lumps are found by women themselves; therefore, regular self-examination is necessary. If you find any of the above symptoms, take immediate action. Remember, breast cancer is curable if identified at any early stage.

FIGURE 13.8 *(Continued)*
Health Protection Plan for Cancer.

STRESS MANAGEMENT

14

Learning to live and get ahead today is nearly impossible without stress. To succeed in an unpredictable world that changes with every new day, working under pressure has become the rule rather than the exception for most people. As a result, stress has become one of the most common problems we face. Current estimates indicate that the annual cost of stress and stress-related diseases in the United States exceeds $100 billion, a direct result of health care costs, lost productivity, and absenteeism.

Although high stress is one of the factors related to 20th-century patterns of life that is detrimental to human health, it also is a factor that can be self-controlled. Most people have accepted stress as a normal part of daily life, and even though everyone has to deal with it, few seem to understand it and know how to cope effectively. Stress should not be avoided entirely, as a certain amount is necessary for optimum health, performance, and well-being. It is difficult to succeed and have fun in life without "hits, runs, and errors."

Just what is stress? Dr. Hans Selye, one of the foremost authorities on stress, defined stress as *the nonspecific response of the human organism to any demand that is placed upon it*. "Nonspecific" indicates that the body reacts in a similar fashion regardless of the nature of the event that leads to the stress response. In simpler terms, *stress is the mental, emotional, and physiological response of the body to any situation that is new, threatening, frightening, or exciting*.

> **Stress is the mental, emotional, and physiological response of the body to any situation that is new, threatening, frightening, or exciting.**

The body's response to stress has been the same ever since humans were first put on the earth. Stress prepares the organism to react to the stress-causing event, also called the *stressor*. The problem, though, is the way in which we react to stress. Many people thrive under stress, whereas others under similar circumstances are unable to handle it. An individual's reaction to a stress-causing agent determines whether stress is positive or negative.

Dr. Selye defined the ways in which we react to stress as either *eustress* or *distress*. In both cases, the nonspecific response is almost the same. In the case of eustress, health and performance continue to improve even as stress increases. Distress, on the other hand, refers to the unpleasant or harmful stress under which health and performance begin to deteriorate. This relationship between stress and performance is illustrated in Figure 14.1.

Stress is a fact of modern life, and every person does need an optimal level of stress that is most conducive to adequate health and performance. When stress levels reach mental, emotional, and physiological limits, however, stress becomes distress and the person no longer functions effectively.

Chronic distress raises the risk for many health disorders, including coronary heart disease, hypertension, eating disorders, ulcers, diabetes, asthma, depression, migraine headaches, sleep disorders, and chronic fatigue and may even play a role in the development of certain types of cancers. Recognizing this turning point and overcoming the problem quickly and efficiently are crucial in maintaining emotional and physiological stability.

SOURCES OF STRESS

During recent years, several instruments have been developed to assess sources of stress in life. One of the instruments used most commonly is the Life Experiences Survey, included in Lab 14A. This survey identifies a person's life changes within the last 12 months that may have an impact on a person's physical and psychological well-being.

The Life Experiences Survey is divided into two sections. Section 1, to be completed by all respondents, contains a list of 47 life events plus three blank spaces for other events experienced but not listed in the survey. Section 2 contains an additional 10 questions designed for students only (students should fill out both sections).

The format of the survey requires the person to rate the extent to which the life events he or she experienced had a positive or negative impact on his or her life at the time these events occurred. The ratings are on a 7-point scale. A rating of −3 indicates an extremely undesirable impact. A rating of zero (0) suggests neither a positive nor a negative impact. A rating of +3 indicates an extremely desirable impact.

After determining the life events that have taken place, the negative and the positive points are added together separately. Both scores should be expressed as positive numbers (for example — positive ratings: 2, 1, 3, 3 = 9 points positive score; negative

FIGURE 14.1

Relationship between stress and health/performance.

ratings: –3, –2, –2, –1, –2 = 10 points negative score). A final "total life change" score can be obtained by adding the positive score and the negative score together as positive numbers (total life change score: 9 + 10 = 19 points).

As negative and positive changes alike can produce nonspecific responses, the total life change score gives a good indication of total life stress. Most research in this area, however, indicates that the negative change score is a better predictor of potential physical and psychological illness than the total change score.

More research is necessary before the role of total change and the role of the ratio of positive to negative stress can be established. Therefore, only the negative score is used as part of the stress profile. To obtain a stress rating, refer to Table 14A.1 in Lab 14A, which presents the various stress categories based on the survey's results.

BEHAVIOR PATTERNS

Common life events are not the only source of stress in life. All too often, individuals bring on stress as a result of their behavior patterns. The two main types of behavior patterns are Type A and Type B. Each type is based on several characteristics that are used in classifying people into one of these behavioral patterns.

Even though several attempts have been made to develop an objective scale to properly identify Type A individuals, these questionnaires are not as valid and reliable as researchers would like them to be. Consequently, the main assessment tool to determine behavioral type is still the Structured Interview. During the Structured Interview a person is asked to reply to several questions that describe Type A and Type B behavior patterns. The interviewer notes not only the responses to the questions but also mental, emotional, and physical behaviors the individual exhibits as he or she replies to each question.

Based on the answers and the behaviors exhibited, the interviewer rates the person along a continuum, ranging from Type A to Type B. Along this continuum, behavioral patterns are classified into five categories: A–1, A–2, X (a mix of Type A and

Type B), B–3, and B–4. The Type A–1 exhibits all of the Type A characteristics, and the B–4 shows a relative absence of Type A behaviors. The Type A–2 does not exhibit a complete Type A pattern, and the Type B–3 exhibits only a few Type A characteristics.

Type A behavior primarily characterizes a hard-driving, overambitious, aggressive, at times hostile and overly competitive person. Type A individuals often set their own goals, are self-motivated, try to accomplish many tasks at the same time, are excessively achievement-oriented, and have a high degree of time urgency.

A Type A person is usually hard-driving, overambitious, aggressive, and, at times, hostile and overly competitive.

In contrast, Type B behavior is characteristic of calm, casual, relaxed, easy-going individuals. Type B people take one thing at a time, do not feel pressured or hurried, and seldom set their own deadlines.

Over the years, experts have indicated that individuals classified as Type A are under too much stress and have a significantly higher incidence of coronary heart disease. Based on these findings, Type A individuals have been counseled to lower their stress level by modifying many of their Type A behaviors.

Most experts agree that Type A behavior is learned. Consequently, if people can learn to identify the sources of stress and make changes in their behavioral responses, they can move along the continuum and respond more like Type B's. The debate, however, has centered on which Type A behaviors should be changed, as not all of them are undesirable.

A Type B person is usually calm, casual, relaxed, and easy-going.

New scientific evidence indicates that not all typical Type A people are at higher risk for disease. Type A individuals who commonly express anger and hostility are the ones at higher risk for disease.

Therefore, many behavioral modification counselors now work on changing primarily the latter behaviors to prevent disease.

Even though personality questionnaires are not as valid and reliable as the structured interview in identifying Type A individuals, Drs. Meyer Friedman and Ray M. Rosenman, two San Francisco scientists/internists, constructed a Type A personality assessment form, adapted from the Structured Interview method, to give people a general idea of Type A behavioral patterns. This assessment form is found in Lab 14B. You can use it to better understand your own behavioral patterns. If you obtain a "high" rating, you probably are a Type A individual.

> *Type C people are usually highly committed to what they are doing, have a great deal of confidence in their ability, and can be in constant control.*

We also know that many individuals perform well under pressure. They typically are classified as Type A but do not demonstrate any of the detrimental effects of stress. Drs. Robert and Marilyn Kriegel came up with the term *Type C* to characterize people with these behaviors.

Type C individuals are just as highly stressed as Type A's but do not seem to be at higher risk for disease than Type B's. The keys to successful Type C performance seem to be commitment, confidence, and control. Type C people are highly committed to what they are doing, have a great deal of confidence in their ability to do their work, and are in constant control of their actions. In addition, they enjoy their work and maintain themselves in top physical condition to be able to meet the mental and physical demands of their work.

Because of the results of recent studies, Type A behavior by itself is no longer viewed as a major risk factor for coronary heart disease. Many experts now believe that emotional stress is far more likely to trigger a heart attack than physical stress. People who are impatient and readily annoyed when they have to wait for someone or something — an employee, a traffic light, in a restaurant line — are especially vulnerable.

Research also is focusing on individuals who have anxiety, depression, and feelings of helplessness when they encounter setbacks and failures in life. It looks as though people who lose control of their lives, those that give up on their dreams in life, knowing that they could and should be doing better, are more likely to have heart attacks than hard-driving people who enjoy their work.

VULNERABILITY TO STRESS

Researchers have identified a number of factors that can affect the way in which people handle stress. How people deal with these factors can actually increase or decrease vulnerability to stress. The questionnaire in Lab 14C, which contains a list of these factors, has been designed to help you determine your vulnerability rating. Many of the items on this questionnaire are related to health, social support, self-worth, and nurturance (sense of being needed). All of the factors are crucial for a person's physical, social, mental, and emotional well-being. The questionnaire will help you identify specific areas in which you can make improvements to help you cope more efficiently.

> *Positive correlations have been found between social support and health outcomes.*

The benefits of physical fitness are discussed extensively in this book. Further, social support, self-worth, and nurturance are essential to cope effectively with stressful life events. These factors render a supportive and protective role in people's lives. The more integrated people are in society, the less vulnerable they are to stress and illness.

Positive correlations have been found between social support and health outcomes. Social support provides vital resources that people can draw upon to weather crises. Knowing that someone else cares, that people are there to lean on, that support is out there, is extremely valuable for survival (or growth) in times of need.

As you take the test, you will notice that many of the items describe situations and behaviors that are within your own control. To make yourself less vulnerable to stress, you will want to improve the behaviors that make you more vulnerable to stress. You should start by modifying the behaviors that are easiest to change before undertaking some of the most difficult ones.

TIME MANAGEMENT

According to Benjamin Franklin, "Time is the stuff life is made of." The present "hurry-up" style of life of the American people is not conducive to wellness. The hassles involved in making it through a routine day often lead to stress-related illnesses. People who fail to manage their time properly will quickly experience chronic stress, fatigue, despair, discouragement, and illness.

Based on a 1990 Gallup Poll, almost 80% of Americans reported that time moves too fast for them, 54% felt they had to get everything done they needed to. The younger the respondents, the more they struggled with lack of time. Almost half wished they had more time for exercise and recreation, hobbies, and family.

Healthy and successful people are good time managers, able to maintain a pace of life within their comfort zone. In a survey of 1954 Harvard graduates from the school of business, only 27% had reached the goals they established in college. Every one had rated himself as a superior time manager, and only 8% of the remaining graduates perceived themselves as superior time managers. The successful graduates attributed their success to "smart work," not necessarily "hard work."

FIVE STEPS TO TIME MANAGEMENT

Trying to achieve one or more goals in a limited time can create a tremendous amount of stress. Many people just don't seem to have enough hours in the day to accomplish their tasks. The greatest demands on our time, nonetheless, frequently are self-imposed: trying to do too much, too fast, too soon. You can follow five basic steps to make better use of your time (also see Lab 14D):

1. **Find the time killers.** Many people do not know how they spend each part of the day. Keep a four- to seven-day log, and record at half-hour intervals the activities you do. Record the activities as you go through your typical day, so you will remember all of them. At the end of each day, decide when you wasted time. You may be shocked by the amount of time you spent on the phone, sleeping (more than 8 hours per night), or watching television.

   Figure 14.2 provides a list of common time killers. Granted, some of these activities (such as eating, sleeping, and recreation) are necessary for health and wellness, but, in excess they'll lead to stress in life.

2. **Set long-range and short range goals.** Setting goals requires some in-depth thinking and helps put your life and daily tasks in perspective. What do I want out of life? Where do I want to be 10 years from now? Next year? Next week? Tomorrow?

3. **Identify your immediate goals, and prioritize them for today and this week.** Each day sit down and determine what you need to accomplish that day and that week. Rank your "today" and "this week" tasks in four categories: (a) top priority, (b) medium priority, (c) low priority, and (d) "trash." Top priority tasks are the most important ones. If you were to reap most of your productivity from 30% of your activities, which would they be? Medium priority activities are those that must be done but can

■ Watching television
■ Listening to radio/music
■ Sleeping
■ Eating
■ Daydreaming
■ Shopping
■ Socializing/parties
■ Recreation
■ Talking on the telephone
■ Worrying
■ Procrastinating
■ Drop-in visitors
■ Confusion (unclear goals)
■ Indecision (what to do next)
■ Interruptions
■ Perfectionism (every detail must be done)

FIGURE 14.2
Common time killers.

wait a day or two. Low priority activities are those to be done only upon completing all top and middle priority activities. Trash are activities that are not worth your time (for example, cruising the hallways).

4. **Use a daily planner.** A daily planner will help you organize and simplify your day. Your priority list, appointments, notes, references, names, places, phone numbers, and addresses all can be accessed conveniently from your coat pocket or purse. Many individuals think that planning daily and weekly activities is a waste of time. A few minutes to schedule your time each day, however, may pay off in hours saved. As you plan your day, be realistic and find your comfort zone. Determine what is the best way to organize your day. Which is the most productive time for work, study, errands? Are you a morning person, or do you get most of your work done when people are quitting for the day? Pick your best hours for top priority activities. Be sure to schedule enough time for exercise and relaxation. Recreation is not necessarily wasted time. You need to take care of your physical and emotional well-being. Otherwise your life will be seriously imbalanced.

5. **Nightly audits.** Take 10 minutes each night to figure out how well you accomplished your goals that day. Successful time managers evaluate themselves daily. This simple task will help you see the entire picture. Cross off the goals you accomplished and carry over to the next day those you did not get done. You also may realize that some goals can be moved down to low priority or be trashed.

TIME MANAGEMENT SKILLS

In addition to these five major steps, the following can help you make better use of your time:

■ **Delegate.** If possible, delegate activities that someone else can do for you. Having another person type your paper while you prepare for an exam might be well worth the expense and your time.

■ **Say "no."** Learn to say no to activities that keep you from getting your top priorities done. You only can do so much in a single day. Nobody has enough time to do everything he or she would like to get done. Don't overload either. Many

people are afraid to say no because they feel guilty if they do. Think ahead, and think of the consequences. Are you doing it to please others? What will it do to your well-being? Can you handle one more task? There comes a point at which you have to balance your activities and look at life and time realistically.

■ **Protect against boredom.** Doing nothing can be a source of stress. People need to feel that they are contributing and that they are a productive member of society. It also is good for self-esteem and self-worth. Set realistic goals, and work toward them each day.

■ **Plan ahead for disruptions.** Even a careful plan of action can be disrupted. An unexpected phone call or visitor can ruin your schedule. Planning your response ahead will help you deal with these saboteurs.

■ **Get it done.** Select only one task at the time, concentrate on it, and see it through. Many people do a little here, a little there, then do something else. In the end, nothing gets done. An exception to working on just one task at a time is when you are doing a difficult task. Rather than "killing yourself," interchange with another activity that is not as hard.

■ **Eliminate distractions.** If you have trouble adhering to a set plan, remove distractions and trash activities from your eye sight. Television, radio, magazines, open doors, or studying in a park can easily distract you and become time killers.

■ **Set aside "overtimes."** Regularly schedule time you did not think you would need as overtime to complete unfinished projects. Most people underschedule rather than overschedule time. The result is usually late night burnouts! If you schedule overtimes and get your tasks done, enjoy some leisure time, get ahead on another project, or work on some of your trash priorities.

■ **Plan time for you.** Set aside special time for yourself daily. Life is not meant to be all work. Use your time to walk, read, or listen to your favorite music.

■ **Reward yourself.** As with any other healthy behavior, positive change or a job well done deserves a reward. We often overlook the value of rewards, even if they are self-given. People practice behaviors that are rewarded and discontinue those that are not.

COPING WITH STRESS

The way in which people perceive and cope with stress seems to be more important in the development of disease than the amount and type of stress itself. For individuals who perceive stress as a definite problem in their lives — when it interferes with their optimal level of health and performance — several excellent stress management techniques have been developed to help them cope more effectively.

The first step, of course, is to recognize that a problem exists. Many people either do not want to believe they are under too much stress or they fail to recognize some of the typical symptoms of distress. Noting some of the stress-related symptoms will help a person respond more objectively and initiate an adequate coping response.

A list of some of the symptoms that people experience when stress becomes distress is given in Figure 14.3. Going through the accompanying list, most of us probably will recognize some of our own bodily responses when stress becomes distress:

> *The way in which people perceive and cope with stress seems to be more important in the development of disease than the amount and type of stress itself.*

When people experience stress-related symptoms, they first should try to identify and remove the stressor or stress-causing agent. This is not as simple as it may seem, because in some situations eliminating the stressor is impossible, or a person may not even know the exact causing agent. If the cause is unknown, keeping a log of the time and days when the symptoms occur, as well as the events that transpire before and after the onset of symptoms, may be helpful.

For instance, a couple noted that every afternoon around six o'clock, the wife became nauseated and experienced abdominal pain. After seeking professional help, the couple was instructed to keep a log of daily events. It soon became clear that the symptoms did not occur on weekends but always started just before the husband came home from work during the week. Following some personal interviews with the couple, it was determined that the wife felt a lack of attention from her husband

COMMON SYMPTOMS OF STRESS

- Headaches
- Muscular aches (mainly neck, shoulders, and back)
- Grinding teeth
- Nervous tick, finger tapping, toe tapping
- Increased sweating
- Increase or loss of appetite
- Insomnia
- Nightmares
- Fatigue
- Dry mouth
- Stuttering
- High blood pressure
- Tightness or pain in the chest
- Impotence
- Hives
- Dizziness
- Depression
- Irritation
- Anger
- Hostility
- Fear, panic, anxiety
- Stomach pain, flutters
- Nausea
- Cold, clammy hands
- Poor concentration
- Pacing
- Restlessness
- Rapid heart rate
- Low-grade infection
- Loss of sex drive
- Rash or acne

FIGURE 14.3
Common symptoms of stress.

and subconsciously responded by becoming ill to the point at which she required personal care and affection from her husband. Once the stressor was identified, appropriate changes in behavior were initiated to correct the situation.

In many instances, however, the stressor cannot be removed. For example, the death of a close family member, first year on the job, an intolerable boss, a change in work responsibility are situations in which little or nothing can be done to eliminate the stress-causing agent. Nevertheless, stress can be managed through relaxation techniques.

The body responds to stress by activating the fight or flight mechanism, which prepares a person to take action by stimulating the vital defense systems. This stimulation originates in the hypothalamus and the pituitary gland in the brain. The hypothalamus activates the sympathetic nervous system, and the pituitary activates the release of catecholamines (hormones) from the adrenal glands.

These hormonal changes increase heart rate, blood pressure, blood flow to active muscles and the brain, glucose levels, oxygen consumption, and strength — all necessary for the body to fight or flee. For the body to relax, one of these actions must take place. If the person fights or flees, the body relaxes and stress is dissipated, but if he or she is unable to take action, the muscles tense up and tighten (see Figure 14.4). This increased tension and tightening can be dissipated effectively with the aid of coping techniques.

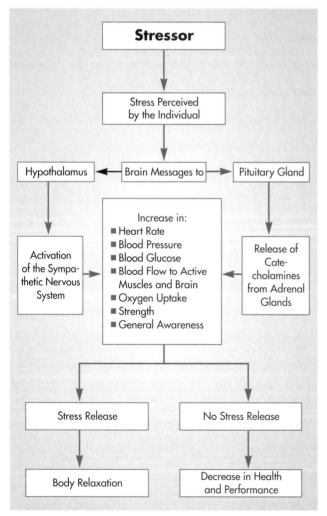

FIGURE 14.4
Physiological response to stress: fight or flight mechanism.

RELAXATION TECHNIQUES

Benefits are reaped immediately after engaging in any of several relaxation techniques. Several months of regular practice may, however, be necessary for complete mastery. The relaxation exercises that follow should not be considered a cure-all or panacea. If these exercises do not prove effective, more specialized textbooks and professional help are called for. In some instances the symptoms a person is experiencing may not be caused by stress but, rather, may be related to a different medical disorder.

Biofeedback

Clinical application of biofeedback in treating various medical disorders has become popular in the last few years. Besides its successful application in managing stress, it is commonly used in treating medical disorders such as essential hypertension, asthma, heart rhythm and rate disturbance, cardiac neurosis, eczematous dermatitis, fecal incontinence, insomnia, and stuttering.

Biofeedback as a treatment modality has been defined as:[2]

> A process in which a person learns to reliably influence physiological responses of two kinds: either responses which are not ordinarily under voluntary control or responses which ordinarily are easily regulated but for which regulation has broken down due to trauma or disease.

In simpler terms, biofeedback is the interaction with the interior self.[4] This interaction allows a person to learn the relationship between the mind and the biological response. The person can actually "feel" how the thought process influences biological responses (e.g., heart rate, blood pressure, body temperature, muscle tension) and how biological responses also influence the thought process.

As an illustration of this process, consider the association between a strange noise in the middle of a dark, quiet night and the heart rate response. At first, the heart rate shoots up because of the stress the unknown noise induces. The individual may even feel the heart palpitating in the chest and, while still uncertain about the noise, attempts not to panic, to prevent an even faster heart rate. Upon realizing all is well, the person can take control and influence the heart rate to come down. The mind now is able to exert almost complete control over the biological response.

Complex electronic instruments usually are required to conduct biofeedback. The process itself entails a three-stage, closed-loop feedback system:

1. A biological response to a stressor is detected and amplified.
2. The response is processed.
3. Results of the response are fed back to the individual immediately.

The person uses this new input and attempts to voluntarily change the physiological response, which, in turn, is detected, amplified, and processed. The results then are fed back to the person. The process continues with the intent of teaching the person to reliably influence for the better the physiological response[1] (see Figure 14.5). The most common methods used to measure physiological responses are heart rate, finger temperature, blood pressure equipment, electromyograms, and electroencephalograms.

Although biofeedback has significant applications in treating various medical disorders, including stress, it requires adequately trained personnel and, in many cases, costly equipment. Therefore, several alternative methods that yield similar results frequently are substituted for biofeedback. For example, research has shown that physical exercise and progressive muscle relaxation, used successfully in stress management, seem to be just as effective as biofeedback in treating essential hypertension.

Physical Activity As A Means of Reducing Stress

Physical activity is one of the simplest tools to control stress. The value of exercise in reducing stress is related to several factors, the main one being a decrease in muscular tension.

For example, a person can be distressed because he or she had a miserable day at work and the job required eight hours of work in a smoke-filled room with an intolerable boss. To make matters worse, it is late and on the way home the car in front is going much slower than the speed limit. The fight or flight mechanism is activated, catecholamines rise, heart rate and blood pressure shoot up, breathing quickens and deepens, muscles tense up, and all systems say "go." No action can be initiated or stress dissipated, though, because the person just cannot hit the boss or the car in front.

A real remedy would be to take action by "hitting" the swimming pool, the tennis ball, the weights, or the jogging trail (Figure 14.6). By engaging in physical activity, a person is able to reduce the muscular tension and metabolize the increased catecholamines that brought about the physiological changes triggering the fight or flight mechanism. Although exercise does not solve problems at work or take care of slow drivers on the road, it certainly can help a person cope with stress, preventing it from becoming a chronic problem.

FIGURE 14.5
Biofeedback mechanism.

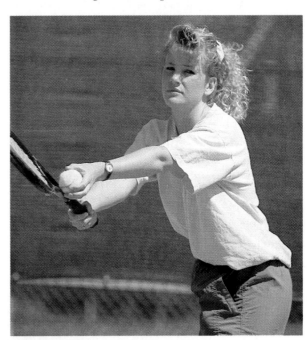

FIGURE 14.6
Physical activity: an excellent tool to control stress.

The early evening hours are becoming the most popular time to exercise for a lot of highly stressed executives. On the way home from work, they stop at the health club or the fitness center. Exercising at this time helps them to dissipate the stress accumulated during the day.

Most people can relate to exercise as a means of managing stress by remembering how good they felt the last time they concluded a strenuous exercise session after a long, difficult day at the office. A fatigued muscle is a relaxed muscle. For this reason, many people have said that the best part of exercise is the shower afterward.

Not only does evening exercise help to get rid of the stress, but it also provides an opportunity to enjoy a better evening. At home, the family will appreciate Dad or Mom coming home more relaxed, leaving work problems behind, and being able to dedicate all energy to family activities.

Research also has shown that physical exercise requiring continuous and rhythmic muscular activity, such as aerobic exercise, stimulates alpha-wave activity in the brain. These are the same wave patterns commonly seen during meditation and relaxation.

> *You cannot hit your boss or the car in front of you, but you can certainly "hit" the swimming pool, the tennis ball, the weights, or the jogging trail.*

Further, during vigorous aerobic exercise lasting 30 minutes or longer, morphine-like substances referred to as endorphines are thought to be released from the pituitary gland in the brain. These substances not only act as painkillers but also seem to induce the soothing, calming effect often associated with aerobic exercise.

Another way that exercise helps to reduce stress is by deliberately diverting stress to various body systems. Dr. Hans Selye explains in his book, *Stress Without Distress*, that when accomplishing one specific task becomes difficult, a change in activity can be as good or better than rest itself. For example, if a person is having trouble with a task and does not seem to be getting anywhere, going jogging or swimming for a while is better than sitting around and getting frustrated. In this way, the mental strain is diverted to the working muscles and one system helps the other to relax.

Other psychologists indicate that when muscular tension is removed from the emotional strain, the emotional strain disappears. In many cases, the change of activity suddenly clears the mind and helps put the pieces together.

Researchers have found that physical exercise gives people a psychological boost because exercise: (a) lessens feelings of anxiety, depression, frustration, aggression, anger, and hostility; (b) alleviates insomnia; (c) provides an opportunity to meet social needs and develop new friendships; (d) allows the person to share common interests and problems; (e) develops discipline; and (f) provides the opportunity to do something enjoyable and constructive that will lead to better health and total well-being.

Beyond the short-term benefits of exercise in reducing stress, another important benefit of a regular aerobic exercise program is the actual strengthening of the cardiovascular system itself. Because the cardiovascular system seems to be most seriously affected by stress, a stronger system should be able to cope more effectively. For instance, good cardiovascular endurance has been shown to lower resting heart rate and blood pressure. Because both heart rate and blood pressure rise in stressful situations, initiating the stress response at a lower baseline will counteract the negative effects of stress. Cardiovascularly fit individuals can cope more effectively and are less affected by the stresses of daily living.

Progressive Muscle Relaxation

Progressive muscle relaxation was developed by Dr. Edmund Jacobsen in the 1930s. This technique enables individuals to relearn the sensation of deep relaxation. The technique involves progressively contracting and relaxing muscle groups throughout the body. As chronic stress leads to high levels of muscular tension, acute awareness of how progressively tightening and relaxing the muscles feels releases the tension on the muscles and teaches the body to relax at will (see Figure 14.7).

Feeling the tension during the exercises also helps the person to be more alert to signs of distress because this tension is similar to that experienced in stressful situations. In everyday life, these feelings then can cue the person to do relaxation exercises.

Relaxation exercises should be done in a quiet, warm, well-ventilated room. The recommended exercises and the duration of the routine vary from one

FIGURE 14.17
Progressive muscle relaxation technique for stress management.

person to the next. Most important is that the individual pay attention to the sensation he or she feels each time the muscles are tensed and relaxed.

The exercises should encompass all muscle groups of the body. An example of a sequence of progressive muscle relaxation exercises is given next. The instructions for these exercises can be read to the person or memorized or tape-recorded. At least 20 minutes should be set aside to complete the entire sequence. Doing them any faster will defeat the purpose of the exercises. Ideally, the sequence should be done twice a day.

The individual performing the exercises must stretch out comfortably on the floor, face up, with a pillow under the knees, and should assume a passive attitude, allowing the body to relax as much as possible. Each muscle group is to be contracted in sequence, taking care to avoid any strain. Muscles should be tightened to only about 70% of the total possible tension to avoid cramping or some type of injury to the muscle itself.

Paying attention to the sensation of tensing up and relaxing is most crucial to produce the relaxation effects. The person holds each contraction about five seconds, and then allows the muscles to go totally limp. The person should take enough time to contract and relax each muscle group before going on to the next. An example of a complete progressive muscle relaxation sequence is:

1. Point your feet, curling the toes downward. Study the tension in the arches and the top of the feet. Hold, and continue to note the tension, then relax. Repeat a second time.

2. Flex the feet upward toward the face and note the tension in your feet and calves. Hold, and relax. Repeat once more.

3. Push your heels down against the floor as if burying them in the sand. Hold, and note the

tension at the back of the thigh. Relax. Repeat once more.

4. Contract the right thigh by straightening the leg, gently raising the leg off the floor. Hold, and study the tension. Relax. Repeat with the left leg; hold and relax. Repeat each leg again.

5. Tense the buttocks by raising your hips ever so slightly off the floor. Hold, and note the tension. Relax. Repeat once again.

6. Contract the abdominal muscles. Hold them tight and note the tension. Relax. Repeat one more time.

7. Suck in your stomach. Try to make it reach your spine. Flatten your lower back to the floor. Hold, and feel the tension in the stomach and lower back. Relax. Repeat once more.

8. Take a deep breath and hold it, then exhale. Repeat. Note your breathing becoming slower and more relaxed.

9. Place your arms at the side of your body and clench both fists. Hold, study the tension, and relax. Repeat a second time.

10. Flex the elbow by bringing both hands to the shoulders. Hold tight and study the tension in the biceps. Relax. Repeat one more time.

11. Place your arms flat on the floor, palms up, and push the forearm hard against the floor. Note the tension on the triceps. Hold, and relax. Repeat once more.

12. Shrug your shoulders, raising them as high as possible. Hold and note the tension. Relax. Repeat once again.

13. Gently push your head backward. Note the tension in the back of the neck. Hold, relax. Repeat one more time.

14. Gently bring the head against the chest, push forward, hold, and note the tension in the neck. Relax. Repeat a second time.

15. Press your tongue toward the roof of your mouth. Hold, study the tension and relax. Repeat once more.

16. Press your teeth together. Hold, and study the tension. Relax. Repeat one more time.

17. Close your eyes tightly. Hold them closed and note the tension. Relax, leaving your eyes closed. Do this one more time.

18. Wrinkle your forehead and note the tension. Hold, and relax. Repeat one more time.

When time is a factor during the daily routine and an individual is not able to go through the entire sequence, he or she may do only the exercises specific to the area that feels most tense. Performing a partial sequence is better than not doing the exercises at all. Completing the entire sequence, of course, yields the best results.

Breathing Techniques For Relaxation

Breathing exercises also can be an antidote to stress. These exercises have been used for centuries in the Orient and India to improve mental, physical, and emotional stamina. In breathing exercises the person concentrates on "breathing away" the tension and inhaling fresh air to the entire body. Breathing exercises can be learned in only a few minutes and require considerably less time than the progressive muscle relaxation exercises.

As with any other relaxation technique, these exercises should be done in a quiet, pleasant, well-ventilated room. Any of the three examples of breathing exercises presented here will help relieve tension induced by stress.

1. **Deep breathing:** Lie with your back flat against the floor, and place a pillow under your knees, feet slightly separated, with toes pointing outward. (The exercise also may be done while sitting up in a chair or standing straight up — see Figure 14.8). Place one hand on your abdomen and the other hand on your chest.

    Slowly breathe in and out so the hand on your abdomen rises when you inhale and falls as you exhale. The hand on the chest should not move much at all. Repeat the exercise about 10 times. Next, scan your body for tension, and

FIGURE 14.8
Breathing exercises for stress management.

compare your present tension with the tension you felt at the beginning of the exercise. Repeat the entire process once or twice more.

2. **Sighing:** Using the abdominal breathing technique, breathe in through your nose to a specific count (e.g., 4, 5, or 6). Now exhale through pursed lips to double the intake count (e.g., 8, 10, 12). Repeat the exercise eight to ten times whenever you feel tense.

3. **Complete natural breathing:** Sit in an upright position or stand straight up. Breathing through your nose, gradually fill your lungs from the bottom up. Hold your breath for several seconds. Now exhale slowly by allowing your chest and abdomen to relax completely. Repeat the exercise eight to ten times.

In breathing exercises, concentrate on "breathing away" the tension and inhaling fresh air to the entire body.

Autogenic Training

Autogenic training is basically a form of self-suggestion, in which people are able to place themselves in an autohypnotic state by repeating and concentrating on feelings of heaviness and warmth in the extremities. This technique was developed by Johannes Schultz, a German psychiatrist, who noted that hypnotized individuals developed sensations of warmth and heaviness in the limbs and torso. The sensation of warmth is caused by dilation of blood vessels, which increases blood flow to the limbs. Muscular relaxation produces the feeling of heaviness.

In this technique, the person lies down or sits in a comfortable position, eyes closed, and progressively concentrates on six fundamental stages:

1. **Heaviness**
    My right (left) arm is heavy.
    Both arms are heavy.
    My right (left) leg is heavy.
    Both legs are heavy.
    My arms and legs are heavy.

2. **Warmth**
    My right (left) arm is warm.
    Both arms are warm.
    My right (left) leg is warm.
    Both legs are warm.
    My arms and legs are warm.

3. **Heart**
   My heartbeat is calm and regular (repeat four or five times).

4. **Respiration**
   My body breathes itself (repeat four or five times).

5. **Abdomen**
   My abdomen is warm (repeat four or five times).

6. **Forehead**
   My forehead is cool (repeat four or five times).

The autogenic training technique is more difficult to master than any of those previously mentioned. The person should not move too fast through the entire exercise, as this may actually interfere with learning and relaxation. Each stage must be mastered before proceeding to the next.

Meditation

Meditation is a mental exercise that can bring about psychological and physical benefits. The objective of meditation is to gain control over one's attention, clearing the mind and blocking out the stressor(s) responsible for the higher tension. This technique can be learned rather quickly and can be used frequently during times of increased tension and stress.

Initially, the person who is learning to meditate should choose a room that is comfortable, quiet, and free of all disturbances (including telephones). After learning the technique, the person will be able to meditate just about anywhere. A time block of approximately 15 minutes, twice a day, is needed to meditate.

1. Sit in a chair in an upright position with the hands resting either in your lap or on the arms of the chair. Close your eyes and focus on your breathing. Allow your body to relax as much as possible. Do not try to consciously relax, because trying means work. Rather, assume a passive attitude and concentrate on your breathing.

2. Allow the body to breathe regularly, at its own rhythm, and repeat in your mind the word "one" every time you inhale, and the word "two" every time you exhale. Paying attention to these two words keeps distressing thoughts from entering into your mind.

3. Continue to breathe about 15 minutes. Because the objective of meditation is to bring about a hypometabolic state, leading to body relaxation, do not use an alarm clock to remind you that the 15 minutes have expired. The alarm will only trigger your stress response again, defeating the purpose of the exercise. Opening your eyes once in a while to keep track of the time is fine, but do not rush or anticipate the end of the 15 minutes. This time has been set aside for meditation, and you need to relax, take your time, and enjoy the exercise.

Stress is not what makes people ill but, rather, the way they react to the stress-causing agent.

WHICH TECHNIQUE IS BEST?

Each person reacts to stress in a different way. Therefore, the best coping strategy to use depends mostly on the individual. Which technique is used does not really matter as long as it works. An individual may want to experiment with all of them to find out which works best. A combination of two or more works best for many people.

All of the coping strategies discussed here help to block out stressors and promote mental and physical relaxation by diverting the attention to a different, nonthreatening action. Some of the techniques are easier to learn and may take less time per session. Regardless of which technique you select, when stress becomes a significant problem in life, the time spent doing stress management exercises (several times a day, as needed) is well worth the effort.

People need to learn to relax and take time out for themselves. Stress is not what makes people ill but, rather, the way they react to the stress-causing agent. Individuals who learn to be diligent and start taking control of themselves find out they can enjoy a better, happier, and healthier life.

LABORATORY EXPERIENCE

LAB 14A
The Life Experiences Survey

Lab Preparation
None required.

LAB 14B
Type A Personality Assessment and Behavioral Objectives for Stress Reduction and Personality Change

Lab Preparation
None required.

LAB 14C
Stress Vulnerability Questionnaire

Lab Preparation
None required.

LAB 14D
Goals and Time Management Skills

Lab Preparation
Read the *Time Management* section in this chapter.

LAB 14E
Stress Management Techniques

Lab Preparation
None required.

REFERENCES

1. Andrasik, F., D. Coleman, and L. H. Epstein. "Biofeedback: Clinical and Research Considerations." In *Behavioral Medicine: Assessment and Treatment Strategies*. Edited by D. M. Doleys, R. L. Meredith, and A. R. Ciminero. New York: Plenum Press, 1982.
2. Blanchard, E. B., and L. H. Epstein. *A Biofeedback Primer*. Reading, MA: Addison-Wesley, 1978.
3. Blue Cross Association. *Stress*. Chicago: Blue Cross, 1974.
4. Brown, B. *New Mind, New Body*. New York: Harper & Row, 1974.
5. Chesney, M. A., J. R. Eagleston, and R. H. Roseman. "Type A Assessment and Intervention." In *Medical Psychology: Contributions to Behavioral Medicine*. Edited by C.K. Prokop and L. A. Bradley. New York: Academic Press, 1981.
6. Gauron, E. F. *Mental Training for Peak Performance*. Lansing, NY: Sport Science Associates, 1984.
7. Girdano, D., and G. Everly. *Controlling Stress and Tension: A Holistic Approach*. Englewood Cliffs, NJ: Prentice Hall, Inc., 1990.
8. Greenberg, J. S. *Comprehensive Stress Management*. Dubuque, IA: Wm. C. Brown Company Publishers, 1990.
9. Kriegel, R. J., and M. H. Kriegel. *The C Zone: Peak Performance Under Stress*. Garden City, NY: Anchor Press/Doubleday, 1984.
10. Luthe, W. "Autogenic Training: Method, Research and Applications in Medicine." *American Journal of Psychotherapy* 17:174-195, 1963.
11. McKay, M., M. Davis, and P. Fanning. *Thoughts and Feelings: The Act of Cognitive Stress Intervention*. Richmond, CA: New Harbinger Publications, 1981.
12. Miller, L. H., and A. D. Smith. "Vulnerability Scale." *Stress Audit*, 1983.
13. Sarason, I. G., J. H. Johnson, and J. M. Siegel. "Assessing the Impact of Life Changes: Development of the Life Experiences Survey." *Journal of Consulting and Clinical Psychology* 46:932- 946, 1978.
14. Schafer, W. *Stress Management for Wellness*. Fort Worth, TX: HBJ College Publishers, 1992.
15. Selye, H. *Stress Without Distress*. New York: Signet, 1974.
16. Selye, H. *The Stress of Life*. New York: McGraw-Hill Book Co., 1978.
17. Smith, J. S. *Creative Stress Management: The 1-2-3 Cope System*. Englewood Cliffs, NJ: Prentice Hall, 1993.
18. Staff. "How Running Relieves Stress." *The Runner* 8(11):38-43, 82, 1986.
19. Turk, D. C., and R. D. Kerns. "Assessment in Health Psychology: A Cognitive-Behavioral Perspective." In *Measurement Strategies in Health Psychology*. Edited by P. Karoly. New York: John Wiley & Sons, 1985.

SMOKING CESSATION

OBJECTIVES

- Understand the detrimental health effects of tobacco use in general.

- Learn the fundamental reasons why people smoke.

- Understand the benefits and the significance of a smoking cessation program.

- Learn how to implement a smoking cessation program, either for yourself (if you smoke), or to help others go through the process of quitting.

People throughout the world have used tobacco for hundreds of years. Before the 18th century, they smoked tobacco primarily in the form of pipes or cigars. Cigarette smoking per se did not become popular until the mid-1800s, and its use started to increase dramatically at the turn of the century.

In 1915, 18 billion cigarettes were consumed in the United States, as compared to 640 billion in 1981. This figure dropped to 538 billion in 1989. Nonetheless, more than 48 million Americans over age 17 still smoke an average of one and one-half packs of cigarettes per day.

The harmful effects of cigarette smoking and tobacco use in general were not exactly known until the early 1960s, when researchers began to show a link between tobacco usage and disease. In 1964, the U. S. Surgeon General issued the first major report presenting scientific evidence that cigarettes were indeed a major health hazard in our society.

Tobacco use in all its forms now is considered a significant threat to life. Estimates indicate that 10% of the 5 billion people presently living on the earth will die as a result of smoking-related illnesses, killing approximately 3 million people each year.

CIGARETTE SMOKING

Illegal drug overdoses kill about 17,500 people per year in the United States. Drug felonies and drug-related murders kill another 1,600 people each year. This brings drug-related deaths to a grand total of 19,100. Citizens and the government have mounted a tremendous campaign to eradicate illegal drug use in America.

A drug-free society certainly would be a great accomplishment for our people and future generations. At the same time, though, cigarettes, a legal drug, kill about 26 times as many people as all illegal drugs combined. Cigarette smoking is the largest

L A B S

preventable cause of illness and premature death in the United States. When considering all related deaths, smoking is responsible for more than 450,000 unnecessary deaths each year — enough deaths to wipe out the entire population of Miami and Miami Beach in a single year.

Death rates from heart disease, cancer, stroke, aortic aneurysm, chronic bronchitis, emphysema, and peptic ulcers have definitely increased. Cigarette smoking by pregnant women has been linked to retarded fetal growth, higher risk for spontaneous abortion, and prenatal death. Smoking also is the most prevalent cause of injury and death from fire. The average life expectancy for a chronic smoker is as much as 18 years shorter than for a nonsmoker, and the death rate among chronic smokers during the most productive years of life, between ages 25 and 65, is twice that of the national average.

According to a 1993 report by U.S. government physicians, each cigarette shortens life by seven minutes. This figure represents a loss of 5 million years of potential life that Americans lose to smoking each year.

Cigarette smoking is the largest preventable cause of illness and premature death in the United States.

According to estimates by the American Heart Association, more than 30%, or 120,000 fatal heart attacks annually, is a result of smoking. The risk for heart attack is 50% to 100% higher for smokers than for non-smokers. The mortality rate following heart attacks also is higher for smokers, as the attacks usually are more severe and the risk for deadly arrhythmias is much greater.

Cigarette smoking affects the cardiovascular system by increasing heart rate, blood pressure, susceptibility to atherosclerosis, and blood clots. Evidence also indicates that smoking decreases high density lipoprotein (HDL) cholesterol, the "good" cholesterol that lowers the risk for heart disease. Finally, the carbon monoxide in smoke hinders the capacity of the blood to carry oxygen to body tissues.

The largest carcinogenic exposure in the workplace is cigarette smoke. The American Cancer Society reports that 83% of lung cancer and 30% of all cancers are attributable to smoking. It kills about 142,000 people each year. Lung cancer (Figure 15.1)

FIGURE 15.1

Normal lung (left) and diseased lung (right). The white growth near the top of the diseased lung is cancer, the dark appearance on the bottom half is emphysema.

Reproduced with permission from "If You Smoke" slide show by Gordon Hewlett.

is the leading killer by cancer, responsible for 30% of all cancer deaths.

Based on a 1990 report by the Environmental Protection Agency (EPA), secondhand smoke also is a killer. Secondhand smoke is responsible for 3,000 or more lung cancer deaths each year.

Although half of all cancers are now curable, the five-year survival rate for lung cancer is less than 13%. Tobacco use also increases the risk for cancer of the oral cavity, larynx, esophagus, bladder, pancreas, and kidneys.

Research presented at the 1990 World Conference on Lung Health also reveals that nonsmokers who live with smokers have a 20% to 30% greater risk of dying from heart disease than do other nonsmokers. Results of this research further suggest that the number of deaths from heart disease attributed to passive smoking is 10 times that of cancer.

Even though many tobacco users are aware of the health consequences of cigarette smoking, they may fail to realize the risk of pipe smoking, cigar smoking, and tobacco chewing. As a group in general, the risk for heart disease and lung cancer is lower than for cigarette smokers. Nevertheless, blood nicotine levels in pipe and cigar smokers have been shown to approach those of cigarette smokers, as nicotine still is absorbed through the membranes of the mouth. Therefore, these tobacco users still have a higher risk for heart disease than nonsmokers do.

Cigarette smokers who substitute pipe or cigar smoking for cigarettes usually continue to inhale the smoke, which actually results in more nicotine and tar brought into the lungs. Consequently, the risk for disease is even higher if pipe or cigar smoke is inhaled. The risk and mortality rates for lip, mouth, and larynx cancer for pipe smoking, cigar smoking, and tobacco chewing actually are higher than for cigarette smoking.

Approximately 450,000 people die each year in the United States from smoking related conditions.

The economic impact of cigarette smoking on American business and industry also is staggering. Companies pay more than $16 billion each year as a direct result of smoking in the workplace, and another $37 billion in lost productivity and earnings because of illness, disability, and death.

Heavy smokers use the health care system, especially hospitals, twice as much as nonsmokers do. The yearly cost to a given company has been estimated to be between $624 and $4,611 per smoking employee. These costs include employee health care, absenteeism, additional health insurance, morbidity/disability and early mortality, on-the-job lost time, property damage/maintenance and depreciation, Workers Compensation, and the impact of second-hand smoke.

Even though the ill effects of tobacco have been well-documented, not enough is being done to discourage and eradicate its use. In the summer of 1985, more than 1,500 people worldwide died in major airplane accidents. These accidents generated a tremendous amount of media attention, and planes were grounded for safety reasons.

Now imagine what the coverage and concern would be if 450,000 people each year were to die in the United States alone because of airplane accidents. People would not even consider flying any more. Most individuals would think of it as a form of suicide. Or think of the public outrage if close to 450,000 Americans were to die annually in a meaningless war, or if a single nonprescription drug would cause more than 138,000 cancer deaths and 120,000 fatal heart attacks. The American public would never tolerate these situations. We probably would mount an intense fight to prevent these deaths.

Yet, are we not committing a form of slow suicide by smoking cigarettes? Isn't tobacco a non-prescription drug available to almost anyone who wishes to smoke, killing more than 450,000 people each year? If cigarettes were invented today, the tobacco industry would be put on trial for mass murder.

We may ask ourselves why a greater campaign is not being waged against all forms of tobacco use. First, to fight an industry that has as great a financial and political influence as the tobacco industry has in the United States is difficult. Tobacco is the sixth largest cash crop in the United States, producing 2.5% of the gross national product. It has influenced elections cleverly by emphasizing the individual's right to smoke, avoiding the fact that so many people die because of its use.

In 1990, Philip Morris, one of the largest tobacco-producing companies in the world, ranked seventh among Fortune 500 companies. Nearly 70% of the profits came from the sale of cigarettes. In 1992, Philip Morris donated about $17 million to "bribing" leading organizations until they no longer question the detrimental effects of tobacco use. Among the organizations receiving donations from Philip Morris in 1992 were: United Way, YMCA, Salvation Army, Pediatric AIDS Foundation, Red Cross, Cystic Fibrosis Foundation, March of Dimes, Easter Seals, Muscular Dystrophy Association, Multiple Sclerosis Society, Hemophilia Foundation, United Cerebral Palsy, American Civil Liberties Union, American Bar Association, Task Force for Battered Women, Boy Scouts, Boys and Girls Club, and Big Brothers and Big Sisters. "We call Colombian drug runners uncivilized scums (for about 19,100 illegal drug-related deaths per year), but we welcome Philip Morris with glee and we call it civic pride."[4]

Each cigarette smoked shortens a person's life by seven minutes.

Second, tobacco had been socially accepted for so many years that many people simply learned to live with it. In the 1980s, however, cigarette smoking no longer was acceptable in many social circles. Nonsmokers and ex-smokers alike are fighting for their right to clean air and health. If every smoker were to give up cigarettes, in one year alone sick time would drop by approximately 90 million days, heart conditions would decrease by 280,000, chronic bronchitis and emphysema would number 1 million fewer cases, and total death rates from cardiovascular disease, cancer, and peptic ulcers would fall off drastically.

Many smokers are unaware of or simply do not care to realize how much cigarette smoke bothers nonsmokers. These smokers think it really is not that bad and if they can put up with it, it should not bother nonsmokers that much. In many instances, smokers think that blowing the smoke off to the side is enough to get it out of the way. As a matter of fact, it is not enough. Smokers do not comprehend this until they quit and later find themselves in that situation. At times, ex-smokers even are bothered by someone else smoking several yards away and all of a sudden come to realize why cigarette smoke is so unpleasant and undesirable to most people.

SMOKELESS TOBACCO

Smokeless tobacco often is promoted as a safe alternative to cigarette smoking. According to the Advisory Committee to the U. S. Surgeon General, smokeless tobacco represents a significant health risk and is just as addictive as cigarette smoking.

Unlike smoking, the use of smokeless tobacco has increased during the last 15 years. Currently, some 15 million Americans use tobacco in this form. The greatest concern is the increase in use of "spit" tobacco, especially by young people.

There are over 2 million people under age 25 who use spit tobacco, including nearly 20% of all males in grades 9 through 12. One-third of those who use spit tobacco started at age 5, and the average starting age was 9. Spit tobacco contains 2.5 times as much nicotine as a similarly priced pack of cigarettes.

Using smokeless tobacco leads to gingivitis, periodontitis, a fourfold increase in oral cancer, and in some cases even premature death. People who chew or dip also have a higher rate of cavities, sore gums, bad breath, and stained teeth. They can't smell or taste as well. Consequently, they frequently add sugar and salt to food. These practices alone increase the risk for overweight and high blood pressure.

Nicotine addiction and its related health risks hold true for smokeless tobacco users. Nicotine blood levels approach those of cigarette smokers, increasing the risk for diseases of the cardiovascular system. Further, research has revealed changes in heart rate and blood pressure similar to those of cigarette smokers.

Using tobacco in any form is addictive and poses a serious threat to health and well-being. Completely eliminating its use in any form is the single most important lifestyle change a tobacco user can make to improve health, quality of life, and longevity.

WHY DO PEOPLE SMOKE?

People typically begin to smoke without realizing its detrimental effects on their health and life in general. Although people start to smoke for many different reasons, the three fundamental instigators are peer pressure, the desire to appear "grown up," and rebellion against authority. Unfortunately, smoking only three packs of cigarettes can lead to physiological addiction, turning the smoking into a nasty habit that has become the most widespread example of drug dependency in the country.

When tobacco leaves are burned, hot air and gases containing tar (chemical compounds) and nicotine are released in the smoke. *More than 1,200 toxic chemicals have been found in tobacco smoke.* Tar contains about 30 chemical compounds that are proven carcinogens.

The drug nicotine has strong addictive properties. Within seconds of inhalation, nicotine affects the central nervous system and can act simultaneously as a tranquilizer and a stimulant. The stimulating effect produces strong physiological and psychological dependency. The physical addiction to nicotine is six to eight times more powerful than the addiction to alcohol, and most likely greater than for some of the hard drugs currently used.

The psychological dependency develops over a longer time. People smoke to help themselves relax, and they also gain a certain amount of pleasure from the ritual of smoking. Smokers automatically associate many activities of daily life with cigarettes. Typical associated activities are: coffee drinking, alcohol drinking, social gatherings, after a meal, talking on the telephone, driving, reading, watching television. In many cases the social rituals of smoking are the most difficult to eliminate. This psychological dependency is so strong that even years after people have stopped smoking, they still may crave cigarettes when they engage in some of these activities.

Most people smoke for a variety of reasons. To find out why people smoke, the National Clearinghouse for Smoking and Health developed a simple "Why-Do-You-Smoke Test" (see Figure 15A.1, Lab 15A). The scores obtained on this test give an indication for each of six factors that describe people's feelings when they smoke. The first three factors point out the positive feelings people derive from smoking. The fourth factor relates to reducing tension and relaxing. The fifth reveals the extent of dependence on cigarettes. The last factor differentiates habit smoking and purely automatic smoking.

WHY-DO-YOU-SMOKE TEST

The "Why-Do-You-Smoke Test," contained in Lab 15A, lists some statements by people describing what they get out of smoking cigarettes. Smokers are to indicate how often they have the feelings described in each statement when smoking. This test, as well as much of the remaining information in this chapter, is presented in the same format as it is given to smokers.

INTERPRETING RESULTS OF THE "WHY-DO-YOU-SMOKE TEST"

The "Why-Do-You-Smoke Test" elicits reasons you smoke. A score of 11 or above on any factor indicates that smoking is an important source of satisfaction for you. The higher you score (15 is the highest), the more important a given factor is in your smoking and the more useful the discussion of that factor can be in your attempt to quit.

If you do not score high on any of the six factors, chances are that you do not smoke much or have not been smoking for very many years. If so, giving up smoking, and staying off, should be fairly easy.

1. *Stimulation.* If you score high or fairly high on this factor, you are one of those smokers who is stimulated by the cigarette; you feel that it helps wake you up, organize your energies, and keep you going. If you try to give up smoking, you may want a safe substitute — a brisk walk or

moderate exercise, for example — whenever you feel the urge to smoke.

2. *Handling.* Handling things can be satisfying, but you can keep your hands busy in many ways without lighting up or playing with a cigarette. Why not toy with a pen or pencil? Try doodling. Play with a coin, a piece of jewelry, or some other harmless object.

3. *Accentuation of pleasure/pleasurable relaxation.* Finding out whether you use the cigarette to feel good — get real, honest pleasure out of smoking (Factor 3) — or to keep from feeling bad (Factor 4) is not always easy. About two-thirds of smokers score high or fairly high on accentuation of pleasure, and about half of those also score as high or higher on reduction of negative feelings. Those who do get real pleasure from smoking often find that honest consideration of the harmful effects of their habit is enough to help them quit. They substitute social and physical activities and find they do not seriously miss their cigarettes.

4. *Reduction of negative feelings, or "crutch."* Many smokers use cigarettes as a kind of crutch in moments of stress or discomfort. Ironically, the heavy smoker — the person who tries to handle severe personal problems by smoking many times a day — is apt to discover that cigarettes do not help in dealing with problems effectively. This kind of smoker may stop smoking readily when everything is going well but may be tempted to start again in a time of crisis. Again, physical exertion or social activity may be useful substitutes for cigarettes, even in times of tension.

5. *Craving or dependence.* Quitting smoking is difficult for people who score high on this factor. The craving for a cigarette begins to build up the moment the cigarette is put out, so tapering off is not likely to work. This smoker must go "cold turkey." If you are dependent on cigarettes, you may try smoking more than usual for a day or two so the taste for cigarettes is spoiled, then isolating yourself completely from cigarettes until the craving is gone.

6. *Habit.* If you are smoking out of habit, you no longer get much satisfaction from the cigarettes. You just light them frequently without even realizing you are doing so. You may have an easy time quitting and staying off if you can break the habitual patterns you have built up. Cutting

down gradually may be effective if you change the way you smoke cigarettes and the conditions under which you smoke them. The key to success is to become aware of each cigarette you smoke. You can do this by asking yourself, "Do I really want this cigarette?" You may be surprised at how many you do not want.

SMOKING CESSATION

Quitting cigarette smoking is not easy. Only about 20% of smokers who try to quit the first time each year succeed. The addictive properties of nicotine and smoke make quitting difficult.

The American Psychiatric Association and the National Institute on Drug Abuse have indicated that nicotine is perhaps the most addictive drug known to humans. Smokers develop a tolerance to nicotine and smoke. They become dependent on both and get physical and psychological withdrawal symptoms when they stop smoking. Even though giving up smoking can be extremely difficult, it by no means is impossible.

During the last several years cigarette smoking in the United States has been declining gradually among smokers of all ages with the exception of young women. Surveys have shown that between 75% and 90% of all smokers would like to quit. Forty percent of the adult population — 53% of men and 32% of women — smoked in 1964 when the U. S. Surgeon General first reported the link between smoking and increased risk for disease and mortality. By 1991, only 25.7%, or 46.3 million adults, smoked. Among men, 24 million (28.1%) were smokers, and 22.2 million (23.5%) women smoked. Approximately 43.5 million Americans have given up cigarettes.

More than 95% of successful ex-smokers have been able to do it on their own, either by quitting cold turkey or by using self-help kits available from organizations such as the American Cancer Society, the American Heart Association, and the American Lung Association. Only 3% of ex-smokers have done so as a result of formal cessation programs. Smokers' information and treatment centers commonly are listed in the yellow pages of the telephone book.

DO-YOU-WANT-TO-QUIT TEST

The most important factor in quitting cigarette smoking is the person's sincere desire to do so. Although some smokers can simply quit, this is not the case in most instances. Those who can quit easily are primarily light or casual smokers. They realize that the pleasure of an occasional cigarette is not worth the added risk for disease and premature death. For heavy smokers, quitting most likely will be a difficult battle. Even though many do not succeed the first time around, the odds of quitting are much better for those who try to stop repeatedly.

To find out a smoker's preparedness to quit, the "Do-You-Want-To-Quit-Test" contained in Lab 15A, Figure 15A.2, developed by the National Clearinghouse for Smoking and Health, will measure a person's attitude toward the four primary reasons people want to quit smoking. The results will give an indication of whether the person is really ready to start the program. On this test, the higher you score in any category, say "health," the more important that reason is to you. A score of 9 or above in one of these categories indicates that this is one of the most important reasons you may want to quit.

1. *Health.* Knowing the harmful consequences of cigarettes, many people have stopped smoking and many others are considering it. If your score on the health factor is 9 or above, the health hazards of smoking may be enough to make you want to quit now. If your score on this factor is low (6 or below), consider the hazards of smoking. You may be lacking important information or may even have incorrect information. If so, health considerations are not playing the role they should be in your decision to keep smoking or to quit.

2. *Example.* Some people stop smoking because they want to set a good example for others. Parents quit to make it easier for their children to resist starting to smoke. Doctors quit to be role models for their patients. Teachers quit to discourage their students from smoking. Sports stars want to set an example for their young fans. Husbands quit to influence their wives to quit, and vice versa. Examples have a significant influence on our behavior. Research shows that almost twice as many high school students smoke if both parents are smokers, compared to those whose parents are nonsmokers or former smokers.

If your score is low (6 or lower), you might not be interested in giving up smoking to set an example for others. Perhaps you do not realize how important your example could be.

3. *Aesthetics*. People who score high, (9 or above) in this category recognize and are disturbed by some of the unpleasant aspects of smoking. The smell of stale smoke on their clothing, bad breath, and stains on their fingers and teeth might be reason enough to consider quitting.

4. *Mastery*. If you score 9 or above on this factor, you are bothered by the knowledge that you cannot control your desire to smoke. You are not your own master. Awareness of this challenge to your self-control may make you want to quit.

BREAKING THE HABIT

The following seven-step plan has been developed as a guide to help you quit smoking. The total program should be completed in four weeks or less. Steps one through four should take no longer than two weeks. A maximum of two additional weeks is allowed for the rest of the program.

Step One

Decide positively that you want to quit. Avoid negative thoughts of how difficult this can be. Think positive. You can do it.

Now prepare a list of the reasons you smoke and why you want to quit (see Figure 15A.3, Lab 15). Make several copies of the list and keep them in places where you commonly smoke. Frequently review the reasons for quitting, as this will motivate and psychologically prepare you for cessation.

When the reasons for quitting outweigh the reasons for smoking, you will have an easier time quitting. Try to read as much information as possible on the detrimental effects of tobacco and the benefits of quitting.

Step Two

Initiate a personal diet and exercise program. About one-third of the people who quit smoking gain weight. This could be caused by one or a combination of several reasons: (a) Food becomes a substitute for cigarettes; (b) appetite increases; and (c) basal metabolism may slow down.

If you start an exercise and weight control program prior to quitting smoking, weight gain should not be a problem. If anything, exercise and lower body weight create more awareness of healthy living and strengthen the motivation for giving up cigarettes (see Figure 15.2).

Even if you gain some weight, the harmful effects of cigarette smoking are much more detrimental to human health than a few extra pounds of body weight. Experts have indicated that, as far as the extra load on the heart is concerned, giving up one pack of cigarettes a day is the equivalent of losing between 50 and 75 pounds of excess body fat!

Step Three

Decide on the approach you will use to stop smoking. You may quit cold turkey or gradually cut down the number of cigarettes you smoke daily. Base your decision on your scores obtained on the "Why-Do-You-Smoke Test." If you scored 11 points or higher in either the "Crutch: Tension Reduction" or the "Craving: Psychological Addiction" categories, your best chance for success is quitting cold turkey. For any of the other four categories, you may choose either approach.

People still argue about which approach is more effective. Quitting cold turkey may cause fewer withdrawal symptoms than gradually tapering off. When cutting down, the fewer the cigarettes you smoke, the more important each one becomes. Therefore, you have a greater chance for relapse and returning to the original number of cigarettes smoked. When the cutting down approach is accompanied by a definite target date for quitting, the

FIGURE 15.2
Starting an exercise program prior to giving up cigarettes motivates toward cessation and helps with weight control during this process.

technique has been shown to be quite effective. Smokers who taper off without a target date for quitting are the most likely to relapse.

Step Four

Keep a daily log of your smoking habit for a few days. This will help you understand the situations in which you smoke. To assist you in doing this, make copies of Figure 15A.4 (Lab 15A) or develop your own form. Keep this form with you, and every time you smoke, record the required information. Keep track of the number of cigarettes you smoke, times of day you smoke them, events associated with smoking, the amount of each cigarette smoked, and a rating of how badly you needed that cigarette. Rate each cigarette from 1 to 3. A 1 means desperately needed, a 2 means moderately needed, and a 3 means no real need. This daily log will assist you in three ways: (a) You will get to know your habit; (b) it will help you eliminate cigarettes you really do not need; (c) it will aid you in finding positive substitutes for situations that trigger your desire to smoke.

Step Five

Set the target date for quitting. If you are going to taper off gradually, read the instructions under the Cutting Down section of this chapter before you proceed to Step 6. In setting the target date, a special date may add a little extra incentive. An upcoming birthday, anniversary, vacation, graduation, family reunion — all are examples of good dates to free yourself from smoking. Dates when you are going to be away from events that trigger your desire to smoke may be especially helpful. Once you have set the date, do not change it. Do not let anyone or anything interfere with this date.

Let your friends and relatives know of your intentions, and ask for their support. Consider asking someone else to quit with you. This way, you can support each other in your efforts to stop. Avoid anyone who will not support you in your effort to quit. Unfortunately, other people can be a prime obstacle when you are attempting to quit. Many smokers can get quite intolerable when they first stop smoking, so some friends and relatives prefer that the person continue to smoke rather than make the extra effort and show increased patience for a few days.

Step Six

Stock up on low-calorie foods — carrots, broccoli, cauliflower, celery, popcorn (butter- and salt-free), fruits, sunflower seeds (in the shell), sugarless gum — and drink plenty of water. Keep the food handy on the day you stop and the first few days following cessation. Substitute this food for a cigarette when you want one.

Step Seven

On your quit day and the first few days thereafter, *do not keep cigarettes handy. Stay away from friends and events that trigger your desire to smoke,* and drink large amounts of water and fruit juices. To replace the old behavior with new behavior, replace smoking time with new, positive substitutes that will make smoking difficult or impossible.

When you want a cigarette, take a few deep breaths and then occupy yourself by doing any of a number of things such as talking to someone else, washing your hands, brushing your teeth, eating a healthy snack, chewing on a straw, doing dishes, playing sports, going for a walk or bike ride, going swimming, and so on. Engage in activities that require the use of your hands. Try gardening, sewing, writing letters, drawing, doing household chores, or washing the car. Visit nonsmoking places such as libraries, museums, stores, or theaters. Plan an outing or a trip away from home. Record your choice of activity or substitute under the Remarks/Substitute column in Figure 15A.4. All of these activities have been shown to keep your mind away from cigarettes.

QUITTING COLD TURKEY

Many people have found that quitting all at once is the easiest way to do it. Most smokers have tried this approach at least once. Even though it may not work the first time, they do not allow themselves to get discouraged, and they succeed eventually. Many times after several attempts, all of a sudden they are able to overcome the habit without too much difficulty.

On the average, as few as three smokeless days are sufficient to break the physiological addiction to nicotine. The psychological addiction may linger on for years but will get weaker as time goes by.

CUTTING DOWN GRADUALLY

Tapering off cigarettes can be done in several ways. You might start by eliminating cigarettes you do not necessarily need (those ranked numbers 3 and 2 on your daily log). You may switch to a brand lower in nicotine/tar every couple of days. You can smoke less of each cigarette. Or you can simply smoke fewer cigarettes each day. Most people prefer a combination of these four suggestions.

When planning your strategy, set a target date for quitting before you start cutting down. Once the date is set, it is not to be changed. The total process until your quit date should not take longer than two weeks. Reduce the total number of cigarettes smoked each day by 10% to 25%. As you smoke less, be careful not to take more puffs or inhale more deeply as you smoke, as this would offset the principle of cutting down.

About three smokeless days are sufficient to break the physiological addiction to nicotine.

As an aid in tapering off, make several copies of Figure 15A.4. (By now you already should have completed the initial daily log of your smoking habit — see Step Four under Breaking the Habit.) Start a new daily log, and every night review your data and set goals for the following day.

Decide which cigarettes will be easiest to give up, what brand you will smoke, the total number of cigarettes to be smoked, and how much of each you will smoke. Write down any comments or situations you may want to avoid, as well as any substitutes you could use to help you in the program. For example, if you always smoke with coffee, substitute juice for coffee. If you smoke while driving, arrange for a ride or take a bus to work. If you smoke with a certain friend at lunch, avoid having lunch with that friend for a week or so. Continue using this log until you have stopped smoking completely.

LIFE AFTER CIGARETTES

When you first quit smoking, you can expect a series of withdrawal symptoms. Among the typical physiological and psychological reactions during the first few days are lower heart rate and blood pressure, headaches, gastrointestinal discomfort, mood changes, irritability, aggressiveness, and difficulty sleeping.

The physiological addiction to nicotine is broken only three days following your last cigarette. Therefore, you should not crave cigarettes as much regularly. For the habitual smoker, the psychological dependency could be the most difficult to break. The first few days may not be as difficult as the first few months. Any of the activities in daily life that have been associated with smoking — either stress or relaxation, joy or unhappiness — may trigger a relapse even months, or at times years, after cessation.

Ex-smokers should realize that even though some harm may have been done already, it is never too late to quit. The greatest early benefit is a lower risk for sudden death. Furthermore, the risk for illness starts to decrease the moment you stop smoking. You will have fewer sore throats and sores in the mouth, less hoarseness, no more cigarette cough, and lower peptic ulcer risk.

Circulation to the hands and feet will improve, as will gastrointestinal and kidney and bladder functions. Everything will taste and smell better. You will have more energy, and you will gain a sense of freedom, pride, and well-being. You no longer will have to worry whether you have enough cigarettes to last you through a day, a party, a meeting, a weekend, a trip.

Quitting cigarette smoking enhances health, boosts energy levels, and gives people a sense of freedom, pride, and well-being.

When you first quit and you think how tough it is and how miserable you feel because you cannot have a cigarette, try the opposite: Think of the benefits and how great it is not to smoke! The ex-smoker's risk for heart disease approaches that of a lifetime nonsmoker 10 years following cessation, and cancer 15 years after cessation.

If you have been successful and stopped smoking, a lot of events can still trigger your urge to smoke. When confronted with these events, people rationalize and think, "One cigarette won't hurt. I've been off for months (years in some cases)" or, "I can handle it. I'll smoke just today." It won't work! Before you know it, you will be back to the regular nasty habit. Be prepared to take action in those situations. Find substitutes. In addition to the many things that have been discussed in this chapter, the list of tips given in Figure 15.3 should help you in retraining yourself to live without cigarettes.

Start thinking of yourself as a nonsmoker — no "buts" about it. Remind yourself of how difficult it has been and how long it has taken you to get to this point. If you have come this far, you certainly can resist "but" small moments of temptation. It will get easier rather than worse as time goes on.

LABORATORY EXPERIENCE

LAB 15A
Smoking Cessation Forms

Lab Preparation
Smokers must prepare themselves to quit smoking. The quitting date must be set 2 weeks from today's date or the last day of classes this semester, whichever comes first. Nonsmokers need no preparation for this lab but should participate to help classmates or friends go through the quitting process.

REFERENCES

1. American Cancer Society. *Cancer Facts & Figures - 1993*. New York: ACS, 1993.
2. American Cancer Society. *Fifty Most Often Asked Questions About Smoking and Health and the Answers*. New York: ACS, 1982.
3. American Cancer Society. *Quitter's Guide: Seven-Day Plan to Help You Stop Smoking Cigarettes*. New York: ACS, 1978.
4. American Cancer Society. *World Smoking & Health*. Atlanta, GA: The Society, 1993.
5. American Heart Association. *Heart at Work: Smoking Reduction Program-Coordinator's Guide*. Dallas, TX: AHA, 1984.
6. American Heart Association. *How to Quit*. Dallas, TX: AHA, 1984.
7. American Heart Association. *Smoking and Heart Disease*. Dallas, TX: AHA, 1981.
8. American Heart Association. *The Good Life: A Guide to Becoming a Nonsmoker*. Dallas, TX: AHA, 1984.
9. Carroll, C. R. *Drugs in Modern Society*. Dubuque, IA: Brown and Benchmark, 1992.
10. Channing L. Bete Co., Inc. *Smoking and Your Heart*. South Deerfield, MA: The Author, 1982.
11. Girdano, D. A., D. Dusek, and G. S. Everly. *Experiencing Health*. Englewood Cliffs, NJ: Prentice Hall, 1985.
12. Halper, M. S. *How to Stop Smoking: A Preventive Medicine Institute/Strang Clinic Health Action Plan*. New York: Holt Rinehart and Winston, 1980.
13. Hodgson, R. J., and P. Miller. *Self-Watching: Addictions, Habits, Compulsions, What to Do*. New York: Facts on File, 1982.
14. National Cancer Institute. *Clearing the Air: A Guide to Quitting Smoking*. Bethesda, MD: NCI, 1979.
15. Public Health Service. *A Self-Test for Smokers*. Rockville, MD: U.S. Department of Health and Human Services, 1983.
16. Public Health Service. *Chronic Obstructive Lung Disease: A Report of the Surgeon General*. Rockville, MD: U.S. Department of Health and Human Services, 1984.
17. Public Health Service. *Why People Smoke Cigarettes*. Rockville, MD: U.S. Department of Health and Human Services, 1982.
18. Public Health Service. *Smoking Tobacco and Health: A Fact Book*. Rockville, MD: U.S. Department of Health and Human Services, 1981.
19. U.S. Office on Smoking and Health. *Smoking and Health: A Report of the Surgeon General*. Washington, DC: U.S. Department of Health, Education and Welfare, 1979.

TIPS TO HELP STOP SMOKING

The following are different ways smokers retrained themselves to live without cigarettes. Any one or several of these methods in combination might be helpful to you. Check the ones you like and from these develop your own retraining program.

1. Before you quit smoking, try wrapping your cigarettes with a sheet of paper like a Christmas present. Every time you want a cigarette, unwrap the pack and write down what you are doing, how you feel, and how important this cigarette is to you. Do this for two weeks and you'll have cut down as well as developed new insights into your smoking.

2. If cigarettes give you an energy boost, try gum, modest exercise, a brisk walk, or a new hobby. Avoid eating new foods that are high in calories.

3. If cigarettes help you relax, try eating, drinking new beverages, or social activities within reasonable bounds.

4. When you crave cigarettes, you must quit suddenly. Try smoking an excess of cigarettes for a day or two before you quit so the taste of cigarettes is spoiled. Or, an opportune time to quit is when you are ill with a cold or influenza and have lost your taste for cigarettes.

5. On a 3" X 5" card, make a list of what you like and dislike about smoking. Add to it and read it daily.

6. Make up a short list of luxuries you have wanted or items you would like to purchase for a loved one. Next to each item, write down the cost. Now convert the cost to "packs of cigarettes." If you save the money each day from packs of cigarettes, you will be able to purchase these items. Use a special "piggy" bank for saving your money or start a "Christmas Club" account at your bank.

7. Never smoke after you get a craving for a cigarette until three minutes have passed since you got the urge. During those three minutes, change your thinking or activity. Telephone an ex-smoker or somebody you can talk to until the craving subsides.

8. Plan a memorable day for stopping. You might choose your vacation, New Year's Day, your birthday, a holiday, the birthday of your child, your anniversary. But don't make the date so distant that you lose momentum.

9. If you smoke under stress at work, pick a date for stopping when you will be away from your work.

10. Decide whether you are going to stop suddenly or gradually. If it is to be gradual, work out a tapering system so that you have intermediate goals on your way to an "I.Q." day.

11. Don't store up cigarettes. Never buy a carton. Wait until one pack is finished before you buy another.

12. Never carry cigarettes about with you at home or at work. Keep your cigarettes as far from you as possible. Leave them with someone or lock them up.

13. Until you quit, make yourself a "smoking corner" that is far from anything interesting. If you like to smoke with others, always smoke alone. If you like to smoke alone, always smoke with others, preferably if they are nonsmokers. Never smoke while watching television.

14. Never carry matches or a lighter with you.

15. Put away your ashtrays or fill them with objects so they cannot be used for ashes. Plant flowers in them or fill them with walnuts. The latter will give you something to do with your hands.

16. Change your brand of cigarettes weekly so that you are always smoking a brand of lower tar and nicotine content than the week before.

17. Never say, "I quit smoking," because your resolution is broken if you have a cigarette. Better to say, "I don't want to smoke." This way you maintain your resolution even if you accidentally have a cigarette.

18. Try to help someone else quit smoking, particularly your spouse.

19. Always ask yourself, "Do I need this cigarette or is this just a reflex?"

20. Each day try to put off lighting your first cigarette.

21. Decide arbitrarily that you will smoke only on even- or odd-numbered hours of the clock.

22. Try going to bed early and rising a half hour earlier than usual to avoid hurrying through breakfast and rushing to work.

23. Keep your hands occupied. Try playing a musical instrument, knitting, or fiddling with hand puzzles.

24. Take a shower. You cannot smoke in the shower.

25. Brush your teeth frequently to get rid of the tobacco taste and stains.

26. If you have a sudden craving for a cigarette, take ten deep breaths, holding the last breath while you strike a match. Exhale slowly, blowing out the match. Pretend the match was a cigarette by crushing it out in an ashtray. Now immediately get busy on some work or activity.

27. Smoke only half a cigarette.

(Continued)

FIGURE 15.3

Tips to help stop smoking.

28. After you quit, start using your lungs. Increase your activities and indulge in moderate exercise, such as short walks before or after a meal.

29. Bet with someone that you can quit. Put the cigarette money in a jar each morning and forfeit it if you smoke. You keep the money if you don't smoke by the end of the week. Try to extend this period for a month.

30. If you gain weight because you are not smoking, wait until you get over the craving before you diet. Dieting is easier then.

31. If you are depressed or have physical symptoms that might be related to your smoking, relieve your mind by discussing this with your physician. It is easier to quit when you know your health status.

32. Visit your dentist after you quit and have your teeth cleaned to get rid of the tobacco stains.

33. If the cost of cigarettes is your motivation for quitting, try purchasing a money order equivalent to a year's supply of cigarettes. Give it to a friend. If you smoke in the next year, he cashes the money order and keeps the money. If you don't smoke, he gives back the money order at the end of the year.

From *TIPS*. American Cancer Society, Texas Division, Inc., with permission.

34. After you quit, never face the confusion of "craving a cigarette" alone. Find someone you can call or visit at this critical time.

35. When you feel irritable or tense, shut your eyes and count backward from ten to zero as you imagine yourself descending a flight of stairs, or imagine that you are looking at the horizon as the sun sets in the west.

36. Get out of your old habits. Seek new activities or perform old activities in a new way. Don't rely on the old ways of solving problems. Do things differently.

37. If you are a "kitchen smoker" in the morning, volunteer your services to schools or nonprofit organizations to get you out of the house.

38. Stock up on light reading materials, crossword puzzles, and vacation brochures that you can read during your coffee breaks.

39. Frequent places where you can't smoke, such as libraries, buses, theatres, swimming pools, department stores, or just going to bed during the first weeks you are off cigarettes.

40. Give yourself time to think and get fit by walking one-half hour each day. If you have a dog, take him for a walk with you.

FIGURE 15.3 *(Continued)*
Tips to help stop smoking.

ADDICTIVE BEHAVIORS AND SEXUALLY TRANSMITTED DISEASES

16

Two of the most serious problems that afflict society as we head into the 21st century are chemical dependency (addictive behavior) and the epidemic of sexually transmitted diseases. Addictive behavior and unprotected sex are extremely destructive behaviors that have ruined and ended millions of lives. People need to understand that, perhaps more so than with any other unhealthy behavior, when addiction and sexually transmitted diseases (especially HIV infection) are at issue, an ounce of prevention is worth a pound of cure. The time to make healthy choices is now.

The information in this chapter will help you make informed decisions before it is too late. Education concerning these subjects may aid in the search for answers, treatment, and, hopefully, a more productive and happier life.

ADDICTION

When most people think of addiction, they probably think of dark/dirty alleys, an addict shooting drugs into the veins, or a "junkie" passed out next to a garbage can after an evening with alcohol. Jacquelyn Small, psychotherapist and author, defines addiction as a problem of imbalance or unease within the body and mind.

Although some addictive behaviors are more detrimental than others, there are many types of addiction, including addictions to food, television, work, compulsive shopping, and even exercise. The most serious type of addiction is chemical dependency to drugs such as tobacco, coffee, alcohol, cocaine, heroin, marijuana, and prescription drugs.

Some people become addicted to food. They eat to release stress or boredom or to reward themselves for every small personal achievement. A great number of people are addicted to television. Estimates indicate that the average adult in the United States spends seven hours a day watching television.

L A B S

Other individuals become so addicted to their jobs that all they think about is work. Although work may start out as an enjoyable activity, when it totally consumes a person's life, work can become an unhealthy behavior. If you find that you are readily irritated, moody, grouchy, constantly tired, not as alert as you used to be, or making more mistakes than usual, you probably are becoming a workaholic and need to slow down or take time off work.

Exercise has enhanced the health and quality of life of millions of people, but a small group of individuals becomes obsessed with exercise, with potential addictive and overuse properties. Compulsive exercisers feel guilty and uncomfortable when they miss a day's workout. Often these individuals continue to exercise even when they have injuries and sickness that require proper rest for adequate recovery. People who exceed the recommended guidelines for fitness development and maintenance (see Chapters 6, 8, and 10) are exercising for reasons other than health — including addictive behavior.

Americans spend more than $100 billion annually on illegal drugs.

Caffeine can become another addiction that produces undesirable side effects. Caffeine doses in excess of 200 to 500 mg can produce an abnormally rapid heart rate, abnormal heart rhythms, higher blood pressure, birth defects in offspring, higher body temperature, and increased secretion of gastric acids leading to stomach problems. It also may induce symptoms of anxiety, depression, nervousness, and dizziness.

The caffeine content of drinks varies according to the product. In 6 ounces of coffee, for example, the content varies from 65 mg for instant coffee to as high as 180 mg for drip coffee. Soft drinks, mainly colas, range in caffeine content from 30 to 60 mg per 12-ounce can.

The previous examples, as well as more serious forms of chemical dependency, are by no means the only types of addiction but are used here to illustrate addictive behaviors. Other examples are gambling, pornography, sex, people, and places.

All forms of addiction are unhealthy. This chapter, however, focuses on three of the most self-destructive forms of addiction in our society: marijuana, cocaine, and alcohol. The fourth, addiction to cigarette smoking and tobacco, is discussed in detail in Chapter 15.

DRUGS AND DEPENDENCE

Approximately 60% of the world's production of illegal drugs is consumed in the United States. Each year Americans spend more than $100 billion on illegal drugs, an amount that surpasses the total dollars taken in from all crops by U. S. farmers. According to the U. S. Department of Education, today's drugs are stronger and more addictive, and they pose a greater risk than ever before.

Drugs lead to physical and psychological dependence. If used regularly, they integrate into the body's chemistry, increasing drug tolerance and forcing the user to constantly increase the dosage to obtain similar results. Drug abuse leads to serious health problems, and more than half of all adolescent suicides are drug-related.

MARIJUANA

Marijuana (pot or grass, as it commonly is referred to) is the most widely used illegal drug in the United States. Estimates indicate that 64% of Americans between ages 18 and 25 and 23% of those age 26 and older have smoked marijuana. Approximately 20 million people in the United States use marijuana regularly. This psychoactive drug is prepared from a mixture of crushed leaves, flowers, small branches, stems, and seeds from the hemp plant *cannabis sativa*. In small doses, marijuana has a sedative effect. Larger doses produce physical and psychic changes.

Studies in the 1960s indicated that the potential effects of marijuana were exaggerated and that the drug was relatively harmless. The drug as it is used today, however, is as much as 10 times stronger than when the initial studies were conducted. Today 90% of the research shows marijuana to be a dangerous and harmful drug.

The main, and most active, psychoactive and mind-altering ingredient in marijuana is thought to be delta-9-tetrahydrocannabinol (THC). In the 1960s, THC content in marijuana ranged from .02% to 2%. Users called the latter "real good grass." Today's THC content averages 4% to 6%, although it has been reported as high as 20%. The THC content in sinsemilla, a seedless variety of high-potency marijuana grown from the seedless female cannabis plant, is approximately 8%.

THC reaches the brain within 30 seconds of inhalation of marijuana smoke, and the psychic and physical changes reach their peak in about two or three minutes. THC then is metabolized in the liver to waste metabolites, but 30% of it remains in the body a week after marijuana was first smoked. Studies indicate that THC is not completely eliminated until 30 days or longer after an initial dose of the drug. For regular users the drug always will remain in the system.

Some of the short-term effects of marijuana are tachycardia (faster heart rate, sometimes as high as 180 beats per minute), dryness of the mouth, reddening of the eyes, stronger appetite, decrease in coordination and tracking (following a moving stimulus), difficulty in concentration, intermittent confusion, impairment of short-term memory and continuity of speech, and interference with the physical and mental learning process during periods of intoxication. Another common effect is the *amotivational syndrome*, a condition characterized by loss of motivation, dullness, apathy, and no interest in the future. This syndrome persists after periods of intoxication but usually disappears a few weeks after the individual stops using the drug. Long-term harmful effects include atrophy of the brain (leading to irreversible brain damage), less resistance to infectious diseases, chronic bronchitis, lung cancer (marijuana smoke may contain as much as 50% more cancer-producing hydrocarbons than cigarette smoke), and possible sterility and impotence.

One of the most common myths about marijuana use is that it does not lead to addiction. Ample scientific evidence, however, clearly shows that regular users of marijuana do develop physical and psychological dependence. Similar to cigarette smoking, when regular users go without the drug, they crave the substance, go through mood changes, are irritable and nervous, and develop an obsession to get more "pot."

COCAINE

Similar to marijuana, cocaine was thought for many years to be a relatively harmless drug. This misconception came to an abrupt halt in 1986 when two well-known athletes, Len Bias (basketball) and Don

Rogers (football), died suddenly following a cocaine overdose. Estimates indicate that between 4 and 8 million Americans use cocaine, 96% of whom had used marijuana prior to that.

Cocaine (2-beta-carbomethoxy-3-betabenozoxy-tropane) is the primary psychoactive ingredient derived from coca plant leaves. Over the years it has been given several different names, including coke, C, snow, blow, toot, flake, Peruvian lady, white girl, and happy dust. The drug usually is sniffed or snorted, but it can be smoked or injected.

Cocaine is an expensive drug. Some users pay more than $2,000 per ounce. Cocaine used in medical therapy sells for about $100 per ounce. Because of the high cost, cocaine is viewed as a luxury drug. Many users are well-educated, affluent, upwardly mobile professionals who are otherwise law-abiding citizens.

Cocaine hallucinations include "coke bugs" or imaginary insects and snakes crawling on or underneath the skin.

Cocaine has become the fastest growing drug problem in the United States. Each day about 5,000 people try cocaine for the first time. The addiction begins with a desire to get high, often at social gatherings, with the assurance that occasional use is harmless. About one in five will continue to use the drug now and then, and for some it is the beginning of a lifetime nightmare.

The popularity of cocaine is based on the almost universal guarantee that users will find themselves in an immediate state of euphoria and well-being. When cocaine is snorted, it quickly is absorbed through the mucous membranes of the nose into the bloodstream.

The drug is usually arranged in fine powder lines one to two inches long. Each line stimulates the autonomic nervous system stimulation for about 30 minutes.

Cocaine seems to alleviate fatigue and raise energy levels, as well as lessen the need for appetite and sleep. Following this stimulation comes a "crash," a state of physiological and psychological depression, often leaving the user with the desire to get more. This can lead to a constant craving for the drug.

Addiction becomes a lifetime illness and, similar to alcoholism, the individual recovers only by completely abstaining from the drug. A single "backslide" can result in renewed addiction.

Light to moderate cocaine use commonly is associated with feelings of pleasure and well-being. Sustained cocaine snorting can lead to a constant runny nose, nasal congestion and inflammation, and perforation of the nasal septum. Long-term consequences of cocaine use in general include loss of appetite, digestive disorders, weight loss, malnutrition, insomnia, confusion, anxiety, and cocaine psychosis. Cocaine psychosis is characterized by paranoia and hallucinations. In one type of hallucination, referred to as formication or "coke bugs," the chronic user perceives imaginary insects or snakes crawling on or underneath the skin.

High doses of cocaine can cause nervousness, dizziness, blurred vision, vomiting, tremors, seizures, high blood pressure, strokes, angina, and cardiac arrhythmias. Those who use freebase (a purer, more potent smokable form of cocaine) have increased risk for lung disease, and intravenous users are at risk for hepatitis, AIDS, and other infectious diseases. Large overdoses of cocaine can precipitate sudden death from respiratory paralysis, cardiac arrhythmias, and severe convulsions. Some individuals lack an enzyme used in metabolizing cocaine, and as few as two to three lines of cocaine may be fatal.

Chronic users who constantly crave the drug often turn to crime, including murder, to sustain their habit. Some users view suicide as the only solution to this sad syndrome.

ALCOHOL

Drinking alcohol has been a socially acceptable behavior for centuries. Alcohol is an accepted accompaniment at parties, ceremonies, dinners, sport contests, the establishment of kingdoms or governments, and the signing of treaties between nations. Alcohol also has been used for medical reasons as a mild sedative or as a pain killer for surgery.

For a short period of 14 years, from 1920 to 1933, by constitutional amendment, the sale and use of alcohol were declared illegal in the United States (Figure 16.1). This amendment was repealed because drinkers and nondrinkers alike questioned the right of government to pass judgment on individual moral standards. In addition, organized crime to smuggle and illegally sell alcohol expanded tremendously.

FIGURE 16.1
The sale of alcohol was illegal in the United States between 1920 and 1933.

The alcohol contained in drinks, known as ethyl alcohol, is a depressant drug that affects the brain and slows down central nervous system activity. As with most drugs that affect the brain, it has strong addictive properties and therefore can be abused easily.

Alcohol is the cause of one of the most significant health-related drug problems in the United States today. An estimated six in ten adults, or more than 100 million Americans 18 years and older, are drinkers. Approximately 10 million of them will develop a drinking problem, including alcoholism, in their lifetime. Another 3 million teenagers are thought to have a drinking problem.

Addiction to alcohol develops slowly. Most people think they are in control of their drinking habits and do not realize they have a problem until they become alcoholics, when they find themselves physically and emotionally dependent on the drug. This addiction is characterized by excessive use and constant preoccupation with drinking. Alcohol abuse, in turn, leads to mental, emotional, physical, and social problems.

Alcohol intake impedes peripheral vision, lowers visual and hearing acuity, decreases reaction time, and impairs concentration and motor performance (including increased swaying and impaired judgment of distance and speed of moving objects). Further, it alleviates fear, increases risk-taking behaviors, stimulates urination, and induces sleep. A single large dose of alcohol also may decrease sexual function. One of the most unpleasant, dangerous, and life-threatening effects of drinking is the *synergistic* action of alcohol when combined with other drugs, particularly central nervous system depressants. The effects of mixing alcohol with another drug can be much greater than the sum of two or more drug actions by themselves. Although each person reacts to a combination of alcohol and other drugs in a different way, these effects range from loss of consciousness to death.

Long-term effects of alcohol abuse are serious and often life-threatening. Some of these detrimental effects are cirrhosis of the liver (scarring of the liver, often fatal); higher risk for oral, esophageal, and liver cancer; cardiomyopathy (a disease affecting the heart muscle); elevated blood pressure; greater risk for strokes; inflammation of the esophagus, stomach, small intestine, and pancreas; stomach ulcers; sexual impotence; malnutrition; brain cell damage leading to loss of memory; psychosis; depression; and hallucinations.

To find out if drinking is a problem in your life, refer to the questionnaire Alcohol Abuse: Are You Drinking Too Much.* In Lab 16A, developed by the American Medical Association. If you respond "yes" twice or more on this questionnaire, you may be jeopardizing your health.

If a person is determined to control the problem, it is not that hard to do. The first and most important step is to want to cut down. If you want to do this but find you cannot, you had better accept the probability that alcohol is becoming a serious problem for you, and you should seek guidance from your physician or from an organization such as Alcoholics Anonymous. The next few suggestions also may help you cut down alcohol intake.

1. **Set reasonable limits for yourself.** Decide not to exceed a certain number of drinks on a given occasion, and stick to your decision. No more than two beers or two cocktails a day is a reasonable limit. You have proven to yourself that you can control your drinking if you set a target such as this and consistently do not exceed it.

2. **Learn to say no.** Many people have "just one more" drink because others in the group are, or because someone puts pressure on them, not because they really want a drink. When you reach the sensible limit you have set for yourself, politely but firmly refuse to exceed it. If you are

being the generous host, pour yourself a glass of water or juice "on the rocks." Nobody will notice the difference.

3. **Drink slowly.** Never gulp down a drink. Choose your drinks for their flavor, not their "kick," and savor the taste of each sip.

4. **Dilute your drinks.** If you prefer cocktails to beer, try having long drinks. Instead of downing your gin or whiskey neat or nearly so, drink it diluted with a mixer such as tonic, water, or soda water, in a tall glass. That way you can enjoy both the flavor and the act of drinking but you will take longer to finish each drink. Also, you can make your two-drink limit last all evening or switch to the mixer by itself.

5. **Do not drink on your own.** Make a point of confining your drinking to social gatherings. You may have a hard time resisting the urge to pour yourself a relaxing drink at the end of a hard day, but many formerly heavy drinkers have found that a cup of coffee or a soft drink satisfies the need as well as alcohol did and that it was just a habit. What may help you really unwind, even with no drink at all, is a comfortable chair, loosened clothing, and perhaps a soothing audio tape, television program, or good book to read.

TREATMENT OF ADDICTION

Treatment of drug addiction (including alcohol) seldom is accomplished without professional guidance and support. Of course, the first step is to recognize the reality of the problem. The questionnaire in Lab 16B will help you recognize possible addictive behavior in yourself or someone you know. If your answers to more than half of these questions are positive, you may have a problem and should speak to your doctor or contact the local mental health clinic for a referral (see the Yellow Pages in your phone book).

SEXUALLY TRANSMITTED DISEASES

Sexually transmitted diseases (STDs) have reached epidemic proportions in the United States. Of the

---

* Source: *Family Medical Guide* by the American Medical Association. New York: Random House, 1982. Reproduced by permission of the AMA.

more than 25 known STDs, some are still incurable. The American Social Health Association stated that 25% of all Americans will acquire at least one STD in their lifetime.

Each year more than 12 million people are newly infected with STDs, including 4.6 million cases of chlamydia, 1.8 million of gonorrhea, 1 million of genital warts, half a million cases of herpes, and almost 100,000 cases of syphilis. Attracting most of the attention because of its life-threatening potential were more than 46,648 new cases of AIDS in 1992 alone.

CHLAMYDIA

Chlamydia is a bacterial infection that spreads during vaginal, anal, or oral sex, or from the vagina to a newborn baby during childbirth. Chlamydia can seriously damage the reproductive system.

This disease is considered to be a major factor in male and female infertility. Because it may have no symptoms, three of four people don't have any symptoms until the infection has become quite serious. The Centers for Disease Control state that about 20% of all college students have chlamydia.

When symptoms are present, they tend to mimic other STDs, so the disease can be mistreated. Symptoms of serious infection include abdominal pain, fever, nausea, vaginal bleeding, and arthritis. It can be treated successfully with oral antibiotics but will not reverse any damage already done to the reproductive system.

GONORRHEA

One of the oldest STDs, gonorrhea, also is caused by a bacterial infection. Gonorrhea is transmitted through vaginal, anal, and oral sex.

Typical symptoms in men include a puslike secretion from the penis and painful urination. Most infected women don't have any symptoms until the infection is fairly serious. At this stage, women develop fever, severe abdominal pain, and pelvic inflammatory disease (see below).

If untreated, gonorrhea can produce infertility, widespread bacterial infection, heart damage, arthritis in men and women, and blindness in children born to infected women. Gonorrhea is treated successfully with penicillin and other antibiotics.

PELVIC INFLAMMATORY DISEASE

Each year approximately 750,000 women have pelvic inflammatory disease (PID). This disease usually is caused by chlamydia and gonorrhea.

Typical symptoms of PID are fever; nausea; vomiting; chills; spotting, heavy bleeding during menstrual periods; and pain in the lower abdomen, during sexual intercourse, between menstrual periods, or urination. Many women do not know they have PID because they have no symptoms.

PID often develops when the STD spreads to the fallopian tubes, uterus, and ovaries. If the woman becomes pregnant, she may have an ectopic or tubal pregnancy. The pregnancy destroys the embryo and can kill the patient.

PID is treated with antibiotics, bed rest, and sexual abstinence. Surgery also may be required to remove infected or scarred tissue or to repair or remove the fallopian tubes or uterus.

GENITAL WARTS

Genital warts are caused by viral infection. They show up anywhere from a month and a half to eight months after exposure. These warts may be flat or raised and usually are found on the penis or around the vulva and the vagina, but they also can appear in the mouth, throat, rectum, on the cervix, or around the anus.

Of sexually active people in the United States, 20% to 30% are infected with the virus that causes this STD. In some cities, nearly half of all sexually active teenagers have genital warts. Similar to chlamydia, the virus is spread through vaginal, anal, or oral sex, or from the vagina to a newborn baby.

Health problems associated with genital warts include increased risk for cancers of the cervix, vulva, or penis and enlargement and spread of the warts leading to obstruction of the urethra, vagina, and anus. Babies born to infected mothers commonly develop warts over their bodies; therefore, Cesarean sections are recommended.

Treatment requires completely removing all warts, which can be done by freezing them with liquid nitrogen, dissolving them with chemicals, or removing them through electrosurgery or laser surgery. Infected patients may have to be treated more than once because genital warts can recur.

HERPES

Herpes also is caused by a viral infection (herpes simplex virus types I and II), and it still has no known cure. Sores appear on the mouth, genitals, rectum, or other parts of the body. The symptoms usually disappear within a few weeks, causing some people to believe they are cured. Herpes is presently incurable, though, and its victims do remain infected. Repeated outbreaks are common.

Herpes is highly contagious and can be transmitted through simple finger contact from the mouth to the genitals. Victims are most contagious during an outbreak. In conjunction with the sores, victims usually have mild fever, swollen glands, and headaches.

SYPHILIS

Another common type of STD, also caused by bacterial infection, is syphilis. Approximately 3 weeks after infection, a painless sore appears where the bacteria entered the body. This sore disappears on its own in a few weeks. If untreated, more sores may appear within 6 months of the initial outbreak but again will disappear by themselves.

A latent stage, during which the victim is not contagious, may last up to 30 years, lulling victims into thinking they are healed. During the last stage of the disease, some people develop paralysis, crippling, blindness, heart disease, brain damage, insanity, and even may die. One of the oldest known STDs, syphilis used to end up killing its victims. Penicillin and other antibiotics now are used in its treatment.

RESPONSIBLE ACTION

If you test positive for any type of STD, you must tell anyone you have had sex with so he or she can be tested and treated if necessary. Unless you do this, you run the risk of being infected again, the disease can cause permanent damage to your partner or partners, and the disease may spread to other individuals.

HIV AND AIDS

AIDS is the most frightening of all STDs because it has no known cure and there seems to be no cure for it in the foreseeable future. AIDS — which stands for acquired immunodeficiency syndrome — is the end stage of infection by the human immunodeficiency virus, or HIV.

HIV is a chronic infectious disease that spreads among individuals who choose to engage in risky behavior such as unprotected sex or the sharing of hypodermic needles. When a person becomes infected with HIV, the virus multiplies, attacks, and destroys white blood cells. These cells are part of the immune system, and their function is to fight off infections and diseases.

As the number of white blood cells killed increases, the body's immune system gradually breaks down or may be destroyed completely. Without the immune system, a person becomes susceptible to opportunistic infections or cancers not ordinarily seen in healthy people.

HIV Disease

HIV is a progressive disease. At first, people who become infected with HIV may not know they are infected. An incubation period of weeks, months, or years may go by during which no symptoms appear. The virus may live in the body ten years or longer before symptoms develop.

As the infection progresses to the point at which certain diseases develop, the person is said to have AIDS. HIV itself doesn't kill. Nor do people die of AIDS. AIDS is the term used to define the final stage of HIV infection. Death is caused by a weakened immune system that is unable to fight off these opportunistic diseases.

Earliest symptoms of the disease include unexplained weight loss, constant fatigue, mild fever, swollen lymph glands, diarrhea, and sore throats. Advanced symptoms include loss of appetite, skin diseases, night sweats, and deterioration of the mucous membranes.

Most of the illnesses AIDS patients develop are harmless and rare in the general population but are fatal to AIDS victims. The two most common fatal conditions in AIDS patients are *pneumocystis carinii pneumonia* (a parasitic infection of the lungs) and *kaposis sarcoma* (a type of skin cancer). The AIDS virus also may attack the nervous system, causing brain and spinal cord damage.

On the average, the individual develops the symptoms that fit the case definition of AIDS about seven to eight years following infection. From that point on, the person may live another two to three years. In essence, from the point of infection, the individual may endure a chronic disease eight to ten years.

The only means to determine whether someone has HIV is through an *HIV antibody test*. Being HIV positive does not necessarily mean the person has AIDS. Several years may go by before the person develops the diseases that fit the case definition of AIDS.

> *Once infected with HIV, a person never will become uninfected. No one should be so ignorant as to believe that it can never happen to him or her!*

Upon HIV infection, the immune system's line of defense against the virus is to form antibodies that bind to the virus. On the average, the body takes three months to manufacture enough antibodies to show up positive in an HIV antibody test. Sometimes this may take six months or longer.

If HIV infection is suspected, a prudent waiting period of three to six months is suggested prior to testing. During this time, and from there on, individuals should refrain from further endangering themselves and others through risky behaviors. Some people choose to be tested to be reassured that their risky behaviors are acceptable. Even if the test turns up negative for HIV, this does not represent a "license" to continue risky behaviors. *Once infected with HIV, a person never will become uninfected.* There is no second chance. Everyone must protect himself or herself against this chronic disease. *No one should be so ignorant as to believe that it can never happen to him or her!*

Although professionals disagree as to how many carriers actually will develop AIDS, sooner or later most HIV-infected individuals will be diagnosed with AIDS. Even if a person has not developed AIDS, the virus can be passed on to others who could easily develop AIDS.

HIV Transmission

HIV is transmitted by the exchange of cellular body fluids including blood, semen, vaginal secretions, and maternal milk. These fluids may be exchanged during sexual intercourse, by using hypodermic needles previously used by infected individuals, between a pregnant woman and her developing fetus, by infection of babies from the mother during childbirth, less frequently during breast feeding, and rarely from a blood transfusion or organ transplant.

The risk of being infected with HIV from a blood transfusion today is very slight. Prior to 1985, several cases of HIV infection came from blood transfusions because the blood was donated by HIV-infected individuals. Today, all individuals who donate blood are tested for HIV.

A myth regarding HIV is that it can be transmitted by donating blood. People cannot get HIV from giving blood. Health professionals use a brand-new needle every time they withdraw blood from a person. These needles are used only once and are destroyed and thrown away immediately after each person has donated blood.

Also, people do not get HIV because of who they are but because of what they do. HIV and AIDS can threaten anyone, anywhere: men, women, children, teenagers, young people, older adults, Whites, Blacks, Hispanics, Orientals, homosexuals, heterosexuals, bisexuals, druggies, Americans, Africans, Europeans. Nobody is immune to HIV.

HIV can be transmitted between males, between females, from male to female, or from female to male. Although HIV and AIDS are basically preventable, almost all of the people who get HIV do so because they choose to engage in risky behaviors.

Risky Behaviors

You cannot tell if people are infected with HIV or have AIDS by simply looking at them or taking their word. Not you, not a nurse, not even a doctor can tell without an HIV antibody test. Therefore, every time you engage in risky behavior, you run the risk of contracting HIV. The two most basic risky behaviors are:

1. **Having unprotected vaginal, anal, or oral sex with an HIV-infected person.** Unprotected sex means having sex without the proper use of a condom. A person should select only latex (rubber or prophylactic) condoms that say "disease prevention" on the package. Although you might have unprotected sex with an infected person and not get the virus, you can also get it by having unprotected sex only once with that infected person.

   Rubbing during sexual intercourse often damages mucous membranes and causes unseen bleeding (even in the mouth). During vaginal, anal, or oral sexual contact, infected blood, semen, or vaginal fluids can penetrate the mucous membranes that line the vagina, the penis, the rectum, the mouth, or the throat. From the membrane, HIV then can travel into the previously uninfected person's blood.

Health experts believe unprotected anal sex is the riskiest type of sex. Even though bleeding is not visible in most cases, anal sex almost always causes tiny tears and bleeding in the rectum. This happens because the rectum does not stretch easily, the mucous membrane is quite thin, and small blood vessels lie directly beneath the membrane. Condoms also are more likely to break during anal intercourse because of the greater friction produced in a smaller cavity. All of these factors greatly enhance the risk of HIV transmission.

Although latex condoms provide for "safer" sex if they are used correctly, they are not 100% foolproof. Abstaining from sex is the only 100% sure way to protect yourself from HIV infection and other STDs.

2. **Sharing hypodermic needles or other drug paraphernalia with someone who is infected.** Following an injection, a small amount of blood remains in the needle and sometimes in the syringe itself. If the person that used the syringe is infected with HIV and someone else uses that same syringe to shoot up, regardless of the drug used (legal or illegal), that small amount of blood is sufficient to spread the virus. All used syringes should be destroyed and disposed of immediately after they are used.

In addition, a person must be cautious when getting acupuncture, getting a tattoo, or having the ears pierced. If the needle used was used previously on someone who is HIV infected and it was not disinfected properly, the person risks getting HIV as well.

Infrequent use of drugs, including alcohol, also heightens the risk of spreading HIV. Otherwise prudent people often act irrationally and engage in risky behaviors when they are under the influence of drugs. Getting high can make you willing to have sex when you really didn't plan to, and thereby run the risk of HIV infection (Figure 16.2).

As pointed out earlier, HIV can be transmitted through a blood transfusion, an organ transplant, pregnancy (mother to fetus), and maternal milk (usually mother to child). Even though the nation's blood supply is quite safe (because all donors are tested for HIV), a very small risk is present in becoming infected from previously tested blood.

Because of the three- to six-month incubation period, donors recently infected with HIV can test negative at the time they donate blood (or an organ). Therefore, people who are planning to have surgery should store their own blood in advance so safe blood will be available if they need it.

Small concentrations of the virus have been found in saliva and teardrops, but there is no record of anyone getting HIV through French-kissing or from someone else's tears, coughs, or sneezes. In principle, if both people have open cuts in the lips, mouth, or gums, HIV could be transmitted through openmouthed kissing, but such a case has never been documented.

The virus cannot be transmitted through perspiration (sweat) either. Sporting activities with no physical contact pose no risk to uninfected individuals, unless they have open wounds through which blood from an infected person can come in direct contact with the open wound of the uninfected person. The skin is an excellent line of defense against HIV. Blood from an infected person cannot penetrate the skin except through an opening in the skin. As an extra precaution, a person should use vinyl or latex gloves when performing work that requires direct contact with someone else's blood or open wound.

VANESSA WAS IN A FATAL CAR ACCIDENT LAST NIGHT. ONLY SHE DOESN'T KNOW IT YET.

FIGURE 16.2
Drug and alcohol use can make people more willing to have unplanned and unprotected sex, thereby, risking HIV infection.

Photo courtesy of the National Institute on Drug Abuse, U.S. Department of Health & Human Services.

Some people fear getting HIV from health care professionals. The chances of getting infected during physical or medical procedures are practically nil. Health care workers take extra care to protect themselves and their patients from HIV.

HIV is not transmitted through casual contact. HIV cannot be caught by spending time, shaking hands, or hugging an infected person; from a toilet seat, dishes, or silverware used by an HIV patient; or by sharing a drink, food, a towel, or clothes with a person who has HIV.

What about dating? Dating and getting to know other people is a normal part of life. Dating, however, does not mean the same thing as having sex. Sexual intercourse as a part of dating can be risky, and one of the risks is AIDS. You can't tell if someone you are dating or would like to date has been exposed to HIV. The good news, though, is that as long as you avoid sexual activity and don't share drug needles, it doesn't matter whom you date.

Another myth regarding HIV transmission is that you can get it from insects or animals. The H in HIV stands for human. You cannot catch HIV from insects or animals. Animals do not get infected with HIV.

HIV and AIDS Statistics

The Centers for Disease Control estimate that 1 million Americans are infected with HIV. Around the world an estimated 12 million people are infected. Because of the lengthy incubation period (seven to eight years to develop AIDS) about 20% of the AIDS patients today are believed to have been infected as teenagers.

By the end of 1992, 253,448 AIDS cases had been diagnosed in the United States (see Figure 16.3) and 171,980 had died from the diseases caused by HIV. The number of deaths is projected to double in three years. Most of the people who die are in the 20- to 45-year-old age group. By the year 2000, deaths from HIV infection are expected to become the third leading cause of death, behind cardiovascular disease and cancer.

FIGURE 16.3
Reported U. S. AIDS cases between 1981 and 1992.

Approximately 66% of all AIDS cases in the United States have occurred in gay or bisexual men. AIDS among heterosexuals, nonetheless, is on the rise. In fact, HIV is now spreading at a faster rate among heterosexuals. Many heterosexuals practice unprotected sex because they don't believe it can happen to their segment of the population. HIV is an epidemic that does not discriminate by sexual orientation. Worldwide, about 75% of the AIDS cases have been reported in heterosexuals.

As with any other serious illness, AIDS patients deserve respect, understanding, and support. Rejection and discrimination are traits of immature, hateful, and ignorant people. Education, knowledge, and responsible behaviors are the best ways to minimize fear and discrimination.

HIV Testing

A person can be tested for HIV in several ways. You may look up your local Public Health Department or AIDS Information Service (or related names) in the phone book. Testing is usually free of charge, and the results are kept confidential. Many states also conduct anonymous testing. Your name is never recorded. You can call several toll-free hotlines for more information on anonymous testing, treatment programs, support services, HIV and AIDS information, and STDs in general. All information discussed during a phone call to these hotlines is kept strictly confidential. The numbers to call are:

- National AIDS Hotline: 1–800–342–AIDS or La Linea Nacional de SIDA: 1–800–344–SIDA, for Spanish speaking people.
- STD Hotline: 1–800–227–8922.
- National Institute on Drug Abuse (NIDA) Information and Treatment Referral: 1–800–662–HELP or 1–800–66–AYUDA for Spanish speaking only. NIDA also provides information on drug abuse and addictive behavior.

HIV Treatment

Even though several drugs are being tested to treat and slow down the disease process, AIDS has no known cure. Approximately 30 different approaches to an AIDS vaccine are being explored, and two have been approved for testing in humans. The best advice at this point is to take a preventive approach.

Although HIV has no cure, medications are available that allow HIV-infected patients to live longer. The sooner the treatment is initiated following infection, the better are the chances for delaying the onset of AIDS.

Developing a vaccine to prevent HIV infection or AIDS seems highly unlikely in the next few years. People should not expect a medical breakthrough. Treatment modalities, however, should continue to improve and allow HIV-infected persons and AIDS patients to live longer and more productive lives.

Presently, several AIDS clinical trials are available in the United States. These projects are co-sponsored by the Centers for Disease Control, the Food and Drug Administration, the National Institute of Allergy and Infectious Diseases, and the National Library of Medicine. The purpose of AIDS clinical trials is to evaluate experimental drugs and various therapies for people at all stages of HIV infection. Interested individuals can call 1–800–TRIALS–A. As with all HIV testing, calls are completely confidential. Eligibility to participate in an AIDS clinical trial varies, and all applicants are evaluated individually. By calling the telephone number given, an interested person will receive information on the purpose and location of the trials (studies) that are open, eligibility requirements and exclusion criteria, and names and telephone numbers of contact persons.

Economic Impact of HIV and AIDS

Federal government spending for AIDS-related projects gradually increased to more than $900 million between 1982 and 1988. Costs continued to escalate to $1.3 billion in 1989, to $4.3 billion in 1992, and are expected to be in excess of $10.4 billion in 1994.

As of 1993, the annual U. S. health care cost to care for an HIV-positive individual who had not reached the AIDS stage was approximately $5,150. The yearly cost to treat an individual who had developed AIDS was about $32,000. The average cost from the onset of AIDS until death was $85,333. Assuming an incubation period of seven years and an additional three years of AIDS, the direct treatment costs per person would average $121,383. This represents more than $30.5 billion to treat the 253,448 AIDS cases reported as of December 1992.

If the estimated 1 million people infected with HIV in the United States develop AIDS, direct health care costs for the disease will equal $121.383 billion. To place this figure in perspective, a person would have to spend $1 million per day for the next 332.5 years to spend the $121.382 billion.

Every American will help pay for these costs through taxes and a more expensive health care system. In the words of Dr. Russell Centanni, Professor of Biology at Boise State University: "Rather sobering for a preventable disease."

GUIDELINES FOR PREVENTING SEXUALLY TRANSMITTED DISEASES

With all the grim news about STDs, there is also some good news: You can do things to prevent their spread, and take precautions to keep yourself from becoming a victim.

The facts are in: The best prevention technique is a mutually monogamous sexual relationship, one in which two people have sexual relationships only with each other. That one behavior, says Dr. James Mason, director of the Centers for Disease Control in Atlanta, will remove you almost completely from any risk for developing an STD.

Unfortunately, in today's society it is becoming much more difficult to know at what point you can truly trust a person. You may be led to believe you are in a monogamous relationship when your partner actually: (a) may be cheating on you and gets infected, (b) ends up having a one night stand with someone who is infected, (c) got the virus several years ago before the present relationship and still doesn't know of the infection, (d) may not be honest with you and chooses not to tell you about the infection, or (e) is shooting up drugs and becomes infected. In any of these cases, HIV can be passed on to you.

Because your future and your life are at stake, and because you may never know if your partner is infected, you should give serious and careful consideration to postponing sex until you believe you have found a lifetime monogamous relationship. In doing so, you will not have to live with the fear of catching HIV or other STDs or deal with an unplanned pregnancy.

As strange as this may seem to some, many people postpone sexual activity until they are married. This is the best guarantee against HIV. Young people should understand that married life will provide plenty of time for fulfilling and rewarding sex.

If you choose to delay sex, do not let peers pressure you into having sex. Some people would have you believe you are not a real man or woman if you don't have sex. Manhood and womanhood are not proven during sexual intercourse but, instead, through mature, responsible, and healthy choices.

Other people lead you to believe that love doesn't exist without sex. Sex in the early stages of a relationship is not the product of love but is simply the fulfillment of a physical, and often selfish, drive. A loving relationship develops over a long time with mutual respect for each other.

Teenagers are especially susceptible to peer pressure leading to premature sexual intercourse. The result: more than a million teen pregnancies per year and a 43% pregnancy rate for all girls at least once as a teenager. Too many young people wish they had postponed sex and silently admire those who do. Sex lasts only a few minutes. The consequences of irresponsible sex, however, may last a lifetime. In some cases, they are fatal.

Then there are those who enjoy bragging about their sexual conquests and mock people who choose to wait. In essence, many of these conquests are only fantasies in an attempt to gain popularity with peers.

Sexual promiscuity never leads to a trusting, loving, and lasting relationship. Mature people respect others' choices. If someone does not respect your choice to wait, he or she certainly does not deserve your friendship or, for that matter, anything else.

There is no greater sex than that between two loving and responsible individuals who mutually trust and admire each other. Contrary to many beliefs, these relationships are possible. They are built upon unselfish attitudes and behaviors.

As you look around, you will find that many believe the same way you do. Seek them out and build your friendships and future around people who respect you for what you are and what you believe. You don't have to compromise your choices or values. In the end you will reap the greater rewards of a choice and lasting relationship, free of AIDS and other STDs.

What about those who do not have — or do not desire — a monogamous relationship? Some other things can be done to lower, but never completely eliminate, the risk for developing STDs in general:

1. Know your partner. The days are gone when anonymous bathhouse or singles-bars sex is safe. Limit your sexual relationships, and always practice safer sex.

2. Limit the number of sexual partners you have. Having one partner lowers your chance of infection. The more partners you have, the greater is your chance for infection.

3. If you are sexually promiscuous, consider having periodic physical checkups. Getting exposed to an STD by a person who does not have any symptoms and who is unaware of the infection is easy. Sexually promiscuous men and women between ages 15 and 35 are considered to be in a particularly high-risk group for developing STDs.

4. Use "barrier" methods of contraception to help prevent the disease from spreading. Condoms, diaphragms, the contraceptive sponge, and spermicidal suppositories, foams, and jellies can all deter the spread of certain STDs. Spermicidal agents may act as a disinfectant as well. Many physicians are especially encouraging promiscuous teenagers to use condoms. Traditionally, teenagers do not use any birth-control methods at all and remain at high risk for STDs.

5. Be responsible enough to abstain from sexual activity if you know you have an infection. Go to a physician or clinic for treatment, and ask your doctor when you can safely resume sexual activity. Abstain until it is safe. Just as you want to be protected in a sexual relationship, you should want to protect your partner as well.

6. Urinate immediately following sexual intercourse. This is not a reliable method, but it may help (especially men) flush bacteria and viruses from the urinary tract.

7. Wash thoroughly immediately after sexual activity. Washing with hot, soapy water will not guarantee safety against STDs, but it can prevent you from spreading certain germs on your fingers and may wash away bacteria and viruses that have not yet entered the body.

8. If you suspect your partner is infected with a STD, ask. He or she may not even be aware of the infection, so look for signs of infection, such as sores, redness, inflammations, a rash, growths, warts, or discharge. If you are unsure, abstain.

9. Consider abstaining from sexual relations if you have any kind of an illness or disease, even a common cold. Any kind of illness makes you more susceptible to other illnesses, and lower immunity can make you extra vulnerable to STDs. The same holds true for times when you are under extreme stress, when you are fatigued, and when you are overworked. Drugs and alcohol also can lower your resistance to disease.

10. Wear loose-fitting clothes made from natural fibers. Tight-fitting clothing made from synthetic fibers (especially underwear and nylon pantyhose) can create conditions that encourage the growth of bacteria and actually can aggravate STDs.

HIV RISK REDUCTION

Based upon recommendations from health experts, observing the following precautions can reduce your risk for getting HIV, and subsequently AIDS:

1. Postpone sex until you and your uninfected partner are prepared to enter into a lifetime monogamous relationship. In his book, *What You Can Do to Avoid AIDS*, Earvin "Magic" Johnson stated:[8]

   > But if I had known what I do now when I was younger, I would have postponed sex as long as I could, and I would have tried to have it the first time with somebody that I knew I wanted to spend the rest of my life with. I certainly want my children to postpone sex. Now the rest of my life may be a lot shorter than I thought it was going to be, and I may not be around to see my son, Andre, grow up and to see what happens to the baby Cookie and I are having in the summer of '92, and, of course, I may not have the long life I want with Cookie.

2. Unless you are in a monogamous relationship and you know your partner is not infected (which you may never know for sure), practice safer sex every single time you have sex. This means you should use a latex condom from start to finish for each sexual act. If you think your partner should use a condom but refuses to do so, say no to sex with that person.

   Many experts believe greater protection can be obtained by placing a small amount of the spermicide nonoxynol–9 inside the condom at its tip and then lubricating the outside with additional spermicide. Nonoxynol–9 is used to kill the man's sperm for birth control purposes. In test tubes, it has been shown to kill STD germs and HIV. This spermicide, however, should not be used in place of a condom because it will not offer the same protection as the condom does by itself.

3. Avoid having multiple and anonymous sexual partners. Keep in mind that anyone you have sex with could be infected with HIV.

4. Don't have sexual contact with anyone who does not practice safer sex.

5. Avoid sexual contact with anyone who has had sex with people at risk for getting HIV, even if they are now practicing safer sex.

6. Don't have sex with prostitutes.

7. If you do have sex with someone who might be infected with HIV or whose history is unknown to you, avoid exchange of body fluids.

8. Don't share toothbrushes, razors, or other implements that could become contaminated with blood with anyone who is, or who might be, infected with HIV.

9. Be cautious regarding procedures such as acupuncture, tattooing, and ear piercing, in which needles or other nonsterile instruments may be used again and again to pierce the skin or mucous membranes. These procedures are safe if proper sterilization methods or disposable needles are followed. Before undergoing the procedure, ask what precautions are being taken.

10. If you are planning to undergo artificial insemination, insist on frozen sperm obtained from a laboratory that tests all donors for infection with HIV. Donors should be tested twice before accepting the sperm — once at the time of donation and again a few months later.

11. If you know you will be having surgery in the near future, and if you are able, consider donating blood for your own use. This will eliminate completely the already small risk of contracting HIV through a blood transfusion. It also will eliminate the more substantial risk for contracting other blood-borne diseases, such as hepatitis, from a transfusion.

Avoiding risky behaviors that destroy quality of life and life itself are critical components of a healthy lifestyle. Learning the facts so you can make responsible choices can protect you and those around you from startling and unexpected conditions. Using alcohol in moderation (or not at all), avoiding substance abuse, and preventing sexually transmitted diseases are key elements in averting both physical and psychological damage.

LABORATORY EXPERIENCE

LAB 16A
Alcohol Abuse: Are You Drinking Too Much?

Lab Preparation
None required.

LAB 16B
Addictive Behavior Questionnaire

Lab Preparation
None required.

LAB 16C
Self-Quiz on HIV and AIDS

Lab Preparation
None required.

REFERENCES

1. "Addiction." *Aerobics News*. Dallas: The Institute for Aerobics Research, July 1987.
2. American Medical Association. *Family Medical Guide*. New York: Random House, 1982.
3. Bennett, E. G., and D. Woolf (Editors). *Substance Abuse*. Albany, NY: Delmar Publishers Inc., 1991.
4. Carroll, C. R. *Drugs in Modern Society*. Dubuque, IA: Brown and Benchmark Publishers, 1992.
5. Centanni, R. J. HIV/AIDS: Into the Second Decade. Boise State University: unpublished manuscript, 1992.
6. Channing L. Bete Co., Inc. *About AIDS and Shooting Drugs*. South Deerfield, MA: The Company, 1986.
7. Hafen, B. Q., A. L. Thygerson, and K. J. Frandsen. *Behavioral Guidelines for Health & Wellness*. Englewood, CO: Morton Publishing Company, 1988.
8. Johnson, E. M. *What You Can Do To Avoid AIDS*. New York: Random House, Inc., 1992.
9. Schlaadt, R. G., and P. T. Shannon. *Drugs*. Englewood Cliffs, NJ: Prentice Hall, 1990.

RELEVANT FITNESS AND WELLNESS ISSUES

17

KEY CONCEPTS

Spirituality
Altruism
Aging
Functional capacity
Personal safety
Prevention Index
Consumer fraud
Behavioral objectives
Quality of life

OBJECTIVES

■ Define spiritual well-being and its relationship to a healthy lifestyle.

■ Describe the relationship between fitness and aging.

■ Discuss the importance and present a plan for accident prevention and personal safety.

■ Learn guidelines for the prevention of consumer fraud.

■ Become familiar with factors to consider when selecting a health/fitness club.

■ Become acquainted with the Prevention Index: a measure of the effort Americans are making to prevent disease and improve total well-being.

■ Review health/fitness accomplishments and chart a wellness program for the future.

Better health, quality of life, and longevity are the three most vital benefits derived from a lifetime physical fitness program. In itself, physical fitness does not always lower the risk for chronic diseases and ensure better health. Nevertheless, a healthy lifestyle is one means to attain the highest potential for total well-being.

In addition to the wellness issues already discussed in this book, four other factors that may directly influence a person's well-being are: (a) spirituality, (b) exercise and aging, and (c) accident prevention and personal safety, and (d) health-promoting behaviors. These components of wellness are the focus of this chapter. Guidelines for preventing consumer fraud and selecting a health/fitness club also are presented. Further, you will have the opportunity to determine how well you achieved your objectives this semester. Finally, you will receive instructions to help you chart a personal wellness program for the future.

SPIRITUAL WELL-BEING

The National Interfaith Coalition on Aging defines spiritual well-being as an affirmation of life in a relationship with God, self, community, and environment that nurtures and celebrates wholeness (Figure 17.1). Because this definition encompasses Christians and non-Christians alike, it assumes that all people are spiritual in nature.

Spiritual health provides a unifying power that integrates the other dimensions of wellness. Basic characteristics of spiritual people include a sense of meaning and direction in life, a relationship to a higher being, freedom, prayer, faith, love, closeness to others, peace, joy, fulfillment, and altruism (service to others).

Religion has been a major part of cultures since the beginning of time. Although not everyone in the United States claims affiliation with a certain religion or denomination, current surveys

L A B S

FIGURE 17.1
Spiritual well-being.

indicate that 94% of the U.S. population believes in God or a universal spirit functioning as God.

People, furthermore, believe to a varying extent that (a) a relationship with God is meaningful; (b) God can grant help, guidance, and assistance in daily living; and (c) mortal existence has a purpose. If we accept any or all of these statements, attaining spirituality will have a definite effect on our happiness and well-being.

SPIRITUALITY AND HEALTH*

The scientific association between spirituality and health is more difficult to establish than that of other lifestyle factors such as alcohol, smoking, physical inactivity, seat belt use, and so on. Several research studies, nonetheless, have reported positive relationships between spiritual well-being, emotional well-being, life satisfaction, and health.

Researchers have found that most successful men and women have strong spiritual values. Furthermore, almost all of these people experienced a crisis early in life. Spiritual beliefs seem to have helped them overcome the crisis and aided in developing better coping techniques to deal with future trauma.

For spiritual people, prayer seems to be the focus of most spiritual experiences. Prayer also has been shown to have an effect on people who are not aware that prayers are being offered in their behalf.

---

* Adapted with permission from Wellness: Guidelines for a Healthy Lifestyle, *Hafen, B. Q. and W. W. K. Hoeger. Englewood, CO: Morton, 1994.*

A nationwide survey of physicians indicated that about half of them believe patients profit from prayer. Approximately 67% said they pray for their patients.

One study indicated a much higher rate of heart attacks among nonreligious people, compared to a religious sample of people who attend church. Other studies suggest that religious support may act as a buffer against disease and that the social support encourages preventive health.

In another study, people around the country were asked to pray daily, during a 10-month period, for a group of almost 200 coronary care unit patients. A second, similar group of patients did not have anyone praying for them. Fewer complications were reported in the group that was prayed for. As compared to the prayed-for group, five times as many patients in the non-prayed for group required antibiotics and three times as many developed pulmonary edema.

Prayer has been shown to have an effect on people who are not aware that prayers are being offered in their behalf.

Altruism, a key attribute of spiritual people, seems to enhance health and longevity. Altruism is defined as *true concern for the welfare of others* (opposite of egoism), or a sincere desire to serve others above one's personal needs. Altruism has been the focus of several studies in recent years. Researchers believe that doing good for others is good for oneself, especially the immune system. Researchers at Harvard found that even watching films of altruistic endeavors enhances the formation of an immune system chemical that helps fight disease.

In a study of more than 2,700 people in Michigan, the investigators found that people who did volunteer work regularly lived longer. People who did not do regular volunteer work (at least once a week) had a 250% higher mortality risk during the course of the study.

Wellness requires a balance between physical, mental, spiritual, emotional, and social well-being. The relationship between spirituality and wellness, therefore, is meaningful in our quest for a better quality of life. As with other wellness parameters, optimum spirituality requires the development of spiritual nature to its fullest potential.

EXERCISE AND AGING

Unlike any previous time in American society, the elderly population constitutes the fastest growing segment of our population. In 1880, less than 3% of the total population, or fewer than 2 million people, were older than 65. By 1980, the elderly population had reached approximately 25 million, more than 11.3% of the population. According to estimates, the elderly will make up more than 20% of the total population by the year 2035.

Historically, older adults have been neglected when developing fitness programs. Fitness is just as important for older people as it is for young people. Although much research remains to be done in this area, studies indicate that older individuals who are physically fit also enjoy better health and a higher quality of life.

The main objective of fitness programs for older adults should be to improve the functional capacity of the participant. A committee of the American Alliance of Health, Physical Education, Recreation, and Dance (AAHPERD) recently defined functional fitness for older adults as *the physical capacity of the individual to meet ordinary and unexpected demands of daily life safely and effectively.* This definition clearly indicates the need for fitness programs that closely relate to activities this population normally encounters. The AAHPERD committee encourages participation in programs that will help develop cardiovascular endurance, localized muscular endurance, muscular flexibility, agility and balance, and motor coordination.*

RELATIONSHIP BETWEEN FITNESS AND AGING

Although previous research studies have documented declines in physiological functioning and motor capacity as a result of aging, no hard evidence at present proves that declines in physical work capacity are related primarily to the aging process. Lack of physical activity — a common phenomenon seen in our society as people age — may be accompanied by decreases in physical work capacity that are greater by far than the effects of aging itself.

Data on individuals who have taken part in systematic physical activity throughout life indicate that these groups of people maintain a higher level of functional capacity and do not experience the typical declines in later years. Dr. George Sheehan, cardiologist and runner, states that, from a functional point of view, the typical American is 30 years older than his or her chronological age indicates. Thus, an active 60-year-old can have a work capacity similar to that of a sedentary 30-year-old.

Sedentary people stop living at age 60 but choose to be buried at age 70.

Unfortunately, unhealthy behaviors precipitate premature aging. For sedentary people, productive life ends at about age 60. Most of these people hope to live to be 65 or 70 and often must cope with serious physical ailments. These people stop living at age 60 but choose to be buried at age 70 (see Figure 17.2).

Scientists believe a healthy lifestyle allows people to live a vibrant life — a physically, intellectually, emotionally, and socially active existence — to age 95. When death comes to active people, it usually comes rather quickly and not as a result of prolonged illness (Figure 17.2). Such are the rewards of a wellness way of life.

PHYSICAL TRAINING IN THE OLDER ADULT

The trainability of elderly men and women alike and the effectiveness of physical activity as a relative modality have been demonstrated in prior research. Older adults who increase their level of physical activity experience significant changes in cardiovascular endurance, strength, and flexibility. The extent of the changes depends on their initial fitness level and the types of activities selected for their training (walking, cycling, strength training, and so on).

Improvements in maximal oxygen uptake in older adults are similar to those of younger people, although older people seem to require a longer training period to achieve these changes. Declines in endurance (maximal oxygen uptake) per decade of

---

* A copy of a recently developed battery of fitness tests for older adults can be obtained from the AAHPERD national office in Reston, Virginia.

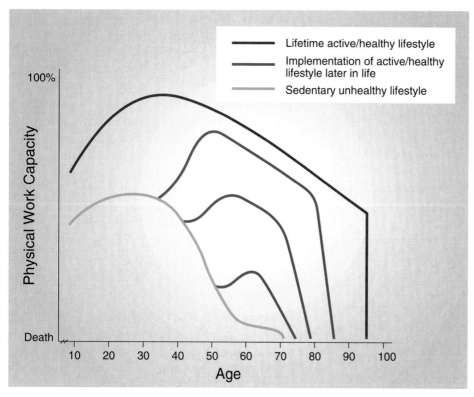

FIGURE 17.2
Relationship between physical work capacity, aging, and lifestyle habits.

life after age 25 seem to be about 9% for sedentary adults and 5% or less in active people.

Results from a recent study on the effects of aging on the cardiovascular system of male exercisers versus non-exercisers showed that the maximal oxygen uptake of regular exercisers was almost twice that of the non-exercisers (see Table 17.1). Between ages 50 and 68, the study revealed a decline in maximal oxygen uptake of only 13% in the active group, compared to 41% in the inactive group. These changes indicate that about one-third of the loss in maximal oxygen uptake results from aging, and two-thirds of the loss comes from inactivity. Blood pressure, heart rate, and body weight also were remarkably better in the exercising group.

In strength development, older adults can increase their strength levels, but the amount of muscle hypertrophy achieved decreases with age. Strength gains as high as 200% have been found in previously inactive adults over age 90. In terms of body composition, inactive adults continue to gain body fat after age 60 despite the tendency toward lower body weight.

Older adults who wish to initiate or continue an exercise program are encouraged strongly to have a complete medical exam, including a stress electro-cardiogram test (see Chapter 12, Figure 12.4). Recommended activities for older adults include calisthenics, walking, jogging, swimming, cycling, and water aerobics.

TABLE 17.1
Effects of Physical Activity and Inactivity on Selected Physiological Parameters in Older Men*

	Exercisers	Nonexercisers
Age (yrs)	68.0	69.8
Weight (lbs)	160.3	186.3
Resting Heart Rate (bpm)	55.8	66.0
Maximal Heart Rate (bpm)	157.0	146.0
Heart Rate Reserve** (bpm)	101.2	80.0
Blood Pressure (mmHg)	120/78	150/90
Maximal Oxygen Uptake (ml/kg/min)	38.6	20.3

* Data from Kash, F. W., J. L. Boyer, S. P. Van Camp, L. S. Verity, and J. P. Wallace. "The Effect of Physical Activity on Aerobic Power in Older men (A Longitudinal Study)." *The Physician and Sports Medicine* 18(4):73–83, 1990.

** Heart rate reserve = maximal heart rate – resting heart rate.

Isometric and other intense weight-training exercises should be avoided. Activities that require all-out effort or require participants to hold their breath (valsalva maneuver) tend to lessen blood flow to the heart and cause a significant increase in blood pressure and the load placed on the heart. Older adults should participate in activities that require continuous and rhythmic muscular activity (about 50% to 70% of functional capacity). These activities do not cause large increases in blood pressure or place an intense overload on the heart.

ACCIDENT PREVENTION AND PERSONAL SAFETY

Most people do not perceive accidents as being a health problem. Even so, accidents are the third leading cause of death in the United States, affecting the total well-being of millions of Americans each year. Accident prevention and personal safety are part of a health enhancement program aimed at achieving a better quality of life. Proper nutrition, exercise, stress management and abstinence from cigarette smoking are of little help if the person is involved in a disabling or fatal accident as a result of distraction, a single reckless decision, or not properly wearing safety seat belts.

Accidents do not just happen. We cause accidents and we are victims of accidents. Although some factors in life, such as earthquakes, tornadoes, and airplane crashes, are completely beyond our control, more often than not, personal safety and accident prevention are a matter of common sense. Most accidents stem from poor judgment and confused mental states. Accidents frequently happen when we are upset, are not paying attention to the task with which we are involved, or are abusing alcohol or other drugs.

Alcohol abuse is the number-one cause of all accidents and alcohol intoxication is the leading cause of fatal automobile accidents. Other commonly abused drugs alter feelings and perceptions, generate mental confusion, and impair judgment and coordination, greatly enhancing the risk for accidental morbidity and mortality.

To help improve your personal safety, you are encouraged to fill out the "Health Protection Plan for Environmental Hazards, Crime Prevention, and Personal Safety" in Lab 17A. You control most actions in your life. By following the recommendations given in this questionnaire, you can further enhance your personal safety and well-being.

THE PREVENTION INDEX

The Prevention Index is an annual measure of the effort Americans are making to prevent disease and accidents and to promote good health and longevity. This nationwide index of the American Public, commissioned by *Prevention Magazine*, has been developed from information collected by Louis Harris and Associates in two national surveys:

1. Self-reported practice of preventive health and safety behaviors based on a national probability sample of 1,250 adults in the continental United States 18 years of age and older.
2. Ratings on the relative importance of each of these behaviors for preventing disease and disability in the general population (on a scale of 1 to 10), as determined by a sample of 103 representative experts in disease prevention and health promotion.

In the Harris national probability survey of adults, 21 of the behaviors were selected for inclusion in the Prevention Index according to the following criteria:

1. A documented relationship between the health behavior and disease or disability, as published in the professional literature.
2. Behaviors that are relevant to the entire adult population.
3. Behaviors that individuals can control or effect (thus the exclusion of important environmental determinants of health such as exposure to air pollution or industrial toxins).

Currently accepted standards of practice for each behavior were determined by thorough review of the professional literature and consultation with experts. In the case of continuous variables (for example, moderate alcohol consumption, exercise, frequency of dental examination), practice was ascertained by the prevailing consensus in the relevant professional literature and from personal consultation with researchers and spokespersons of professional organizations. For behaviors with no clear consensus on a minimum compliance level (for example, taking steps to control stress or restricting cholesterol intake), practice was defined in terms of always engaging in the behavior (taking steps to control stress) or trying a lot (restricting cholesterol intake). The 1993 percentages of the adult population practicing these 21 major health-promoting behaviors are given in Table 17.2.

A detailed description of the development and computation of the Prevention Index and related analyses is presented in the technical report, "The Prevention Index: A Report Card on the Nation's Health," available from *Prevention Magazine*. And you can score your own prevention profile by taking the test provided in Lab 17B.

TABLE 17.2
Prevention Index 1993 Results

Health-Promoting Behavior	% of Adults Practicing
1. Annual blood pressure test	84
2. Annual dental exam	76
3. Limit sodium in the diet	51
4. Limit fat in the diet	58
5. Consume adequate fiber	64
6. Limit cholesterol in the diet	49
7. Adequate vitamins/minerals	60
8. Limit sugar in the diet	46
9. Maintain proper weight	21
10. Frequent strenuous exercise	40
11. Do not smoke	70
12. Control stress	70
13. Sleep 7-8 hours per night	62
14. Socialize regularly	85
15. Drink alcohol moderately	90
16. Wear seat belts	71
17. Obey speed limit	53
18. Avoid driving after drinking	83
19. Smoke detector in home	89
20. Avoid smoking in bed	92
21. Avoid home accidents	83
Average	66.5

Data from Consumers' Survey conducted for *Prevention Magazine* by Louis Harris & Associates, Inc. "Summary Report — The Prevention Index 1993: A Report Card On The Nation's Health". (Emmaus, PA: *Prevention Magazine*, 1993).

AN EDUCATED WELLNESS CONSUMER

The rapid growth in fitness and wellness programs during the last two decades has spurred the promotion of fraudulent products that deceive consumers into "miraculous," quick, and easy ways toward total well-being. Quackery and fraud have been defined as the conscious promotion of unproven claims for profit.

Today's market is saturated with "special" foods, diets, supplements, pills, cures, equipment, books, and videos that promise quick, dramatic results. Advertisements for these products often are based on testimonials, unproven claims, secret research, half-truths, and quick-fix statements that the uneducated consumer wants to hear. In the meantime, the organization or enterprise making the claims stands to make a large profit from the consumers' willingness to pay for astonishing and spectacular solutions to problems related to their unhealthy lifestyle.

Television, magazine, and newspaper advertisements are not necessarily reliable. For instance, one piece of equipment sold through television and newspaper advertisements promised to "bust the gut" through five minutes of daily exercise that appeared to include the abdominal muscle group. This piece of equipment consisted of a metal spring that attached to the feet on one end and was held in the hands on the other end. According to handling and shipping distributors, the equipment was selling like "hotcakes" and companies could barely keep up with the consumer's demands.

Three problems became apparent to the educated consumer. First, there is no such thing as spot-reducing; therefore, the claims could not be true. Second, five minutes of daily exercise burn hardly any calories, therefore, have no effect on weight loss. Third, the intended abdominal (gut) muscles were not really involved during the exercise. The exercise engaged mostly the gluteal and lower back muscles. This piece of equipment now can be found at garage sales for about a tenth of its original cost!

Although people in the United States tend to be firm believers in the benefits of physical activity and positive lifestyle habits as a means to promote better health, most do not reap these benefits because they simply do not know how to put into practice a sound fitness and wellness program that will give them the results they want. Unfortunately, many uneducated wellness consumers are targets of deception by organizations making fraudulent claims for their products.

Even though deceit is all around us, we can protect ourselves from consumer fraud. The first step, of course, is education. You have to be an informed consumer of the product you intend to purchase. If you do not have or cannot find the answers, seek the advice of a reputable professional. Ask someone who understands the product but does not stand to profit from the transaction. As examples, a physical educator or an exercise physiologist can advise you regarding exercise equipment; a registered dietitian can provide information on nutrition and weight control programs; a physician can offer advice on nutritive supplements. Also, be alert to those who bill themselves as "experts." Look for qualifications degrees, professional experience, certifications, reputation.

People willing to pay for astonishing solutions to problems related to their unhealthy lifestyle are frequently the victims of consumer fraud.

Another clue to possible fraud is that if it sounds too good to be true, it probably is. Quick-fix, miraculous, special, secret, mail orders only, money-back guarantee, and testimonials often are heard in advertisements of fraudulent promotions. When claims are made, ask where the claims are published. Newspapers, magazines, and trade books are apt to be unreliable sources of information. Refereed scientific journals are the most reliable sources of information. When a researcher submits information for publication in a refereed journal, at least two qualified and reputable professionals in the field conduct blind reviews of the manuscript. A blind review means the author does not know who will review the manuscript and the reviewers do not know who submitted the manuscript. Acceptance for publication is based on this input and relevant changes.

If you have questions or concerns about a health product, you may write to the National Council Against Health Fraud (NCAHF), P. O. Box 1276, Loma Linda, CA 92354. The purpose of this organization is to monitor deceitful advertising, investigate complaints, and offer the public information regarding fraudulent health claims.

HEALTH/FITNESS CLUB MEMBERSHIPS

As you follow a lifetime wellness program, you also may want to consider joining a health/fitness facility. If you have mastered the contents of this book and if your choice of fitness activity is one you can pursue on your own (walking, jogging, cycling), you may not need to join a health club. Barring injuries, you may continue your exercise program outside the walls of a health club for the rest of your life. You also can conduct strength-training and stretching programs within the walls of your own home (see Chapters 8 and 10).

To stay up to date on fitness and wellness developments, you probably should buy a reputable and updated fitness/wellness book every 4 to 5 years. You also might subscribe to a credible health, fitness, nutrition, or wellness newsletter (see Table 17.3) to stay current.

If you are contemplating membership in a fitness facility:

■ Examine all exercise options in your community: health clubs/spas, YMCAs, gyms, colleges, schools, community centers, senior centers, and the like.

■ Check to see if the facility's atmosphere is pleasurable and nonthreatening to you. Will you

TABLE 17.3
Reliable Sources of Health, Fitness, Wellness, and Nutrition Information

Newsletter	Yearly Issues	Approximate Annual Cost
Consumer Reports Health Letter P.O. Box 56356 Boulder, CO 80323-2148	12	$24.00
Executive Health's Good Health Report P.O. Box 8880 Chapel Hill, NC 27515	12	$34.00
Tufts University Diet & Nutrition Letter P.O. Box 57857 Boulder, CO 80322-7857	12	$20.00
University of California Berkeley *Wellness Letter* P.O. Box 420148 Palm Coast, FL 32142	12	$20.00

feel comfortable with the instructors and other people who go there? Is it clean and well kept up? If the answer is no, this may not be the right place for you.

■ Analyze costs versus facilities, equipment, and programs. Take a look at your personal budget. Will you really use the facility? Will you exercise there regularly? Many people obtain memberships and permit dues to be automatically withdrawn from a local bank account, yet seldom attend the fitness center.

■ Find out what types of facilities are available: running track, basketball/tennis/racquetball courts, aerobic exercise room, strength-training room, pool, locker rooms, saunas, hot tubs, handicapped access, and so on.

■ Check the aerobic and strength-training equipment available. Does the facility have treadmills, bicycle ergometers, Stair Masters, cross-country skiing simulators, free weights, Universal Gym, Nautilus? Make sure the facilities and equipment meet your activity interests.

■ Consider the location. Is the facility close, or do you have to travel several miles to get there? Distance often discourages participation.

■ Check on times the facility is accessible. Is it open during your preferred exercise time (for example early morning or late evening)?

■ Work out at the facility several times before becoming a member. Are people standing in line to use the equipment, or is it readily available during your exercise time?

■ Inquire about the instructors' qualifications. Do the fitness instructors have college degrees or professional certifications from organizations such as the American College of Sports Medicine (ACSM) or the International Dance Exercise Association (IDEA)? These organizations have rigorous standards to ensure professional preparation and quality of instruction.

■ Consider the approach to fitness (including all health-related components of fitness). Is it well-rounded? Do the instructors spend time with members or do members constantly have to seek them out for help and instruction?

■ Ask about supplementary services. Does the facility provide or contract out for regular health and fitness assessments (cardiovascular endurance, body composition, blood pressure, blood chemistry analysis). Are wellness seminars (nutrition, weight control, stress management) offered? Do these have hidden costs?

A final consideration is that of purchasing your own exercise equipment. Many people buy expensive equipment only to find out they really do not enjoy that mode of activity. Stationary bicycles (lower body only) and rowing ergometers were among the most popular pieces of equipment sold in the 1980s. Many of them are seldom used and now are stored away in basements. Actually try out the piece of equipment several times before you buy it.

Quality also is important. Some cheaper brands of equipment may not be durable, so your investment would be wasted. Ask for references — people or clubs that have used the equipment extensively. Are they satisfied? Have they enjoyed the activity (the equipment)? You also may want to talk with professionals at colleges, sports medicine clinics, or health clubs.

SELF-EVALUATION AND BEHAVIORAL OBJECTIVES FOR THE FUTURE

The main objective of this book is to provide the information and experiences necessary to implement your personal fitness and wellness program. If you have implemented the programs in this book, including exercise, you should be convinced that a wellness lifestyle is the only way to attain a higher quality of life.

Most people who engage in a personal fitness and wellness program experience this new quality of life after only a few weeks of training and practicing healthy lifestyle patterns. In some instances, however, especially individuals who have led a poor lifestyle for a long time, a few months may be required to establish positive habits and feelings of well-being. In the end, though, everyone who applies the principles of fitness and wellness will reap the desired benefits.

SELF-EVALUATION

Through various laboratory experiences, you have had an opportunity to assess different fitness and wellness components and write behavioral objectives to improve your quality of life. You should now take the time to evaluate how well you have achieved your own objectives. Ideally, if time allows and facilities and technicians are available, you should reassess at least the health-related components of physical fitness. If you are unable to reassess these components, subjectively determine how well you accomplished your objectives. You will find a self-evaluation form in part A of Lab 17C.

BEHAVIORAL OBJECTIVES FOR THE FUTURE

The real challenge will come now that you are about to finish this course: a lifetime commitment to fitness and wellness. Adhering to a program in a structured setting is a lot easier, but from now on you will be on your own. Realizing that you may not have achieved all of your objectives during this course, or perhaps you need to reach beyond your current achievements, a final assignment should be conducted to help you chart the future. To complete this assignment, you are directed to the Wellness Compass given in Figure 17C.1, in Part B of Lab 17C. This compass provides a list of various wellness components, each illustrating a scale from 5 to 1. A "5" indicates a low or poor rating; a "1" indicates an excellent or "wellness" rating for that component. Using the Wellness Compass, rate yourself for each component according to the following instructions:

1. Color in red a number from 5 to 1 to indicate where you stood on each component at the beginning of the semester. For example, if at the start of this course, you rated poor in cardiovascular endurance, color the number 5 in red.
2. Color in blue a second number from 5 to 1 to indicate where you stand on each component at the present time. If your level of cardiovascular endurance improved to average by the end of the semester, color the number 3 in blue. If you were not able to work on a given component, simply color in blue on top of the previous red.
3. Select one or two components you intend to work on in the next two months. Developing new behavioral patterns takes time, and trying to work on too many components at once most likely will lower your chances for success.

Start with components in which you think you will have a high chance for success. Next, color in yellow the intended objective (number) to accomplish by the end of this period. If your objective in the next two months is to achieve a "good" level of cardiovascular endurance, color the number 2 in yellow. When you achieve this level, you may later color the number 1, also in yellow, to indicate your next objective.

After you have completed the previous exercise, write behavioral objectives for the two components you intend to work on during the next two months (use part B of Lab 17C). As you write and work on these objectives, keep in mind the following guidelines:

1. **You should set both general and specific objectives.** The general objective is the ultimate goal you intend to achieve. The specific objectives are the steps required to reach this general objective. For example, a general objective might be to achieve recommended body weight. Several specific objectives could be: (a) to lose an average of one pound (or one fat percentage point) per week (b) to monitor body weight before breakfast every morning (c) to assess body composition every two weeks (d) to limit fat intake to less than 30% of total calories (e) to eliminate all pastries from the diet during this time and (f) to exercise in the proper target zone for 30 minutes, five times per week.

2. **Whenever possible, objectives (general and specific) should be measurable.** For example, "to lose weight" is not measurable. In the previous general objective, recommended body weight implies lowering your body weight (fat) to the recommended percent body fat standards given in Chapter 3 (Table 3.7). If this person is a 19-year-old female, the high fitness recommended fat percent would be in the range of 17% to 27%.

To be more descriptive, the general objective could be reworded as: Reduce body weight to 22% body fat. The sample specific objectives given in Item 1 also are measurable. For instance, you can figure out easily whether you are losing a pound (a percentage point) per week; you can conduct a nutrient analysis to assess the average fat intake; or you can monitor your weekly exercise sessions to make sure you are meeting this specific objective.

3. **Objectives must be realistic.** If you currently weigh 170 pounds and your target weight at 22% is 120 pounds, it would be unsound, if not impossible, to implement a weight loss program to lose 50 pounds in two months. This program would not allow implementation of adequate behavior modification techniques and ensure weight maintenance at the target weight.

4. **Objectives can be either short-term or long-term.** If the general objective is to attain recommended body weight and you are 50 pounds overweight, setting a general short-term objective of losing 10 pounds and writing specific objectives to accomplish this goal is best. Then the task will not seem as overwhelming and will be easier to do.

5. **Set a specific date to achieve your objective.** To simply state "I will lose weight" is not time-specific. With a deadline, a task is much easier to work toward.

6. **Educate yourself about the objective you plan to work on.** You cannot lose weight if you do not know the principles governing weight loss and maintenance. This is the reason only three in ten individuals achieve the target weight loss and only one in those three is able to keep it off thereafter.

7. **Think positive, and reward yourself for your accomplishments.** As difficult as some tasks may seem, where there's a will, there's a way. If you prepare a plan of action according to these guidelines, you should be able to achieve your objective. Reward yourself for your accomplishments. Buy yourself new clothing, exercise shoes, or something special you have wanted for some time.

8. **Seek support from those around you.** Losing weight is difficult if you share meal planning and cooking with a roommate who enjoys foods that are high in fat and sweets. It can be even worse if the roommate also has a weight problem and does not desire or have the willpower to lose weight. Surround yourself with people who will help and encourage you along the way. If necessary, plan and prepare your own meals.

9. **Recognize that you will face obstacles and you will make mistakes.** Making mistakes is human and does not mean failure. Failure comes only to those who give up. Use your mistakes and learn from them by creating a plan that will help you get around self-defeating behaviors in the future.

10. **Monitor your progress regularly.** You will not always be meeting the specific objectives. If you are not, you will need to evaluate your objectives and perhaps make changes in the general or the specific objectives, or both. People are different, and you may not be able to progress as fast as someone else. Be flexible with yourself, and reconsider your plan of action.

THE FITNESS/WELLNESS EXPERIENCE AND A CHALLENGE FOR THE FUTURE

Patty Neavill is a typical example of someone who often tried to change her life around but was unable to do so because she did not know how to implement a sound exercise and weight control program. At age 24 and at 240 pounds, she was discouraged with her weight, level of fitness, self-image, and quality of life in general. She had struggled with her weight most of her life. Like thousands of other people, she had made many unsuccessful attempts to lose weight.

Patty put her fears aside and decided to enroll in a fitness course. As part of the course requirement, a battery of fitness tests was administered at the beginning of the semester. Patty's cardiovascular fitness and strength ratings were poor, her flexibility classification was average, and her percent body fat was 41.

Following the initial fitness assessment, Patty met with her course instructor, who prescribed an exercise and nutrition program like the one in this book. Patty fully committed to carry out the prescription. She walked/jogged five times a week. She enrolled in a weight training course that met twice a week. Her daily caloric intake was set in the range of 1,500 to 1,700 calories.

Determined to further increase her level of activity, Patty also signed up for recreational volleyball and basketball courses. Besides fun, these classes provided four additional hours of activity per week.

She took care to meet the minimum required servings from the basic food groups each day, which contributed about 1,200 calories to her diet. The remainder of the calories came primarily from complex carbohydrates.

At the end of the 16-week semester, Patty's cardiovascular fitness, strength, and flexibility ratings had all improved to the good category, she lost 50 pounds, and her percent body fat had decreased to 22.5!

Patty was tall. At 190 pounds, most people would have thought she was too heavy. Her percent body fat, however, was lower than the average for college female physical education major students (about 23% body fat).

A thank-you note from Patty to the course instructor at the end of the semester read:

Thank you for making me a new person. I truly appreciate the time you spent with me. Without your kindness and motivation, I would have never made it. It is great to be fit and trim. I've never had this feeling before, and I wish everyone could feel like this once in their life.

Thank you,

Your trim Patty!

Patty never had been taught the principles governing a sound weight loss program. In Patty's case, not only did she need this knowledge, but, like most Americans who never have experienced the process of becoming physically fit, she needed to be in a structured exercise setting to truly feel the joy of fitness.

Even more significant, Patty maintained her aerobic and strength-training programs. A year after ending her calorie-restricted diet, her weight increased by 10 pounds, but her body fat decreased from 22.5% to 21.2%. As you may recall from Chapter 4, this weight increase is related mostly to changes in lean tissue, lost during the weight reduction phase.

In spite of only a slight drop in weight during the second year following the calorie-restricted diet, the two year follow-up revealed a further decrease in body fat, to 19.5%. Patty understood the new quality of life reaped through a sound fitness program, and, at the same time, she finally learned how to apply the principles that regulate weight maintenance.

If you have read and successfully completed all of the assignments set out in this book, including a regular exercise program, you should be convinced of the value of exercise and healthy lifestyle habits in achieving a new quality of life (Figure 17.3).

FIGURE 17.3
Fitness and healthy lifestyle habits lead to improved health, quality of life, and wellness.

Perhaps this new quality of life was best explained by Dr. George Sheehan, when he wrote:

> For every runner who tours the world running marathons, there are thousands who run to hear the leaves and listen to the rain, and look to the day when it is all suddenly as easy as a bird in flight. For them, sport is not a test but a therapy, not a trial but a reward, not a question but an answer.

The real challenge will come now: a lifetime commitment to fitness and wellness. To make the commitment easier, enjoy yourself and have fun along the way. Implement your program based on your interests and what you enjoy doing most. Then adhering to your new lifestyle will not be difficult.

Your activities over the last few weeks or months may have helped you develop positive "addictions" that will carry on throughout life. If you truly experience the feelings Dr. Sheehan expressed, there will be no looking back. If you don't get there, you won't know what it's like. Fitness and wellness is a process, and you need to put forth a constant and deliberate effort to achieve and maintain a higher quality of life. Improving the quality of your life, and most likely your longevity, is in your hands. Only you can take control of your lifestyle and thereby reap the benefits of wellness.

LABORATORY EXPERIENCE

(All three of these laboratories may be conducted as homework assignments)

LAB 17A
Health Protection Plan for Environmental Hazards, Crime Prevention, and Personal Safety

Lab Preparation
None required.

LAB 17B
The Prevention Index

Lab Preparation
None required.

LAB 17C
Self-Evaluation and Behavioral Objectives for the Future

Lab Preparation
None required.

REFERENCES

1. Clark, B., W. Osness, W. W. K. Hoeger, M. Adrian, D. Raab, & R. Wiswell. Tests for fitness in older adults: AAHPERD fitness task force. *Journal of Physical Education, Recreation, and Dance* 60(3):66-71, 1989.
2. Gordon, E. and E. Golanty. *Health & Wellness*. Boston: Jones and Bartlett Publishers, Inc., 1985.
3. Hafen, B. Q., and W. W. K. Hoeger. *Wellness: Guidelines for a Healthy Lifestyle*. Englewood, CO: Morton Publishing Company, 1994.
4. Hafen, B. Q., A. L. Thygerson, and K. J. Frandsen. *Behavioral Guidelines for Health & Wellness*. Englewood, CO: Morton Publishing Company, 1988.
5. Hagberg, J. M., J. E. Graves, M. Limacher, et al. "Cardiovascular Responses of 70-79 Year Old Men and Women to Exercise Training." *Journal of Applied Physiology* 66:2589-2594, 1989.
6. Kash, F. W., J. L. Boyer, S. P. Van Camp, L. S. Verity, and J. P. Wallace. "The Effect of Physical Activity on Aerobic Power in Older Men (A Longitudinal Study)." *The Physician and Sports Medicine* 18(4):73-83, 1990.
7. Kemper, D. W., J. Giuffre, and G. Drabinski. *Pathways: A Success Guide for a Healthy Life*. Boise, ID: Healthwise, Inc., 1985.
8. Osness, W., M. Adrian, B. Clark, W. W. K. Hoeger, D. Raab, & R. Wiswell. The AAHPERD fitness task force, history and philosophy. *Journal of Physical Education, Recreation, and Dance* 60(3):64-65, 1989.
9. *Prevention Magazine*. The Prevention Index 1993: A Report Card on The Nation's Health. Emmaus, PA: *Prevention Magazine*, 1993.

LABS

LAB 1A CLEARANCE FOR EXERCISE PARTICIPATION

Name: _____ Date: _____ Grade: _____

Instructor: _____ Course: _____ Section: _____

NECESSARY LAB EQUIPMENT None.

OBJECTIVE To determine the safety of exercise participation.

INTRODUCTION While exercise testing and/or exercise participation is relatively safe for most apparently healthy individuals under the age of forty-five, the reaction of the cardiovascular system to increased levels of physical activity cannot always be totally predicted. Consequently, there is a small but real risk of certain changes occurring during exercise testing and/or participation. Some of these changes may include abnormal blood pressure, irregular heart rhythm, fainting, and in rare instances a heart attack or cardiac arrest. Therefore, it is imperative that you provide honest answers to this questionnaire. Exercise may be contraindicated under some of the conditons listed below, while others may simply require special consideration. **If any of the conditions apply, you should consult your physician before you participate in an exercise program.** You should also promptly report to your instructor any exercise-related abnormalities that you may experience during the course of the semester.

A. Have you ever had or do you now have any of the following conditions:

☐ 1. A myocardial infarction.

☐ 2. Coronary artery disease.

☐ 3. Congestive heart failure.

☐ 4. Elevated blood lipids (cholesterol and triglycerides).

☐ 5. Chest pain at rest or during exertion.

☐ 6. Shortness of breath.

☐ 7. An abnormal resting or stress electrocardiogram.

☐ 8. Uneven, irregular, or skipped heartbeats (including a racing or fluttering heart).

☐ 9. A blood embolism.

☐ 10. Thrombophlebitis.

☐ 11. Rheumatic heart fever.

☐ 12. Elevated blood pressure.

☐ 13. A stroke.

☐ 14. Diabetes.

☐ 15. A family history of coronary heart disease, syncope, or sudden death before age sixty.

☐ 16. Any other heart problem that makes exercise unsafe.

B. Do you suffer from any of the following conditions:

☐ 1. Arthritis, rheumatism, or gout.

☐ 2. Chronic low back pain.

☐ 3. Any other joint, bone, or muscle problems.

☐ 4. Any respiratory problems.

☐ 5. Obesity (more than 30 percent overweight).

☐ 6. Anorexia.

☐ 7. Bulimia.

☐ 8. Mononucleosis.

☐ 9. Any physical disability that could interfere with safe exercise participation.

C. Do any of the following conditions apply:

☐ 1. Do you smoke cigarettes?

☐ 2. Are you taking any prescription drug?

☐ 3. Are you forty-five years or older?

D Do you have any other concern regarding your ability to safely participate in an exercise program? If so, explain:

_____

_____

Student's Signature: _____ Date: _____

LAB 1B HEART RATE AND BLOOD PRESSURE ASSESSMENT

Name: _____ Date: _____ Grade: _____

Instructor: _____ Course: _____ Section: _____

NECESSARY LAB EQUIPMENT Stopwatches, stethoscopes, and blood pressure sphygmomanometers.

OBJECTIVE To determine resting heart rate and blood pressure.

PREPARATION The instructions to determine heart rate and blood pressure are given at the end of Chapter 1. Many factors can affect heart rate and blood pressure. Such factors as excitement, nervousness, stress, food, smoking, pain, temperature, and physical exertion can all significantly alter heart rate and blood pressure. Therefore, whenever possible, readings should be taken in a quiet, comfortable room following a few minutes of rest in the recording position. Avoid any form of exercise several hours prior to the assessment. Wear exercise clothing, including a shirt with short or loose-fitting sleeves to allow for the placement of the blood pressure cuff around the upper arm.

Resting Heart Rate and Blood Pressure

Determine your resting heart rate and blood pressure in the right and left arms while sitting comfortably in a chair.

Resting Heart Rate: _____ bpm   Rating:* _____

Blood Pressure:	Right Arm	Risk Rating**	Left Arm	Risk Rating
Systolic	_____	_____	_____	_____
Diastolic	_____	_____	_____	_____

Standing, Walking, Jogging Heart Rate and Blood Pressure

Have one individual measure your heart rate and another individual your blood pressure immediately after standing for one minute, after walking for one minute, and after jogging in place for one minute. For blood pressure assessment use the arm with the highest reading in the sitting position.

Activity	Heart Rate (bpm)	Systolic/Diastolic Blood Pressure (mmHg)
Standing	_____	_____ / _____
Walking	_____	_____ / _____
Jogging	_____	_____ / _____

Conclusions. Draw conclusions based on your observed resting and activity heart rates and blood pressures.

_____

_____

_____

_____

*See Table 1.3, Chapter 1
**See Table 1.4, Chapter 1

LAB 1C   WELLNESS LIFESTYLE QUESTIONNAIRE*

Name: _____ Date: _____ Grade: _____

Instructor: _____ Course: _____ Section: _____

NECESSARY LAB EQUIPMENT   None required.

OBJECTIVE   To evaluate your present wellness lifestyle.

INSTRUCTIONS   Please circle the appropriate answer to each question and total your points as indicated at the end of the questionnaire. Circle 5 if the statement is ALWAYS true, 4 if the statement is FREQUENTLY true, 3 if the statement is OCCASIONALLY true, 2 if the statement is SELDOM true, 1 if the statement is NEVER true.

1. I am able to identify the situations and factors that overstress me.   5 4 3 2 1

2. I eat only when I am hungry.   5 4 3 2 1

3. I don't take tranquilizers or other drugs to relax.   5 4 3 2 1

4. I support efforts in my community to reduce environmental pollution.   5 4 3 2 1

5. I avoid buying foods with artificial colorings.   5 4 3 2 1

6. I rarely have problems concentrating on what I'm doing because of worrying about other things.   5 4 3 2 1

7. My employer (school) takes measures to ensure that my work (study) place is safe.   5 4 3 2 1

8. I try not to use medications when I feel unwell.   5 4 3 2 1

9. I am able to identify certain bodily responses and illnesses as my reactions to stress.   5 4 3 2 1

10. I question the use of diagnostic x-rays.   5 4 3 2 1

11. I try to alter personal living habits that are risk factors for heart disease, cancer, and other life-style diseases.   5 4 3 2 1

12. I avoid taking sleeping pills to help me sleep.   5 4 3 2 1

13. I try not to eat foods with refined sugar or corn sugar ingredients.   5 4 3 2 1

14. I accomplish goals I set for myself.   5 4 3 2 1

15. I stretch or bend for several minutes each day to keep my body flexible.   5 4 3 2 1

16. I support immunization of all children for common childhood diseases.   5 4 3 2 1

17. I try to prevent friends from driving after they drink alcohol.   5 4 3 2 1

18. I minimize extra salt intake.   5 4 3 2 1

19. I don't mind when other people and situations make me wait or lose time.   5 4 3 2 1

20. I walk four or fewer flights of stairs rather than take the elevator.   5 4 3 2 1

* Edlin and Golanty: Health & Wellness, fourth edition, © 1992, Boston: Jones and Bartlett Publishers. Reprinted by permission.

21. I eat fresh fruits and vegetables.   5 4 3 2 1

22. I use dental floss at least once a day.   5 4 3 2 1

23. I read product labels on foods to determine their ingredients.   5 4 3 2 1

24. I try to maintain a normal body weight.   5 4 3 2 1

25. I record my feelings and thoughts in a journal or diary.   5 4 3 2 1

26. I have no difficulty falling asleep.   5 4 3 2 1

27. I engage in some form of vigorous physical activity at least three times a week.   5 4 3 2 1

28. I take time each day to quiet my mind and relax.   5 4 3 2 1

29. I am willing to make and sustain close friendships and intimate relationships.   5 4 3 2 1

30. I obtain an adequate daily supply of vitamins from my food or vitamin supplements.   5 4 3 2 1

31. I rarely have tension or migraine headaches, or pain in the neck or shoulders.   5 4 3 2 1

32. I wear a safety belt when driving.   5 4 3 2 1

33. I am aware of the emotional and situational factors that lead me to overeat.   5 4 3 2 1

34. I avoid driving my car after drinking any alcohol.   5 4 3 2 1

35. I am aware of the side effects of the medicines I take.   5 4 3 2 1

36. I am able to accept feelings of sadness, depression, and anxiety, knowing that they are almost always transient.   5 4 3 2 1

37. I would seek several additional professional opinions if my doctor recommended surgery for me.   5 4 3 2 1

38. I agree that nonsmokers should not have to breathe the smoke from cigarettes in public places.   5 4 3 2 1

39. I agree that pregnant women who smoke harm their babies.   5 4 3 2 1

40. I feel I get enough sleep.   5 4 3 2 1

41. I ask my doctor why a certain medication is being prescribed and inquire about alternatives.   5 4 3 2 1

42. I am aware of the calories expended in my activities.   5 4 3 2 1

43. I am willing to give priority to my own needs for time and psychological space by saying "no" to others' requests of me.   5 4 3 2 1

44. I walk instead of drive whenever feasible.   5 4 3 2 1

45. I eat a breakfast that contains about one-third of my daily need for calories, proteins, and vitamins.   5 4 3 2 1

46. I prohibit smoking in my home.   5 4 3 2 1

47. I remember and think about my dreams.   5 4 3 2 1

48. I seek medical attention only when I have symptoms or feel that some (potential) condition needs checking, rather than have routine yearly checkups.   5 4 3 2 1

49. I endeavor to make my home accident free.   5 4 3 2 1

50. I ask my doctor to explain the diagnosis of my problem until I understand all that I care to.   5 4 3 2 1

51. I try to include fiber or roughage (whole grains, fresh fruits and vegetables, or bran) in my daily diet.   5 4 3 2 1

52. I can deal with my emotional problems without alcohol or other mood-altering drugs.   5 4 3 2 1

53. I am satisfied with my school/work.   5 4 3 2 1

LAB
1C

54. I require children riding in my car to be in infant seats or in shoulder harnesses.   5 4 3 2 1

55. I try to associate with people who have a positive attitude about life.   5 4 3 2 1

56. I try not to eat snacks of candy, pastries, and other "junk" foods.   5 4 3 2 1

57. I avoid people who are "down" all the time and bring down those around them.   5 4 3 2 1

58. I am aware of the calorie content of the foods I eat.   5 4 3 2 1

59. I brush my teeth after meals.   5 4 3 2 1

60. (for women only) I routinely examine my breasts.   5 4 3 2 1

(for men only) I am aware of the signs of testicular cancer.   5 4 3 2 1

LAB
1C

How to Score

Enter the numbers you've circled next to the question number and total your score for each category. Then determine your degree of wellness for each category using the wellness status key.

Emotional health	Fitness and body care	Environmental health	Stress	Nutrition	Medical self-responsibility
6_____	15_____	4_____	1_____	2_____	8_____
12_____	20_____	7_____	3_____	5_____	10_____
25_____	22_____	17_____	9_____	13_____	11_____
26_____	24_____	32_____	14_____	18_____	16_____
36_____	27_____	34_____	19_____	21_____	35_____
40_____	33_____	38_____	28_____	23_____	37_____
47_____	42_____	39_____	29_____	30_____	41_____
52_____	44_____	46_____	31_____	45_____	48_____
55_____	58_____	49_____	43_____	51_____	59_____
57_____	59_____	54_____	53_____	56_____	60_____
Total_____	Total_____	Total_____	Total_____	Total_____	Total_____

Wellness Status

To assess your status in each of the six categories, compare your total score in each to the following key: 0-34 Need improvement; 35-44 Good; 45-50 Excellent.

LAB 2A   NUTRIENT ANALYSIS

Name: _____ Date: _____ Grade: _____

Instructor: _____ Course: _____ Section: _____

NECESSARY LAB EQUIPMENT   List of "Nutritive Value of Selected Foods," Appendix A. An IBM-PC or Apple IIe computer, if the computer software for use with this book is used. Otherwise, only a small calculator is needed.

OBJECTIVE   To evaluate your present diet using the Recommended Daily Allowances (RDA).

INSTRUCTIONS   To conduct the following nutritional analysis, you need a record of all foods eaten during a three-day period (use the list of "Nutritive Value of Selected Foods" given in Appendix A). This information should be recorded prior to this lab session in the forms provided in Figure 2A.1. After recording the nutritive values for each day, add up the values in each column and record the totals at the bottom of the form This work should also be done before the lab session. During your lab, you should proceed to compute an average for the three days. The percentages for carbohydrates, fat, saturated fat, and the protein requirements can be computed by using the instructions at the bottom of Figure 2A.2. The results can then be compared against the Recommended Daily Allowances (RDA).

The analysis can be simplified by using the computer software for this lab. Up to seven days may be analyzed when using the software and Figure 2A.3 should be used instead of 2A.1. Further, you only need to record the code for each food and the amount of servings eaten (.5 for half a serving, 2 for twice the standard serving, and so forth).

LAB 2A

Date: _____

Foods	Amount	Calories	Protein (gm)	Fat (total) (gm)	Sat. Fat (gm)	Chol-esterol (mg)	Carbo-hydrates (gm)	Cal-cium (mg)	Iron (mg)	Sodium (mg)	Vit. A (I.U.)	Vit. B₁ (mg)	Vit. B₂ (mg)	Niacin (mg)	Vit. C (mg)
Totals															

FIGURE 2A.1
Daily nutrient intake.

Date: _____

Foods	Amount	Calories	Protein (gm)	Fat (total) (gm)	Sat. Fat (gm)	Chol- esterol (mg)	Carbo- hydrates (gm)	Cal- cium (mg)	Iron (mg)	Sodium (mg)	Vit. A (I.U.)	Vit. B_1 (mg)	Vit. B_2 (mg)	Niacin (mg)	Vit. C (mg)
Totals															

LAB 2A

FIGURE 2A.1 (Continued)
Daily nutrient intake.

LAB
2A

Date: _____

Foods	Amount	Calories	Protein (gm)	Fat (total) (gm)	Sat. Fat (gm)	Cholesterol (mg)	Carbohydrates (gm)	Calcium (mg)	Iron (mg)	Sodium (mg)	Vit. A (I.U.)	Vit. B$_1$ (mg)	Vit. B$_2$ (mg)	Niacin (mg)	Vit. C (mg)
Totals															

FIGURE 2A.1 (Continued)
Daily nutrient intake.

Name: _____

Day	Calories	Protein (gm)	Fat (gm)	Sat. Fat (gm)	Cholesterol (mg)	Carbohydrates (gm)	Calcium (mg)	Iron (mg)	Sodium (mg)	Vit. A (I.U.)	Thiamin Vit. B_1 (mg)	Riboflavin Vit. B_2 (mg)	Niacin (mg)	Vit. C (mg)
One														
Two														
Three														
Totals														
Average[a]														
Percentages[b]														
Recommended Dietary Allowances*														
Men 15–18 yrs.	See below[c]	See below[d]	<30%[e]	<10%[e]	<300[e]	50%>[e]	1,200	12	2,400[e]	5,000	1.5	1.8	20	60
Men 19–24 yrs.			<30%[e]	<10%[e]	<300[e]	50%>[e]	1,200	10	2,400[e]	5,000	1.5	1.7	19	60
Men 25–50 yrs.			<30%[e]	<10%[e]	<300[e]	50%>[e]	800	10	2,400[e]	5,000	1.5	1.7	19	60
Men 51+ yrs.			<30%[e]	<10%[e]	<300[e]	50%>[e]	800	10	2,400[e]	5,000	1.2	1.4	15	60
Women 15–18 yrs.			<30%[e]	<10%[e]	<300[e]	50%>[e]	1,200	15	2,400[e]	4,000	1.1	1.3	15	60
Women 19–24 yrs.			<30%[e]	<10%[e]	<300[e]	50%>[e]	1,200	15	2,400[e]	4,000	1.1	1.3	15	60
Women 25–50 yrs.			<30%[e]	<10%[e]	<300[e]	50%>[e]	800	15	2,400[e]	4,000	1.1	1.3	15	60
Women 51+ yrs.			<30%[e]	<10%[e]	<300[e]	50%>[e]	800	10	2,400[e]	4,000	1.0	1.2	13	60
Pregnant			<30%[e]	<10%[e]	<300[e]	50%>[e]	1,200	30	2,400[e]	4,000	1.5	1.6	17	70
Lactating			<30%[e]	<10%[e]	<300[e]	50%>[e]	1,200	15	2,400[e]	6,000	1.6	1.8	20	95

[a]Divide totals by 3 or number of days assessed.
[b]Percentages: Protein and Carbohydrates = multiply average by 4 and divide by average calories, Fat and Saturated Fat = multiply average by 9 and divide by average calories.
[c]Use Table 4.1 (Chapter 4) for all categories.
[d]Protein intake should be .8 grams per kilogram of body weight. Pregnant women should consume an additional 15 grams of daily protein, while lactating women should have an extra 20 grams.
[e]Based on recommendations by nutrition experts.

FIGURE 2A.2
Three-day nutritional analysis.

LAB
2A

Date: _____

Name: _____ Age: _____ Weight: _____

Sex: Male-M, Female-F (Pregnant-P, Lactating-L, Neither-N)

Activity Rating: Sedentary (limited physical activity)   = 1
                   Moderate physical activity   = 2
                   Hard labor (strenuous physical activity)   = 3

Number of days to be analyzed: _____   Day: _____

No.	Code*	Food	Amount
1			
2			
3			
4			
5			
6			
7			
8			
9			
10			
11			
12			
13			
14			
15			
16			
17			
18			
19			
20			
21			
22			
23			
24			
25			
26			
27			
28			
29			
30			
31			

*When done, to advance to the next day or end, type 0 (zero).

FIGURE 2A.3
Daily nutrient intake form for computer software use.

LAB 2B ACHIEVING A BALANCED DIET

HOMEWORK ASSIGNMENT

Name: _____ Date: _____ Grade: _____

Instructor: _____ Course: _____ Section: _____

Assignment: This laboratory experience should be carried out as a homework assignment to be completed over the next seven days.

LAB RESOURCES "Food Guide Pyramid" chart and list of "Nutritive Value of Selected Foods" (Figure 2.11 in Chapter 2 and Appendix A).

OBJECTIVE Meet the minimum daily required servings of the basic food groups and monitor total daily fat intake.

INSTRUCTIONS Keep a seven-day record of your food consumption using the Food Guide Pyramid and the form given in Figure 2B.1. Whenever you have something to eat, record the food code from the Nutritive Value of Selected Foods list contained in Appendix A, the number of calories, grams of fat, and the servings in the corresponding spaces provided for each food group. If a particular food item is not listed in the Nutritive Value of Selected Foods list, the information can be obtained from the food container itself or some of the references given at the end of the list of foods in Appendix A.

Record all information immediately after each meal, because it will be easier to keep track of foods and amounts eaten. If twice the amount of a particular serving is eaten, the calories and grams of fat must doubled and two servings should be recorded under the respective food group.

At the end of the day, the diet is evaluated by checking whether the minimum required servings for each food group were met, and by the total amount of fat consumed. If you meet the required servings, you are well on your way to achieving a well-balanced diet. Additionally, fat intake should not exceed 30% of the total daily caloric consumption. If you are on a diet, you may want to reduce fat intake to less than 20% of total daily calories (see information under *Losing Weight the Sound and Sensible Way* and Table 4.3 in Chapter 4).

LAB
2B

Name: _____

No.	Code*	Food	Amount	Calories	Fat (gm)	Bread, Cereal, Rice & Pasta	Vegetable	Fruit	Milk, Yogurt & Cheese	Meat, Poultry, Fish, Dry Beans, Eggs, & Nuts
						Food Groups (servings)				
1										
2										
3										
4										
5										
6										
7										
8										
9										
10										
11										
12										
13										
14										
15										
16										
17										
18										
19										
20										
21										
22										
23										
24										
25										
26										
27										
28										
29										
30										
Totals										
Recommended Amount				**	***	6–11	3–5	2–4	2–3	2–3
Deficiencies										

*See list of nutritive value of selected foods in Appendix A.

**Compute using Table 4.1 in Chapter 4.

***Multiply the recommended amount of calories by .30 (30%) and divide by 9 to obtain the recommended amount of grams of fat (if on a diet, multiply by .20 or .10 — see Table 4.3 in Chapter 4).

FIGURE 2B.1   Daily diet record form.

LAB 3A   HYDROSTATIC WEIGHING FOR BODY COMPOSITION ASSESSMENT

Name: _____ Date: _____ Grade: _____

Instructor: _____ Course: _____ Section: _____

NECESSARY LAB EQUIPMENT Hydrostatic or underwater weighing tank and residual volume spirometer (if no spirometer is available, predicting equations can be used to determine this volume — see Figure 3.2).

OBJECTIVE Determine body density and percent body fat.

LAB PREPARATION Bring a swimsuit and towel to this lab. A six- to eight-hour fast and bladder and bowel movements are recommended prior to underwater weighing.

INSTRUCTIONS Follow the procedure outlined in Figure 3.2. If time is a factor, only assess the body composition of one or two subjects in the course and compute the results using the form provided with this lab. A sample of the computations is provided on the back of this page.

Subject Name: _____ I.D. _____

Age: _____   Weight: _____ lbs   Height: _____ inches × 2.54 = cm

Water Temperature: _____ °C   Water Density (WD)*: _____ gr/ml

Residual Volume (RV)*: _____ lt

Body Weight (BW) in kg = weight in pounds ÷ 2.2046

BW in kg = _____ ÷ 2.2046 = _____ Kg

Gross Underwater Weights:

1. _____ kg   2. _____ kg   3. _____ kg   4. _____ kg   5. _____ kg

6. _____ kg   7. _____ kg   8. _____ kg   9. _____ kg   10. _____ kg

Average of Three Heaviest Underwater Weights (AUW): _____ kg

Tare Weight (TW): _____ kg

Net Underwater Weight (UW) = AUW − TW

Net Underwater Weight (UW) = _____ − _____ = _____ kg

Body Density (BD):

$$BD = \frac{BW}{\dfrac{BW - UW}{WD} - RV - .1} \qquad\qquad BD = \frac{}{\dfrac{-}{} - - .1} =$$

Percent Body Fat (%Fat):

$$\%Fat = \frac{495}{BD} - 450 \qquad\qquad \%Fat = \frac{495}{} - 450 = \%$$

*See Figure 3.2, Chapter 3

299

Subject Name:_____Jane Doe_____   I.D._____123456789_____

Age: __20__   Weight: __148.5__ lbs   Height: __67__ inches × 2.54 = 170.2 cm

Water Temperature: __33__ °C   Water Density (WD): __.99473__ gr/ml

Residual Volume (RV): __1.37__ lt

Body Weight (BW) in kg = weight in pounds ÷ 2.2046

BW in kg = __148.5__ ÷ 2.2046 = __67.36__ kg

Gross Underwater Weights:

   1. _6.15_ Kg   2. _6.12_ Kg   3. _6.24_ Kg   4. _6.26_ Kg   5. _6.21_ Kg

   6. _6.29_ Kg   7. _6.27_ Kg   8. _6.28_ Kg   9. _____ Kg   10. _____ Kg

Average of Three Heaviest Underwater Weights (AUW): _____6.28_____ Kg

Tare Weight (TW): _5.154_ Kg

Net Underwater Weight (UW) = AUW − TW

Net Underwater Weight (UW) = 6.28 − 5.154 = 1.126 kg

Body Density (BD):

$$BD = \frac{BW}{\frac{BW - UW}{WD} - RV - .1}$$

$$BD = \frac{67.36}{\frac{67.36 - 1.126}{.99473} - 1.37 - .1} = 1.03448$$

Percent Body Fat (%Fat):

$$\%Fat = \frac{495}{BD} - 450$$

$$\%Fat = \frac{495}{1.03448} - 450 = 28.5\%$$

FIGURE 3A.1.
Sample computation for percent body fat according to hydrostatic weighing.

LAB 3B

ANTHROPOMETRIC MEASUREMENTS FOR BODY COMPOSITION ASSESSMENT AND RECOMMENDED BODY WEIGHT DETERMINATION

Name: _____ Date: _____ Grade: _____

Instructor: _____ Course: _____ Section: _____

NECESSARY LAB EQUIPMENT Skinfold calipers and standard measuring tapes.

OBJECTIVE To assess percent body fat using skinfold thickness or girth measurements.

INSTRUCTIONS If skinfold calipers are available, use the skinfold thickness technique to assess your percent body fat. If calipers are unavailable, estimate the percent fat according to the girth measurements technique (you may wish to use both techniques and compare the results). Compute your recommended body weight according to your current and the recommended percent body fat guidelines provided in Table 3.7.

I. Percent Body Fat According to Skinfold Thickness

Men	
Chest (mm):	_____
Abdomen (mm):	_____
Thigh (mm):	_____
Total (mm):	_____
Percent Fat:	_____

Women	
Triceps (mm):	_____
Suprailium (mm):	_____
Thigh (mm):	_____
Total (mm):	_____
Percent Fat:	_____

II. Percent Fat According to Girth Measurements

Men	
Waist (inches):	_____
Wrist (inches):	_____
Difference:	_____
Body Weight:	_____
Percent Fat:	_____

Women

Upper Arm (cm):	_____	Constant A =	_____
Age:	_____	Constant B =	_____
Hip (cm):	_____	Constant C =	_____
Wrist (cm):	_____	Constant D =	_____

$BD^* = A - B - C + D$

$BD =$ _____ $-$ _____ $-$ _____ $+$ _____ $=$ _____

Percent Fat = $(495 \div BD) - 450 = (495 \div$ _____ $) - 450 =$ _____

*Body density

III. Recommended Body Weight Determination

A. Body Weight (BW): _____

B. Current Percent Fat (%F)*: _____

C. Fat Weight (FW) = BW $\times$ %F

   FW = _____ $\times$ _____ = _____

D. Lean Body Mass (LBM) = BW – FW = _____ – _____ = _____

E. Age: _____

F. Desired Fat Percent (DFP – *see* Table 3.7): _____

G. Recommended Body Weight (RBW) = LBM ÷ (1.0 – DFP*)

   RBW = _____ ÷ (1.0 – _____) = _____

*Express percentages in decimal form (e.g., 25% = .25)

IV. Percent Body Fat Objective

1. Indicate what percent body fat you would like to achieve by the end of the semester: _____

2. Briefly state how you are planning to achieve this objective:

   _____

   _____

   _____

   _____

   _____

LAB 3B

LAB 3C   WEIGHT AND HEALTH: DISEASE RISK ASSESSMENT

Name: _____ Date: _____ Grade: _____

Instructor: _____ Course: _____ Section: _____

NECESSARY LAB EQUIPMENT   Scale and standard measuring tapes.

OBJECTIVE   Determine disease risk based on the waist-to-hip ratio and the body mass index (BMI)

INSTRUCTIONS   Determine your height, waist, and hip measurements in inches. Record your body weight in pounds. Compute your waist-to-hip ratio and BMI as indicated below.

I. Waist-to-Hip Ratio

Waist (inches):   _____

Hip (inches):   _____

Ratio (waist ÷ hip):   _____   Disease Risk: _____

Recommended Standards

Waist-to-Hip Ratio		
Men	**Women**	**Disease Risk**
≤0.95	≤0.80	Very Low
0.96–0.99	0.81–0.84	Low
≥1.00	≥0.85	High

II. Body Mass Index

Weight (pounds):   _____

Height (inches):   _____

BMI = Weight × 705 ÷ Height ÷ Height

BMI = _____ × 705 ÷ _____ ÷ _____

BMI = _____   Disease Risk: _____

Recommended Standards

BMI	Disease Risk
<20.00	Moderate to Very High
20.00 to 21.99	Low
22.00 to 24.99	Very Low
25.00 to 29.99	Low
30.00 to 34.99	Moderate
35.00 to 39.99	High
≥ 40.00	Very High

LAB 4A ESTIMATION OF DAILY CALORIC REQUIREMENT

Name: _____ Date: _____ Grade: _____

Instructor: _____ Course: _____ Section: _____

NECESSARY LAB EQUIPMENT Tables 4.1 and 4.2 from Chapter 4.

OBJECTIVE To determine an estimated daily caloric requirement with exercise for weight maintenance and or reduction.

Computation Form for Daily Caloric Requirement

A. Current body weight _____

B. Caloric requirement per pound of body weight (use Table 4.1) _____

C. Typical daily caloric requirement without exercise to maintain body weight (A × B) _____

D. Selected physical activity (e.g., jogging)* _____

E. Number of exercise sessions per week _____

F. Duration of exercise session (in minutes) _____

G. Total weekly exercise time in minutes (E × F) _____

H. Average daily exercise time in minutes (G ÷ 7) _____

I. Caloric expenditure per pound per minute (cal/lb/min) of physical activity (use Table 4.2) _____

J. Total calories burned per minute of physical activity (A × I) _____

K. Average daily calories burned as a result of the exercise program (H × J) _____

L. Total daily caloric requirement with exercise to maintain body weight (C + K) _____

M. Number of calories to subtract from daily requirement to achieve a negative caloric balance** _____

N. Target caloric intake to lose weight (L − M) _____

* If more than one physical activity is selected, you will need to estimate the average daily calories burned as a result of each additional activity (steps D through K) and add all of these figures to L above.

** Subtract 500 calories if the total daily requirement with exercise (L) is below 3,000 calories. As many as 1,000 calories may be subtracted for daily requirements above 3,000 calories.

LAB 4B
BEHAVIORAL OBJECTIVES FOR EXERCISE, NUTRITION, AND WEIGHT MANAGEMENT

Name: _____ Date: _____ Grade: _____

Instructor: _____ Course: _____ Section: _____

NECESSARY LAB EQUIPMENT   None.

OBJECTIVE   The participant will prepare a plan to initiate a lifetime exercise, nutrition, and weight management program.

LAB PREPARATION   Chapters 2, 3 and 4 must be read prior to this lab.

Please Answer All of the Following:

1. State your own feelings regarding your current body weight.

   _____

   _____

   _____

2. If you suffer from eating disorders, indicate what type of professional advice you will seek to help you overcome this condition.

   _____

   _____

   _____

3. Is your present diet adequate according to the nutritional analysis?   _____ Yes   _____ No

   3A. If your answer to the previous question was "no," state what general dietary changes are necessary to achieve a balanced diet and/or lose weight (e.g., increase or decrease caloric intake, decrease fat intake, increase intake of complex carbohydrates, etc.).

   _____

   _____

   _____

   3B. Specifically list foods that will help you to meet the recommended dietary allowances in areas where you may have deficiencies (*see* Figure 2.13 and the "Nutritive Value of Selected Foods" list in Appendix A).

   _____

   _____

   _____

   3C. List foods that you should avoid to help you achieve better nutrition and/or a balanced diet.

   _____

   _____

   _____

LAB
4B

307

4. Indicate your feelings about participating in an exercise program.

_____

_____

_____

5. Will you commit to participate in a combined aerobic and strength-training program?* _____ Yes _____ No

If your answer is "yes," proceed to the next question.

If you answered "no," please review Chapters 2, 3 and 4 again and read Chapters 5, 6, 7, and 8.

6. List aerobic activities that you enjoy or may enjoy doing.

_____

7. Select one or two aerobic activities in which you will participate regularly.

_____

8. List facilities available to you where you can carry out the aerobic and strength-training program.

_____

_____

_____

9. Indicate days and times that you will set aside for your aerobic and strength-training program (four to six days should be used for aerobic exercise and three nonconsecutive days for strength-training).

Monday: _____

Tuesday: _____

Wednesday: _____

Thursday: _____

Friday: _____

Saturday: _____

Sunday: A complete day of rest once a week is recommended to allow your body to fully recover from exercise.

* Flexibility programs are necessary for the development and maintenance of good health and adequate fitness but are not effective in the achievement of weight loss. Stretching exercises should be conducted regularly either to warm up or cool down in conjunction with your aerobic and strength-training program (see Chapters 9 and 10).

WEIGHT MANAGEMENT:
BEHAVIOR MODIFICATION PROGRESS FORM

Name: _____ Date: _____ Grade: _____

Instructor: _____ Course: _____ Section: _____

NECESSARY LAB EQUIPMENT None required.

OBJECTIVE To monitor behavioral improvements for weight management.

INSTRUCTIONS Read the section on *tips for behavior modification and adherence to a lifetime weight management program* in Chapter 4. On a weekly basis, go through the list of strategies given below and provide a "Yes" or "No" answer to each statement. If you are able to answer "Yes" to most questions, you have succeeded in implementing positive weight management behaviors.

Strategy Date:														
1. I made a commitment to change															
2. I set realistic goals															
3. I exercise regularly															
4. I have healthy eating patterns															
5. I avoid automatic eating															
6. I stay busy															
7. I plan meals ahead of time															
8. I cook wisely															
9. I do not serve more food than I should eat															
10. I eat slowly and at the table only															
11. I avoid social binges															
12. I avoid refrigerator and cookie-jar raids															
13. I avoid eating out. If I do, I eat low fat meals															
14. I practice stress management															
15. I monitor behavior changes															
16. I reward my accomplishments															
17. I think positive															

LAB 4B

LAB 5A | CARDIOVASCULAR ENDURANCE ASSESSMENT

Name: _____ Date: _____ Grade: _____

Instructor: _____ Course: _____ Section: _____

NECESSARY LAB EQUIPMENT

1.5 -Mile Run: School track or premeasured course and a stopwatch.

1.0-Mile Walk Test: School track or premeasured course and a stopwatch.

Step Test: A bench or gymnasium bleachers 16¼ inches high, a metronome, and a stopwatch..

Astrand-Ryhming Test: A bicycle ergometer which allows for regulation of workloads in kilopounds per meter (or watts) and a stopwatch.

12-Minute Swim Test: Swimming pool and a stopwatch.

OBJECTIVE   To assess maximal oxygen uptake (Max VO₂) and cardiovascular endurance classification.

LAB PREPARATION   Wear appropriate exercise clothing including jogging shoes and a swimsuit if required. Be prepared to take the 1.0-Mile Walk Test, the Step Test, the Astrand-Ryhming Test, the 1.5-Mile Run Test, and/or the 12-Minute Swim Test. If more than one test will be conducted, perform them in the order just listed and allow at least 15 minutes between tests. Avoid vigorous physical activity twenty-four hours prior to this lab.

LAB 5A

I. 1.5-Mile Run Test

1.5-Mile Run Time: _____ minutes and _____ seconds

Max VO₂ (see Table 5.2, Chapter 5):   ml/kg/min

Cardiovascular Fitness Classification (Table 5.8): _____

II. 1.0-Mile Walk Test

Weight (W) = _____ lbs

Age (A)   = _____

Gender (G) = _____ (females = 0, males = 1)

Time   = _____ minutes and _____ seconds

   Time in minutes (T) = min. + (sec ÷ 60)

   T =   + (÷ 60) =   min

Heart Rate (HR) = _____ bpm

$Max\ VO_2 = 132.853 - (.0769 \times W) - (.3877 \times A) + (6.315 \times G) - (3.2649 \times T) - (.1565 \times HR)$

$Max\ VO_2 = 132.853 - (.0769 \times \underline{\quad}) - .3877 \times \underline{\quad}) + (6.315 \times \underline{\quad}) - (3.2649 \times \underline{\quad}) - (.1565 \times \underline{\quad})$

$Max\ VO_2 = 132.853 - (\quad\quad) - (\quad\quad) + (\quad\quad) - (\quad\quad) - (\quad\quad)$

$Max\ VO_2 = $ ml/kg/min

Cardiovascular Fitness Classification (Table 5.8): _____

III. Step Test.

Fifteen second recovery heart rate: _____ beats

Max VO_2 (Table 5.3): _____ ml/kg/min

Cardiovascular Fitness Classification (Table 5.8): _____

IV. Astrand-Ryhming Test.

Weight (W)   = _____ lbs

Body weight (BW) in kilograms = (W ÷ 2.2046)   = _____ kg

Workload   = _____ kpm

Exercise heart rates

	30-second pulse count	Heart Rate in bpm*
First minute:	_____	_____
Second minute:	_____	_____
Third minute:	_____	_____
Fourth minute:	_____	_____
Fifth minute:	_____	_____
Sixth minute:	_____	_____

*Use Table 5.4

Average heart rate for the fifth and sixth minutes   = _____ bpm

Maximal oxygen uptake in liters per minute (Table 5.5)   = _____ L/min

Correction factor (Table 5.6)   = _____

Corrected maximal oxygen uptake in liters per minute
  (Max VO_2 in L/min × correction factor)   = _____ L/min

Maximal oxygen uptake in milliliters per kilogram per minute
  (Corrected Max VO_2 in L/min × 1000 ÷ by BW in kg)   = _____ × 1000 ÷

Max VO_2 = _____ ml/kg/min

Cardiovascular Fitness Classification (Table 5.8): _____

V. 12-Minute Swim Test

Distance swum in 12-minutes: _____ yards

Cardiovascular Fitness Classification (Table 5.7): _____

VI. University of Houston Non-Exercise Test (See sample computation in Figure 5.14, Chapter 5)

Age (A) = _____

Physical Activity Rating (PAR) (see Figure 5.13) = _____

Percent Fat (N-Ex % Fat) Model

Men   Max VO_2 = 56.370 − (.289 × A) − (.552 × %Fat) + (1.589 × PAR)

Women   Max VO_2 = 50.513 − (.289 × A) − (.552 × %Fat) + (1.589 × PAR)

Max VO_2 = _____ − (.289 × _____) − (.552 × _____) + (1.589 × _____)

Max VO_2 = _____ ml/kg/min

Body Mass Index (N-Ex BMI) Model

BMI = Weight in pounds × 705 ÷ Height in inches ÷ Height in inches

BMI = _____ × 705 ÷ _____ ÷

BMI = _____

Men   Max VO_2 = 67.350 − (.381 × A) − (.754 × BMI) + (1.951 × PAR)

Women   Max VO_2 = 56.363 − (.381 × A) − (.754 × BMI) + (1.951 × PAR)

Max VO_2 = _____ − (.381 × _____) − (.754 × _____) + (1.951 × _____)

Max VO_2 = _____ ml/kg/min

Cardiovascular Fitness Classification (Table 5.8): _____

VII. Cardiovascular Endurance Objectives

1. Indicate what cardiovascular endurance classification you would like to achieve by the end of the semester:

   _____

2. Briefly state how you are planning to achieve this objective (also refer to Lab 4B, questions 6, 7, 8, and 9):

   _____

   _____

   _____

   _____

LAB 6A — ADVANTAGES AND DISADVANTAGES OF ADDING EXERCISE TO YOUR LIFESTYLE

Name: _____ Date: _____ Grade: _____

Instructor: _____ Course: _____ Section: _____

NECESSARY LAB EQUIPMENT None required.

OBJECTIVE Determine personal factors that may help you add exercise to your lifestyle.

INSTRUCTIONS The basic question for you is: are you willing to give exercise a try? The first step is to decide positively that you will try. Based on your personal feelings and the information learned in this course, prepare a list of the advantages and disadvantages of adding exercise to your lifestyle. When the reasons for exercise outweigh the reasons for not exercising, it will become easier to give exercise a try.

Advantages of Starting an Exercise Program

1. _____
2. _____
3. _____
4. _____
5. _____
6. _____
7. _____
8. _____

Disadvantages of Starting an Exercise Program

1. _____
2. _____
3. _____
4. _____
5. _____
6. _____
7. _____
8. _____

LAB 6B   EXERCISE READINESS QUESTIONNAIRE

Name: _____ Date: _____ Grade: _____

Instructor: _____ Course: _____ Section: _____

NECESSARY LAB EQUIPMENT   None required.

OBJECTIVE   Determine your preparedness to start an exercise program.

INSTRUCTIONS   Carefully read each statement and circle the number that best describes your feelings in each statement. Please be completely honest with your answers.

Exercise Readiness Questionnaire

	Strongly Agree	Mildly Agree	Mildly Disagree	Strongly Disagree
1. I can walk, ride a bike (or a wheelchair), swim, or walk in a shallow pool.	4	3	2	1
2. I enjoy exercise.	4	3	2	1
3. I believe exercise can help decrease the risk for disease and premature mortality.	4	3	2	1
4. I believe exercise contributes to better health.	4	3	2	1
5. I have previously participated in an exercise program.	4	3	2	1
6. I have experienced the feeling of being physically fit.	4	3	2	1
7. I can envision myself exercising.	4	3	2	1
8. I am contemplating an exercise program.	4	3	2	1
9. I am willing to stop contemplating and give exercise a try for a few weeks.	4	3	2	1
10. I am willing to set aside time at least three times a week for exercise.	4	3	2	1
11. I can find a place to exercise (the streets, a park, a YMCA, a health club).	4	3	2	1
12. I can find other people who would like to exercise with me.	4	3	2	1
13. I will exercise when I am moody, fatigued, and even when the weather is bad.	4	3	2	1
14. I am willing to spend a small amount of money for adequate exercise clothing (shoes, shorts, leotards, or swimsuit).	4	3	2	1
15. If I have any doubts about my present state of health, I will see a physician before beginning an exercise program.	4	3	2	1
16. Exercise will make me feel better and improve my quality of life.	4	3	2	1

Scoring Your Test:

This questionnaire allows you to examine your readiness for exercise. You have been evaluated in four categories: mastery (self-control), attitude, health, and commitment. Mastery indicates that you can be in control of your exercise program. Attitude examines your mental disposition toward exercise. Health provides evidence of the wellness benefits of exercise. Commitment shows dedication and resolution to carry out the exercise program. Write the number you circled after each statement in the corresponding spaces below. Add the scores on each line to get your totals. Scores can vary from 4 to 16. A score of 12 and above is a strong indicator that that factor is important to you, and 8 and below is low. If you score 12 or more points in each category, your chances of initiating and adhering to an exercise program are good. If you fail to score at least 12 points in three categories, your chances of succeeding at exercise may be slim. You need to be better informed about the benefits of exercise, and a retraining process may be required.

Mastery: 1._____ + 5. _____ + 6. _____ + 9. _____ = _____

Attitude: 2._____ + 7. _____ + 8. _____ + 13. _____ = _____

Health: 3._____ + 4. _____ + 15. _____ + 16. _____ = _____

Commitment: 10._____ + 11. _____ + 12. _____ + 14. _____ = _____

LAB
6B

LAB 6C   CARDIOVASCULAR EXERCISE PRESCRIPTION

Name: _____ Date: _____ Grade: _____

Instructor: _____ Course: _____ Section: _____

NECESSARY LAB EQUIPMENT   None required.

OBJECTIVE   To write your own cardiovascular exercise prescription.

Intensity of Exercise

1. Estimate your own maximal heart rate (MHR)

   MHR = 220 minus age (220 – age)

   MHR = 220 – _____ = _____ bpm

2. Resting Heart Rate (RHR) = _____ bpm

3. Heart Rate Reserve (HRR) = MHR – RHR

   HRR = _____ – _____ = _____ beats

4. Training Intensities (TI) = HRR × TI + RHR

   50 Percent TI = _____ × .50 + _____ = _____ bpm

   70 percent TI = _____ × .70 + _____ = _____ bpm

   85 Percent TI = _____ × .85 + _____ = _____ bpm

5. Cardiovascular Training Zone. The optimum cardiovascular training zone is found between the 70 and 85 percent training intensities. However, individuals who have been physically inactive or are in the poor or fair cardiovascular fitness categories should use a 50 percent training intensity during the first few weeks of the exercise program.

   Cardiovascular Training Zone: _____ (70% TI) to _____ (85% TI)

   Rate of Perceived Exertion (see Figure 6.2, Chapter 6): _____ to _____

Mode of Exercise

Select any activity or combination of activities that you enjoy doing. The activity has to be continuous in nature and must get your heart rate up to the cardiovascular training zone and keep it there for as long as you exercise. Indicate your preferred mode(s) of exercise:

   1. _____   2. _____   3. _____

   4. _____   5. _____   6. _____

Cardiovascular Exercise Program

The following is your weekly program for cardiovascular endurance development. If you are in the average, good, or excellent fitness category, you may start at week five. After completing this twelve-week program, in order for you to maintain your fitness level, you should exercise in the 70 to 85 percent training zone for about twenty to thirty minutes, a minimum of three times per week, on nonconsecutive days. You should also recompute your target zone periodically because you will experience a significant reduction in resting heart rate with aerobic training (approximately ten to twenty beats in about eight to twelve weeks).

Week	Duration (min.)	Frequency	Training Intensity	10-Sec. Pulse Count*
1	15	3	Approximately 50%	
2	15	4	Approximately 50%	
3	20	4	Approximately 50%	_____ beats
4	20	5	Approximately 50%	
5	20	4	About 70%	
6	20	5	About 70%	
7	30	4	About 70%	_____ beats
8	30	5	About 70%	
9	30	4	Between 70% and 85%	
10	30	5	Between 70% and 85%	
11	30–40	5	Between 70% and 85%	_____ to _____ beats
12	30–40	5	Between 70% and 85%	

*Fill out your own 10-sec. pulse count under this column.

LAB 6D   EXERCISE HEART RATE AND CALORIC COST OF PHYSICAL ACTIVITY

Name: _____ Date: _____ Grade: _____

Instructor: _____ Course: _____ Section: _____

NECESSARY LAB EQUIPMENT A school track (or premeasured course) and a stopwatch. Each student should also bring a watch with a second hand.

OBJECTIVE To monitor exercise heart rate and determine the caloric cost of physical activity based on exercise heart rate.

LAB PREPARATION Wear exercise clothing, including jogging shoes. Do not engage in vigorous physical activity prior to this lab. Read the information on predicting caloric expenditure from exercise heart rates in Chapter 6.

Procedure

1. Cardiovascular Training Zone. Look up your cardiovascular training zone at 70 and 85 percent of heart rate reserve in Lab 6C. Record this information in beats per minute (bpm) and in 10-second pulse counts in the blank spaces provided below.

                              Beats/minute   10-sec. count

   70 percent intensity =   _____   _____

   85 percent intensity =   _____   _____

2. Resting Heart Rate (HR) and Body Weight (BW). Determine your resting HR prior to exercise and your body weight in kilograms (divide pounds by 2.2046).

   Resting HR: _____ bpm

   BW: _____ lbs ÷ 2.2046 = _____ kg

3. Walking HR, Oxygen Uptake (VO_2), and Caloric Expenditure. Walk two laps around a 400-meter (440-yard) track at an average speed of 75 to 100 meters per minute. Try to maintain a constant speed around the track. You can monitor your speed by starting the walk at the beginning of the 100-meter straightway and making sure that you have walked at least 75 meters and no more than 100 meters in one minute. As soon as you complete the two laps (800 meters), notice the time it required to walk this distance and immediately check your exercise HR by taking a 10-second pulse count. Record this information in the spaces provided below. Do not record the time until after you have checked your pulse. Exercise HR will remain at the same rate for about fifteen seconds following cessation of exercise. Therefore, you need to check your pulse as soon as you finish the walk, after noticing the 800-meter walk time.

   10-sec. pulse count: _____ beats

   800-meter time: _____ min. and _____ sec.

   HR in bpm = 10-sec pulse count × 6

   HR in bpm = _____ × 6 = _____ bpm

   800-meter time in minutes = min. + (sec. ÷ 60)

   800-meter time in minutes = _____ + (_____ ÷ 60) = _____ min.

   Speed in meters per minute (mts/min.) = 800 ÷ 800-meter time in min.

   Speed in mts/min. = 800 ÷ _____ = _____ mts/min.

   VO_2 in ml/kg/min at this walking speed (Use Table 6.3) = _____ ml/kg/min.

VO_2 in L/min = VO_2 in ml/kg/min × BW in kg ÷ 1000

VO_2 in L/min = _____ × _____ ÷ 1000 = _____ L/min

Caloric expenditure for 800-meter walk = VO_2 in L/min × 5 × 800-meter time in min.

Caloric expenditure for 800-meter walk = _____ × 5 × _____ = _____ calories

4. Slow-Jogging HR, VO_2, and Caloric Expenditure. Slowly jog 800 meters (two laps) around the track. Try to maintain the same slow-jogging pace throughout the two laps. Do NOT jog fast or sprint. This is not a speed test and is intended to be a slow jog only. As soon as you complete the 800 meters, notice the time it required to complete the distance and immediately check your exercise HR by taking another 10-second pulse count. Record this information below.

10-sec. pulse count: _____ beats

800-meter time: _____ min. and _____ sec.

HR in bpm = 10-sec pulse count × 6

HR in bpm = _____ × 6 = _____ bpm

800-meter time in minutes = min. + (sec. ÷ 60)

800-meter time in minutes = _____ + (_____ ÷ 60) = _____ min.

Speed in mts/min. = 800 ÷ 800-meter time in min.

Speed in mts/min. = 800 ÷ _____ = _____ mts/min.

VO_2 in ml/kg/min at this slow-jogging speed (Use Table 6.3) = _____ ml/kg/min

VO_2 in L/min = VO_2 in ml/kg/min × BW in kg ÷ 1000

VO_2 in L/min = _____ × _____ ÷ 1000 = _____ L/min

Caloric expenditure for 800-meter slow jog = VO_2 in L/min × 5 × 800-meter time in min.

Caloric expenditure for 800-meter slow jog = _____ × 5 × _____ = _____ calories

5. Fast-Jogging HR, VO_2, Caloric Expenditure and Recovery HR. Jog another 800 meters at a faster speed around the track. Again try to maintain the same jogging pace throughout the two laps. Do NOT sprint. Your HR should not exceed 180 bpm on this test. As soon as you complete the 800 meters, notice your time for the two laps and check your 10-second pulse count. Record this information below. You should also check your two- and five-minute recovery HRs after the run and record these rates below.

10-sec. pulse count: _____ beats

800-meter time: _____ min. and _____ sec.

HR in bpm = 10-sec pulse count × 6

HR in bpm = _____ × 6 = _____ bpm

800-meter time in minutes = min. + (sec. ÷ 60)

800-meter time in minutes = _____ + (_____ ÷ 60) = _____ min.

Speed in mts/min. = 800 ÷ 800-meter time in min.

Speed in mts/min. = 800 ÷ _____ = _____ mts/min.

VO_2 in ml/kg/min at this fast-jogging speed (Use Table 6.3) = _____ ml/kg/min

VO_2 in L/min = VO_2 in ml/kg/min × BW in kg ÷ 1000

VO_2 in L/min = _____ × _____ ÷ 1000 = _____ L/min

Caloric expenditure for 800-meter fast jog = VO_2 in L/min × 5 × 800-meter time in min.

Caloric expenditure for 800-meter fast jog = _____ × 5 × _____ = _____ calories

Recovery HRs

	10-sec. count	bpm
Two minutes	_____	_____
Five minutes*	_____	_____

6. Resting, Exercise, and Recovery HRs. Plot your resting, exercise, and recovery HRs on the graph provided below.

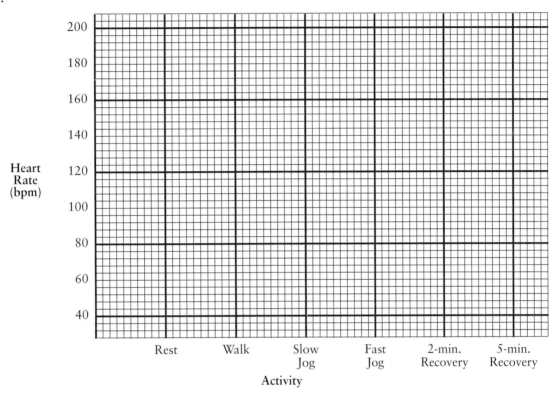

7. Training Exercise HR and Equivalent Caloric Expenditure. This part of the lab should be completed outside your regular lab time, during the next two or three days prior to turning in the assignment. According to the previous exercise HRs (numbers 3, 4, and 5 above), try to select a walking or jogging speed that will allow you to maintain your exercise HR in the appropriate cardiovascular training zone. Using a 400-meter track, walk or jog for twenty minutes at the selected speed and again try to maintain a constant speed throughout the exercise time. At the end of the twenty minutes check your 10-second pulse count and estimate the distance covered in meters. Record this information below and estimate the VO_2 and caloric expenditure.

10-sec. pulse count: _____ beats

HR in bpm = 10-sec pulse count × 6

HR in bpm = _____ × 6 = _____ bpm

Approximate distance covered in twenty minutes: _____ meters

Speed in mts/min. = distance in meters ÷ 20 minutes

Speed in mts/min. = _____ ÷ 20 = _____ mts/min.

VO_2 at this speed (see Table 6.3) = _____ ml/kg/min

VO_2 in L/min = VO_2 in ml/kg/min × BW in kg ÷ 1000

*Your five-minute recovery HR should be below 120 bpm. If it is above 120, you have most likely overexerted yourself and, therefore, need to decrease the intensity of exercise (and/or duration when exercising for long periods of time). If your five-minute recovery HR is still above 120 after decreasing the intensity of exercise, you should consult a physician regarding this condition.

VO$_2$ in L/min = _____ × _____ ÷ 1000 = _____ L/min

Caloric expenditure for 20-min. walk/jog = VO$_2$ in L/min × 5 × 20 min.

Caloric expenditure for 20-min. walk/jog = _____ × 5 × 20 = _____ calories

Using the previous information, how many calories would you have burned if you had maintained this pace for:

10 minutes (VO$_2$ in L/min × 5 × 10) = _____ × 5 × 10 = _____ calories

30 minutes (VO$_2$ in L/min × 5 × 30) = _____ × 5 × 30 = _____ calories

60 minutes (VO$_2$ in L/min × 5 × 60) = _____ × 5 × 60 = _____ calories

PREDICTING CALORIC EXPENDITURE ACCORDING TO EXERCISE HR

Research indicates that there is a linear relationship between HR and VO$_2$, as long as the HR ranges from about 110 to 180 bpm. If you were able to obtain two exercise HRs in this range and the equivalent oxygen uptakes (in L/min), you can easily predict your VO$_2$ and caloric expenditure for any given HR in the specified range. Plot your two exercise HRs and the corresponding VO$_2$ values on the graph provided below. Next, draw a line between these two points on the graph and extend the line to 110 and 180 bpm. You may now look up the VO$_2$ for any HR by finding the desired HR on the Y axis, then going across to the reference line and straight down to the X axis, where you will find the corresponding VO$_2$ in L/min. To obtain the caloric expenditure in calories per minute, simply multiply the VO$_2$ by 5. You may also predict your maximal VO$_2$ (in L/min) by extending the line up to your maximal HR. The maximal HR is estimated by subtracting your age from 220. To convert the maximal VO$_2$ to ml/kg/min, multiply the L/min value by 1,000 and divide by body weight in kilograms.

Using the results from your lab and the graph below, indicate the VO$_2$ in L/min and the caloric expenditure at the following HRs:

	VO$_2$ (L/min)	Caloric Expenditure (calories per minute)
120 bpm	_____	_____
150 bpm	_____	_____
170 bpm	_____	_____

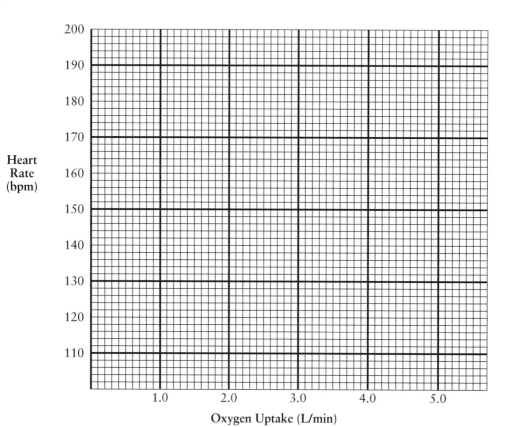

Heart Rate (bpm)

Oxygen Uptake (L/min)

LAB 6D

LAB 7A   MUSCULAR STRENGTH AND ENDURANCE ASSESSMENT

Name: _____ Date: _____ Grade: _____

Instructor: _____ Course: _____ Section: _____

NECESSARY LAB EQUIPMENT   A sixteen-station, fixed resistance, Universal Gym Apparatus and a metronome are required for the Muscular Strength and Endurance Test (two-and-one-half and five-pound weights, also obtainable from Universal Gym Equipment, Inc., are recommended to get to within one pound of the actual resistance to be lifted). A metronome, gymnasium bleachers, and a stopwatch are needed for the Muscular Endurance Test. A Lafayette hand grip dynamometer model 78010 is recommended for the Hand Grip Test.

OBJECTIVE   To determine the participant's muscular strength and/or endurance and the respective fitness classification.

LAB PREPARATION   Wear exercise clothing and avoid strenuous strength training forty-eight hours prior to this lab.

I. Muscular Strength and Endurance Test

Perform the Muscular Strength and Endurance Test according to the procedure outlined in Figure 7.5 in Chapter 7. Record the results and percentile ranks (use Table 7.1) in the appropriate blanks provided below.

Body Weight: _____ lb.s

Lift	Percent of Body Weight		Resistance (pounds)	Repetitions	Percentile Rank
	Men	Women			
Lat Pull-Down	.70	.45			
Leg Extension	.65	.50			
Bench Press	.75	.45			
Abdominal Crunch	NA*	NA			
Leg Curl	.32	.25			
Arm Curl	.35	.18			

*Not applicable, no resistance required. Use same test described in Figure 7.6.

Total: _____

Average Percentile Rank (divide total by six): _____

Overall Strength/Endurance Fitness Category (see Figure 7.5): _____

II. Muscular Endurance Test

Conduct this test using the guidelines provided in Figure 7.6 in Chapter 7. Record your results and percentile ranks (use Table 7.2).

Exercise	Metronome Cadence	Results (Repetitions)	Percentile Rank
Bench Jumps	none		
Modified Dips (Men)	56 bpm		
Modified Push-Ups (Women)	56 bpm		
Abdominal Crunch	60 bpm		

Total: _____

Average Percentile Rank (divide total by three): _____

Overall Muscular Endurance Fitness Category (see Figure 7.6): _____

III. Hand Grip Strength Test

The instructions for the Hand Grip Strength Test are provided in Figure 7.7. Perform the test according to the instructions and look up your results in Table 7.3.

Hand Used: ☐ Right   ☐ Left

Reading: _____ lbs.

Fitness Category (see Figure 7.7): _____

IV. Muscular Strength and Endurance Objectives

1. Indicate what muscular strength and endurance classification you would like to achieve by the end of the semester: _____

2. Indicate what muscular endurance classification you would like to achieve by the end of the semester:

_____

3. Briefly state how you are planning to achieve these objectives (also refer to Lab 4B, questions 8 and 9):

_____

_____

_____

_____

LAB 8A   SAMPLE STRENGTH-TRAINING PROGRAM

Name: _____ Date: _____ Grade: _____

Instructor: _____ Course: _____ Section: _____

NECESSARY LAB EQUIPMENT Free weights, strength-training machines, or no equipment if the "Strength-Training Exercises Without Weights" program is selected.

OBJECTIVE To introduce the participant to a sample strength-training exercise program, which may be carried out throughout life.

LAB PREPARATION Wear exercise clothing and prepare to participate in a sample strength-training exercise session. All of the strength-training exercises are illustrated in Chapter 8.

INSTRUCTIONS Select one of the three strength-training exercise programs. Perform all of the recommended exercises and, with the exception of the abdominal curl-up exercise, determine the resistance required to do approximately ten repetitions maximum (for "Strength-Training Exercises Without Weights," simply indicate the total number of repetitions performed). For the abdominal curl-up exercise, perform or build up to about twenty repetitions.

I. Strength-Training Exercises Without Weights

Exercise	Repetitions
Step-Up or High Jumper (select and circle one)	_____
Push-Up	_____
Abdominal Curl-Up (Crunch)	_____
Leg Curl	_____
Modified Dip	_____
Pull-Up or Arm Curl (select one)	_____
Heel Raise	_____
Leg Abduction and Adduction	_____

II. Universal Gym® Equipment Strength-Training Exercises

Exercise	Repetitions	Resistance
Arm Curl or Upright Rowing (select and circle one)	_____	_____
Leg Press, Squat, or Leg Extension (select one)	_____	_____
Abdominal Curl-Up or Abdominal Crunch (select one)	_____	_____
Bench Press, Chest Press, Shoulder Press, or Seated Overhead Press (select one)	_____	_____
Leg Curl	_____	_____
Lat Pull-Down or Bent-Arm Pullover (select one)	_____	_____
Heel Raise	_____	_____
Tricep Extension or Dip (select one)	_____	_____
Seated Back	_____	_____

III. Nautilus® Strength-Training Exercises

Exercise	Repetitions	Resistance
Multi-Biceps (Arm Curl)	_____	_____
Abdominal Crunch	_____	_____
Leg Extension	_____	_____
Bench Press, Leg Press, or Chest Press (select and circle one)	_____	_____
Leg Curl	_____	_____
Lower Back	_____	_____
Rowing Torso	_____	_____
Duo Hip and Back	_____	_____
Pullover	_____	_____
Rotary Torso	_____	_____
Multi-Triceps (Triceps Extension)	_____	_____

LAB 8A

LAB 9A · MUSCULAR FLEXIBILITY ASSESSMENT

Name: _____ Date: _____ Grade: _____

Instructor: _____ Course: _____ Section: _____

NECESSARY LAB EQUIPMENT Acuflex I, Acuflex II, and Acuflex III Flexibility Testers* or homemade flexibility testing equipment as described in Figures 9.3, 9.4, and 9.5 in Chapter 9.

OBJECTIVE To assess muscular flexibility and the respective fitness categories.

LAB PREPARATION The procedures for the flexibility tests* administered in this lab are explained in Chapter 9 (Figures 9.3, 9.4, and 9.5). It is important that you warm up properly before you perform any of these tests. Do gentle stretching exercises specific to the tests that will be administered. Wear loose exercise clothing for this lab.

I. Modified Sit-and-Reach Test

Trials: 1. _____ in.   2. _____ in.

Average Score: _____ in.   Percentile Rank: _____

Fitness Classification: _____

II. Total Body Rotation Test

Right Side   Left Side   (circle one)

Trials: 1. _____ in.   2. _____ in.

Average Score: _____ in.   Percentile Rank: _____

Fitness Classification: _____

III. Shoulder Rotation Test

Biacromial Width: _____ in.   Rotation Score: _____

Final Score = Rotation score – biacromial width

Final Score = _____ – _____ = _____ in.   Percentile Rank: _____

Fitness Classification: _____

IV. Overall Flexibility Rating

Test	Percentile Rank
Modifed Sit-and-Reach:	_____
Total Body Rotation (right, left — circle one):	_____
Shoulder Rotation:	_____

Total: _____

Average Percentile Rank (divide total by 3): _____

Overall Flexibility Classification: _____

* The Acuflex I, II, and III Flexibility Testers can be obtained from Figure Finder Collection, Novel Products, Inc., P.O. Box 408, Rockton, IL 61072-0408, Phone (800) 323-5143.

V. Flexibility Objectives

1. Indicate what flexibility classification you would like to achieve by the end of the semester: _____

2. Briefly state how you are planning to achieve this objective.

_____

_____

_____

_____

LAB 9A

LAB 9B POSTURE EVALUATION

Name: _____ Date: _____ Grade: _____

Instructor: _____ Course: _____ Section: _____

NECESSARY LAB EQUIPMENT A plumb line, two large mirrors set at about an eighty-five-degree angle, and a Polaroid camera (the mirrors and the camera are optional — *see* "Posture Evaluation" in Chapter 9).

OBJECTIVE To determine current body alignment.

LAB PREPARATION To conduct the posture analysis, men should wear shorts only and women shorts and a tank top. Shoes should also be removed for this test.

LAB ASSIGNMENT The class should be divided in groups of four students each. The group should carefully study the posture form given in this lab and then proceed to fill out the form for each member according to the instructions given under "Posture Evaluation" in Chapter 9. If no mirrors and camera are available, three members of the group are to rate the fourth person's posture while he/she first stands with the side of the body and then with the back to the plumb line. A final score is obtained by totaling the points given for each body segment and looking up the posture rating according to the total score in Table 9.5.

Results

Total Score: _____

Posture Improvement

Indicate which areas of your posture need to be corrected and what steps you can take to make improvements.

_____

_____

_____

_____

LAB
9B

	Good — 5	Fair — 3	Poor — 1	Score
HEAD Left Right	head erect, gravity passes directly through center	head twisted or turned to one side slightly	head twisted or turned to one side markedly	
SHOULDERS Left Right	shoulders level horizontally	one shoulder slightly higher	one shoulder markedly higher	
SPINE Left Right	spine straight	spine slightly	spine markedly curved laterally	
HIPS Left Right	hips level horizontally	one hip slightly higher	one hip markedly higher	
KNEES and ANKLES	feet pointed straight ahead, legs vertical	feet pointed out, legs deviating outward at the knee	feet pointed out markedly, legs deviate markedly	
NECK and UPPER BACK	neck erect, head in line with shoulders, rounded upper back	neck slightly forward, chin out, slightly more rounded upper back	neck markedly forward, chin markedly out, markedly rounded upper back	
TRUNK	trunk erect	trunk inclined to rear slightly	trunk inclined to rear markedly	
ABDOMEN	abdomen flat	abdomen protruding	abdomen protruding and sagging	
LOWER BACK	lower back normally curved	lower back slightly hollow	lower back markedly hollow	
LEGS	legs straight	knees slightly hyper-extended	knees markedly hyper-extended	

Total Score

LAB 9A

* Adapted with permission from *The New York Physical Fitness Test: A Manual for Teachers of Physical Education.* New York State Education Department (Division of HPER), 1958.

FIGURE 9B.1
Posture Analysis Form*

SAMPLE FLEXIBILITY DEVELOPMENT PROGRAM

Name: _____ Date: _____ Grade: _____

Instructor: _____ Course: _____ Section: _____

NECESSARY LAB EQUIPMENT Minor implements such as a chair, a table, an elastic band (surgical tubing or a wood or aluminum stick), and a stool or steps.

OBJECTIVE To introduce the participant to a sample stretching exercise program, which may be carried out throughout life.

LAB PREPARATION Wear exercise clothing and prepare to participate in a sample stretching exercise session. All of the flexibility exercises are illustrated in Chapter 10.

INSTRUCTIONS Perform all of the recommended flexibility exercises given in Chaper 10. Use a combination of slow-sustained and proprioceptive neuromuscular facilitation stretching techniques. Indicate the technique(s) used for each exercise, and, where applicable, the number of repetitions performed and the length of time that the final degree of stretch was held.

Stretching Exercises

Exercise	Stretching Technique	Repetitions	Length of Final Stretch
Lateral Head Tilt	_____	_____	NA*
Arm Circles	_____	_____	NA
Side Stretch	_____	_____	_____
Body Rotation	_____	_____	_____
Chest Stretch	_____	_____	_____
Shoulder Hyperextension	_____	_____	_____
Shoulder Rotation	_____	_____	NA
Quad Stretch	_____	_____	_____
Heel Cord Stretch	_____	_____	_____
Adductor Stretch	_____	_____	_____
Sitting Adductor Stretch	_____	_____	_____
Sit-and-Reach Stretch	_____	_____	_____
Triceps Stretch	_____	_____	_____

*Not Applicable

LAB 10B EXERCISES FOR THE PREVENTION AND REHABILITATION OF LOW BACK PAIN

Name: _____ Date: _____ Grade: _____

Instructor: _____ Course: _____ Section: _____

NECESSARY LAB EQUIPMENT A chair.

OBJECTIVE To introduce the participant to an exercise program for the prevention and rehabilitation of low back pain.

LAB PREPARATION Wear exercise clothing and prepare to participate in the lab session. All of the exercises for this lab are illustrated in Chapter 10.

I. Stretching Exercises

Perform all of the recommended exercises for the prevention and rehabilitation of low back pain given in Chapter 10. Indicate the number of repetitions performed for each exercise.

Exercise	Repetitions
Single-Knee to Chest	_____
Double-Knee to Chest	_____
Upper and Lower Back Stretch	_____
Sit-and-Reach Stretch	_____
Gluteal Stretch	_____
Back Extension	_____
Trunk Rotation and Lower Back Stretch	_____
Pelvic Tilt	_____
Abdominal Crunch	_____

II. Proper Body Mechanics

Perform the following tasks using the proper body mechanics given in Figure 10.3 in Chapter 10 (check each item off as you perform the task):

_____ Standing (Carriage) Position

_____ Sitting Position

_____ Bed Posture

_____ Resting Position for Tired and Painful Back

_____ Lifting an Object

III. "Rules To Live By — From Now On"

Read the eighteen "Rules To Live By — From Now On" given in Figure 10.4, Chapter 10, and indicate below those rules that you need to work on to improve posture and body mechanics and prevent low back pain.

_____

_____

_____

_____

ASSESSMENT OF SKILL-RELATED COMPONENTS OF FITNESS

Name: _____ Date: _____ Grade: _____

Instructor: _____ Course: _____ Section: _____

NECESSARY LAB EQUIPMENT

Agility: Free-throw area of a basketball court (or any smooth area twelve by nineteen feet with sufficient running space around it), four plastic cones, and a stopwatch.

Balance: Any flat, smooth floor (not carpeted) and a stopwatch.

Coordination: A cardboard with six circles drawn on it as explained in Chapter 11 (*see* test procedures for the coordination test), three full cans of soda pop (12 oz.), and a stopwatch.

Power: A flat, smooth surface, and a ten-foot-long tape measure (or two standard cloth measuring tapes, each sixty inches long).

Reaction Time: A standard yardstick with a shaded "concentration zone" drawn on the first two inches of the stick.

Speed: A school track or premeasured fifty-yard straightway.

LAB PREPARATION
Wear exercise clothing, including running shoes. Do not exercise strenuously several hours prior to this lab.

INSTRUCTIONS
Perform all six tests for the fitness-related components as outlined in Chapter 11. Report the results below and answer the questions given at the end of this lab.

Skill-Related Fitness: **Test Results**

Agility   Trials: 1. ____ ____ . ____   2. ____ ____ . ____

Balance   Trials: 1. ____ ____ . ____   2. ____ ____ . ____

Coordination   Trials: 1. ____ ____ . ____   2. ____ ____ . ____

Power   Trials: 1. ____ ____   2. ____ ____   3. ____ ____

Reaction Time Trials: 1. ____ ____ . ____   2. ____ ____ . ____   3. ____ ____ . ____

        4. ____ ____ . ____   5. ____ ____ . ____   6. ____ ____ . ____   7. ____ ____ . ____

        8. ____ ____ . ____   9. ____ ____ . ____   10. ____ ____ . ____   11. ____ ____ . ____

        12. ____ ____ . ____   Average (6 middle scores) = ____ ____ . ____

Speed   Trial: 1. ____ ____ . ____

Skill-Related Fitness Classifications*

Fitness Component (test)	Percentile Rank	Classification
Agility (SEMO test)	_____	_____
Balance (One foot stand)	_____	_____
Coordination (Soda pop test)	_____	_____
Power (Standing long jump)	_____	_____
Reaction Time (Yardstick test)	_____	_____
Speed (Fifty-yard dash)	_____	_____

*Use Tables 11.1 and 11.2

Interpretation of Test Results

1. What conclusions can you draw from your test results?

   _____

   _____

   _____

   _____

2. Briefly state how you could improve your test results and what activities you could engage in to obtain the desired results?

   _____

   _____

   _____

   _____

LAB 11A

3. Did you ever participate in organized sports or have you found success in a particular game or sport?

   _____ Yes   _____ No

   3a. If your answer to number 3 above is positive, list those sports, games, or events where you enjoy(ed) success.

   _____

   3b. Is there a relationship between those sports, games, or events where you enjoyed particular success and your test results in this lab?

   _____

   _____

   _____

LAB 12A SELF-ASSESSMENT OF CARDIOVASCULAR RISK

Name: _____ Date: _____ Grade: _____

Instructor: _____ Course: _____ Section: _____

NECESSARY LAB EQUIPMENT Basic lab equipment to repeat the cardiovascular endurance, body composition, and blood pressure tests.

OBJECTIVE To assess your current risk for coronary heart disease (CHD).

INSTRUCTIONS The disease process for cardiovascular disease starts early in life, primarily as a result of poor lifestyle habits. Studies have shown beginning stages of atherosclerosis and elevated blood lipids in children as young as ten years old. Consequently, the purpose of this lab is to establish a baseline CHD risk profile and to point out the "zero risk" level for each coronary risk factor.

You may want to repeat the blood pressure, cardiovascular endurance, and body composition tests to obtain current values for this lab experience. If time does not allow for reassessment of these parameters, use the results obtained in labs 1B, 5A, and 3A or 3B. In addition, if you have had a blood chemistry analysis performed recently that included total cholesterol, HDL-cholesterol, triglycerides, and glucose levels, you may use the results for this lab.

Self-Assessment Coronary Heart Disease Risk Factor Analysis

			Score
1. Physical Activity	Do you participate in a regular aerobic exercise program (brisk walking, jogging, swimming, bicycling, aerobics, etc.) for more than 20 minutes:		
	Once a week or less	8	
	Two times per week	3	[ ]
	Three or more times per week	0	

2. Resting and Stress Electrocardiograms (ECG)	Add scores for both ECGs				
	ECG	Resting	Stress		
	Normal	(0)	(0)	....	0
	Equivocal	(1)	(4)	....	1-5
	Abnormal	(3)	(8)	....	3-11 [ ]

3. HDL-Cholesterol (If unknown, answer question 6)	Men	Women		Score
	≥ 45	≥ 55	....	0
	35-44	45-54	....	3
	≤ 34	≤ 44	....	6 [ ]

4. LDL-Cholesterol (If unknown, answer question 6)	≤ 130	....	0
	131-159	....	3
	≥ 160	....	6 [ ]

5. Triglycerides (If unknown, answer question 6)	≤ 125	....	0
	126-499	....	1
	≥ 500	....	2 [ ]

Subtotal Risk Score: [ ]

Self-Assessment Coronary Heart Disease Risk Factor Analysis *(continued)*

Subtotal Risk Score (from previous page): ☐

6. Diet (Do not answer if questions 3, 4 and 5 have been answered)

Does your regular diet include (high score if all apply):
One or more daily servings of red meat; 7 or more eggs/week; daily butter, cheese, whole milk, sweets and alcohol 10-14
Four to six servings of red meat/week, 4-6 eggs per week, margarine, 1 or 2% milk, some cheese, sweets, and alcohol 4-10
Fish, poultry, red meat less than three times/week, less than 3 eggs/week, skim milk and skim milk products, moderate sweets and alcohol 0-3   ☐

7. Diabetes/Glucose

≤120 0
121-128 1
129-136 .... 1.5
137-144 2
145-149 .... 2.5
≥150 3
Diabetics add another 3 points 3   ☐

8. Blood Pressure

Score applies to each reading
(e.g. 144/88 score = 4)

Systolic		Diastolic		
≤120	(0)	≤80	(0)	0
121-130	(1)	81-90	(1)	1-2
131-140	(2)	91-98	(2)	2-4
141-150	(3)	99-106	(3)	3-6
≥151	(4)	≥107	(4)	4-8 ☐

9. Percent Body Fat

Men	Women	
12-17%	18-22%	0
18-22%	23-27%	1
23-27%	28-32%	2
≥28%	≥33%	3 ☐

10. Smoking

Lifetime nonsmoker 0
Ex-smoker over one year 0
Ex-smoker less than one year 1
Smoke less than 1 cigarette/day 1
Nonsmoker, but live or work in smoking environment 2
Pipe, cigar smoker, or chew tobacco 2
Smoke 1-9 cigarettes/day 3
Smoke 10-19 cigarettes/day 4
Smoke 20-29 cigarettes/day 5
Smoke 30-39 cigarettes/day 6
Smoke 40 or more cigarettes/day 8   ☐

LAB 12A

Subtotal Risk Score: ☐

Self-Assessment Coronary Heart Disease Risk Factor Analysis *(continued)*

Subtotal Risk Score (from previous page): [   ]

11.	Tension and Stress	Are you:	
		Sometimes tense...	0
		Often tense	1
		Nearly always tense	2
		Always tense	3 [ ]

12. Personal History — Have you ever had a heart attack, stroke, coronary disease, or any known heart problem:

- During the last year 8
- 1-2 years ago 5
- 2-5 years ago 3
- More than 5 years ago.. 2
- Never suffered from heart disease.................................... 0 [   ]

13. Family History — Have any of your blood relatives (parents, uncles, brothers, sisters, grandparents) suffered from cardiovascular disease (heart attack, strokes, bypass surgery):

- One or more before age 51 6
- One or more between 51 and 60 3
- One or more after age 60.. 1
- None have suffered from cardiovascular disease................ 0 [   ]

14. Age

- 29 or younger 0
- 30-39.. 1
- 40-49.. 2
- 50-59.. 3
- ≥60 .... 4 [   ]

Total Risk Score: [   ]

Risk Categories

Very Low ....5 or less points
Low ....Between 6 and 15 points
Moderate ....Between 16 and 25 points
High ....Between 26 and 35 points
Very High............................36 or more points

Lifestyle Changes

Briefly indicate behaviors that you need to modify to decrease your current risk for cardiovascular disease.

_____

_____

_____

CANCER PREVENTION: ARE YOU TAKING CONTROL?

Name: _____ Date: _____ Grade: _____

Instructor: _____ Course: _____ Section: _____

NECESSARY LAB EQUIPMENT None required.

OBJECTIVE To encourage healthy lifestyle practices that will help decrease the risk for cancer.

LAB PREPARATION Students are encouraged to read Chapter 13 prior to filling out this questionnaire.

ARE YOU TAKING CONTROL?

Today, scientists think most cancers may be related to lifestyle and environment—what you eat, drink, if you smoke and where you work and play. So the good news is you can help reduce your own cancer risk by taking control of things in your daily life.

10 Steps To A Healthier Life and Reduced Cancer Risk	Yes	No
1. **Are you eating more cabbage-family vegetables?** They include broccoli, cauliflower, brussels sprouts, all cabbages and kale.	☐	☐
2. **Are high-fiber foods included in your diet?** Fiber occurs in whole grains, fruits and vegetables including peaches, strawberries, potatoes, spinach, tomatoes, wheat and bran cereals, rice, popcorn and whole-wheat bread.	☐	☐
3. **Do you choose foods with Vitamin A?** Fresh foods with beta-carotene like carrots, peaches, apricots, squash and broccoli are the best source, not vitamin pills.	☐	☐
4. **Is Vitamin C included in your diet?** You'll find it naturally in lots of fresh fruits and vegetables like grapefruit, cantaloupe, oranges, strawberries, red and green peppers, broccoli and tomatoes.	☐	☐
5. **Do you exercise and monitor calorie intake to avoid weight gain?** Walking is ideal exercise for many people.	☐	☐
6. **Are you cutting overall fat intake?** This is done by eating lean meat, fish, skinned poultry and low-fat dairy products.	☐	☐
7. **Do you limit salt-cured, smoked, nitrite-cured foods?** Choose bacon, ham, hot dogs or salt-cured fish only occasionally if you like them a lot.	☐	☐
8. **If you smoke, have you tried quitting?**	☐	☐
9. **If you drink alcohol, are you moderate in your intake?**	☐	☐
10. **Do you respect the sun's rays?** Protect yourself with sunscreen—at least # 15, wear long sleeves and a hat, especially during midday hours—11 a.m. to 3 p.m.	☐	☐

If you answer yes to most of these questions, **Congratulations.** You are taking control of simple lifestyle factors that will help you feel better and reduce your cancer risk.

*Courtesy of the Texas Division of the American Cancer Society.

EARLY WARNING SIGNS OF POSSIBLE SERIOUS ILLNESS

Name: _____ Date: _____ Grade: _____

Instructor: _____ Course: _____ Section: _____

NECESSARY LAB EQUIPMENT   None required.

OBJECTIVE   To alert the reader regarding early warning signs of possible serious illness.

Figure 13A.1. *Early Warning Signs of Possible Serious Illness Questionnaire**

Many serious illnesses begin with apparently minor or localized symptoms that, if they are recognized early, can alert you to act in time for the disease to be cured or controlled. In most cases, of course, nothing is seriously wrong. **If you experience any of the following symptoms, discuss the problem with your physician without delay.** Only check conditions that apply.

☐   1. Rapid loss of weight—more than about 4 kg (10 lbs) in ten weeks—without apparent cause.

☐   2. A sore, scab, or ulcer, either in the mouth, or on the body, that fails to heal within a period of about three weeks.

☐   3. A skin blemish or mole that begins to bleed or itch, or that changes color, size, or shape.

☐   4. Severe headaches that develop for no obvious reason.

☐   5. Sudden attacks of vomiting, without preceding nausea.

☐   6. Fainting spells for no apparent reason.

☐   7. Visual problems such as seeing "haloes" around lights, or intermittently blurred vision, especially in dim light.

☐   8. Increasing difficulty with swallowing.

☐   9. Hoarseness without apparent cause that lasts for a week or more.

☐   10. A "smoker's" cough or any other nagging cough that has been getting worse.

☐   11. Blood in coughed-up phlegm, or sputum.

☐   12. Constantly swollen ankles.

☐   13. A bluish tinge to the lips, the insides of the eyelids, or the nailbeds.

☐   14. Extreme shortness of breath for no apparent reason.

☐   15. Vomiting of blood or a substance that resembles coffee grounds.

☐   16. Persistent indigestion or abdominal pain.

☐   17. A marked change in normal bowel habits, such as alternating attacks of diarrhea and constipation.

☐   18. Bowel movements that look black and tarry.

☐   19. Rectal bleeding.

☐   20. Unusually cloudy, pink, red, or smoky-looking urine.

☐   21. In men, discomfort or difficulty when urinating.

☐   22. In men, discharge from the tip of the penis.

☐   23. In women, a lump or unusual thickening of a breast or any alteration in breast shape such as flattening, bulging, or puckering of skin.

☐   24. In women, bleeding or unusual discharge from the nipple.

☐   25. In women, vaginal bleeding or "spotting" that occurs between usual menstrual periods or after menopause.

*Reproduced with permission from Family Medical Guide by The American Medical Association. New York: Random House, 1982.

Name: _____ Date: _____ Grade: _____

Instructor: _____ Course: _____ Section: _____

NECESSARY LAB EQUIPMENT None required.

OBJECTIVE To determine your potential risk for certain types of cancer.

INTRODUCTION Carefully read the questions concerning each cancer site and its specific risk factors contained in Figure 13.8 and under the "Other Cancer Sites" heading in Chapter 13. Be honest in your responses. Copy all "yes" statements in the spaces provided below. A "yes" answer in any A category does not necessarily mean that there is a problem, but those symptoms should be brought to the attention of a physician as soon as possible. You can be alert to the symptoms, but only a trained person can evaluate them. A "yes" answer in categories B and C are important medical information that your physician should have. A "yes" answer in any D cagetory indicates that certain lifestyle changes should be made to decrease your risk for cancer. You are also advised to discuss any risk factors that you may have for the "Other Cancer Sites" with your physician (record below the applicable risk factors, warning signals, and prevention techniques that apply to you).

Skin and Lymph Nodes

A. Do you now have . . .? (for physician evaluation)

_____

_____

_____

B. Has a member of your family ever had . . .? (for physician attention)

_____

_____

C. Have you ever had . . .? (for physician record)

_____

_____

D. Do you . . .? (for personal action)

_____

_____

Head and Neck

A. Do you now have . . .? (for physician evaluation)

_____

_____

_____

B. Has a member of your family ever had . . .? (for physician attention)

_____

_____

C. Have you ever had . . .? (for physician record)

_____

_____

D. Do you . . .? (for personal action)

_____

_____

Respiratory System

A. Do you now have . . .? (for physician evaluation)

_____

_____

_____

B. Has a member of your family ever had . . .? (for physician attention)

_____

_____

_____

C. Have you ever had . . .? (for physician record)

_____

_____

_____

D. Do you . . .? (for personal action)

_____

_____

Urinary Tract

A. Do you now have . . .? (for physician evaluation)

_____

_____

_____

B. Has a member of your family ever had . . .? (for physician attention)

_____

_____

_____

C. Have you ever had . . .? (for physician record)

_____

_____

_____

D. Do you . . .? (for personal action)

_____

_____

_____

Gastrointestinal Tract

A. Do you now have . . .? (for physician evaluation)

_____

_____

_____

B. Has a member of your family ever had . . .? (for physician attention)

_____

_____

_____

C. Have you ever had . . .? (for physician record)

_____

_____

_____

D. Do you . . .? (for personal action)

_____

_____

_____

Male Reproductive System

A. Do you now have . . .? (for physicians evaluation)

_____

_____

_____

B. Does not apply

C. Have you ever had . . .? (for physician record)

_____

_____

_____

D. Do you . . .? (for personal action)

_____

_____

_____

LAB
13C

Female Reproductive System

A. Do you now have . . .? (for physician evaluation)

_____

_____

_____

B. Has a member of your family ever had . . .? (for physician attention)

_____

_____

_____

C. Have you ever had . . .? (for physician record)

_____

_____

_____

D. Do You . . .? (for personal action)

_____

_____

_____

Cancer of the Breast

A. Do you now have . . .? (for physician evaluation)

_____

_____

_____

B. Has a member of your family ever had . . .? (for physician attention)

_____

_____

_____

C. Have you ever had . . .? (for physician record)

_____

_____

_____

D. Do you . . .? (for personal action)

_____

_____

Pancreatic Cancer

Risk Factors:

_____

_____

Warning Signals:

_____

_____

Preventive Measures:

_____

_____

Oral Cancer

Risk Factors:

_____

_____

Preventive Measures:

_____

_____

Thyroid Cancer

Risk Factors:

_____

_____

Warning Signals:

_____

_____

Preventive Measures:

_____

_____

LAB
13C

Liver Cancer

Risk Factors:

_____

_____

Warning Signals:

_____

_____

Preventive Measures:

_____

_____

Leukemia

Risk Factors:

_____

_____

Warning Signals:

_____

_____

Preventive Measures:

_____

_____

LAB 14A THE LIFE EXPERIENCES SURVEY

Name: _____ Date: _____ Grade: _____

Instructor: _____ Course: _____ Section: _____

NECESSARY LAB EQUIPMENT   None required.

OBJECTIVE   To determine stressful life experiences within the last twelve months that may have an impact on your physical and psychological well-being.

INTRODUCTION   The Life Experiences Survey (Figure 14A.1.) contains a list of events that sometimes bring about change in the lives of those who experience them and that necessitate social readjustment. Please check events that you have experienced in the past twelve months. Be sure that all check marks are directly across from the items to which they correspond (only check those that apply).

Also, for each item checked, please indicate the extent to which you viewed the event as having a positive or negative impact on your life at the time the event occurred. That is, indicate the type and extent of impact that the event had. A rating of -3 would indicate an extremely negative impact. A rating of 0 suggests no impact either positive or negative. A rating of $+3$ would indicate an extremely positive impact. After determining the life events that have taken place, sum the negative and the positive points separately (e.g., positive ratings: 3, 2, 1, 2 = 11 points positive score; negative ratings: -1, -3, -1, -3, -2, -3 = 13 negative points score). A final "total life change" score is obtained by adding both the positive and negative scores together as positive numbers (e.g., total life change score: 11 + 13 = 24 points). The various stress ratings for The Life Experiences Survey are given in Table 14A.1. Your negative score is the best indicator of stress (distress or negative stress) in your life.

Table 14A.1.
Stress Ratings for the Life Experiences Survey*

Category	Negative Score		Total Score	
	Men	Women	Men	Women
Poor	$\geqslant 13$	$\geqslant 15$	$\geqslant 27$	$\geqslant 27$
Fair	7-12	8-14	17-26	18-26
Average	6	7	16	17
Good	1-5	1-6	5-15	6-16
Excellent	0	0	1-4	1-5

*Adapted from Sarason, 1. G. et al. "Assessing the Impact of Life Changes: Development of the Life Experiences Survey." *Journal of Consulting and Clinical Psychology* 46: 932-946, 1978.

Life Experiences Survey Results

	Points	Stress Category
Negative Score:	_____	_____
Positive Score:	_____	_____
Total Score:	_____	_____

LAB 14A

Section I

1. Marriage	−3	−2	−1	0	+1	+2	+3
2. Detention in jail or comparable institution	−3	−2	−1	0	+1	+2	+3
3. Death of spouse	−3	−2	−1	0	+1	+2	+3
4. Major change in sleeping habits (much more or much less sleep)	−3	−2	−1	0	+1	+2	+3
5. Death of close family member:							
a. mother	−3	−2	−1	0	+1	+2	+3
b. father	−3	−2	−1	0	+1	+2	+3
c. brother	−3	−2	−1	0	+1	+2	+3
d. sister	−3	−2	−1	0	+1	+2	+3
e. grandmother	−3	−2	−1	0	+1	+2	+3
f. grandfather	−3	−2	−1	0	+1	+2	+3
g. other (specify)	−3	−2	−1	0	+1	+2	+3
6. Major change in eating habits (much more or much less food intake)	−3	−2	−1	0	+1	+2	+3
7. Foreclosure on mortgage or loan	−3	−2	−1	0	+1	+2	+3
8. Death of close friend	−3	−2	−1	0	+1	+2	+3
9. Outstanding personal achievement	−3	−2	−1	0	+1	+2	+3
10. Minor law violations (traffic tickets, disturbing the peace, etc.)	−3	−2	−1	0	+1	+2	+3
11. Male: Wife/girlfriend's pregnancy	−3	−2	−1	0	+1	+2	+3
12. Female: Pregnancy	−3	−2	−1	0	+1	+2	+3
13. Changed work situation (different work responsibility, major change in working conditions, working hours, etc.)	−3	−2	−1	0	+1	+2	+3
14. New job	−3	−2	−1	0	+1	+2	+3
15. Serious illness or injury of close family member:							
a. father	−3	−2	−1	0	+1	+2	+3
b. mother	−3	−2	−1	0	+1	+2	+3
c. sister	−3	−2	−1	0	+1	+2	+3
d. brother	−3	−2	−1	0	+1	+2	+3
e. grandfather	−3	−2	−1	0	+1	+2	+3
f. grandmother	−3	−2	−1	0	+1	+2	+3
g. spouse	−3	−2	−1	0	+1	+2	+3
h. other (specify)	−3	−2	−1	0	+1	+2	+3
16. Sexual difficulties	−3	−2	−1	0	+1	+2	+3
17. Trouble with employer (in danger of losing job, being suspended, demoted, etc.)	−3	−2	−1	0	+1	+2	+3
18. Trouble with in-laws	−3	−2	−1	0	+1	+2	+3
19. Major change in financial status (a lot better off or a lot worse off)	−3	−2	−1	0	+1	+2	+3

LAB 14A

(Continued)

From Sarason, I.G., et al. Assessing the Impact of Life Changes: Development of the Life Experiences Survey. *Journal of Consulting and Clinical Psychology* 46:932-946, 1978. Copyright 1978 by the American Psychological Association. Reprinted by permission of the publisher and author.

FIGURE 14A.1
The life experiences survey.

20. Major change in closeness of family members (increased or decreased closeness)	−3	−2	−1	0	+1	+2	+3
21. Gaining a new family member (through birth, adoption, family member moving in, etc.)	−3	−2	−1	0	+1	+2	+3
22. Change of residence	−3	−2	−1	0	+1	+2	+3
23. Marital separation from mate (due to conflict)	−3	−2	−1	0	+1	+2	+3
24. Major change in church activities (increased or decreased attendance)	−3	−2	−1	0	+1	+2	+3
25. Marital reconciliation with mate	−3	−2	−1	0	+1	+2	+3
26. Major change in number of arguments with spouse (a lot more or a lot less arguments)	−3	−2	−1	0	+1	+2	+3
27. Married Male: Change in wife's work outside the home (beginning work, ceasing work, changing to a new job, etc.)	−3	−2	−1	0	+1	+2	+3
28. Married Female: Change in husband's work (loss of job, beginning new job, retirement, etc.)	−3	−2	−1	0	+1	+2	+3
29. Major change in usual type and/or amount of recreation	−3	−2	−1	0	+1	+2	+3
30. Borrowing more than $10,000 (buying home, business etc.)	−3	−2	−1	0	+1	+2	+3
31. Borrowing less than $ 10,000 (buying car, TV, getting school loan, etc.)	−3	−2	−1	0	+1	+2	+3
32. Being fired from job	−3	−2	−1	0	+1	+2	+3
33. Male: Wife/girlfriend having abortion	−3	−2	−1	0	+1	+2	+3
34. Female: Having abortion	−3	−2	−1	0	+1	+2	+3
35. Major personal illness or injury	−3	−2	−1	0	+1	+2	+3
36. Major change in social activities, e.g., parties, movies, visiting (increased or decreased participation)	−3	−2	−1	0	+1	+2	+3
37. Major change in living conditions of family (building new home, remodeling, deterioration of home, neighborhood, etc.)	−3	−2	−1	0	+1	+2	+3
38. Divorce	−3	−2	−1	0	+1	+2	+3
39. Serious injury or illness of close friend	−3	−2	−1	0	+1	+2	+3
40. Retirement from work	−3	−2	−1	0	+1	+2	+3
41. Son or daughter leaving home (due to marriage, college, etc.)	−3	−2	−1	0	+1	+2	+3
42. Ending of formal schooling	−3	−2	−1	0	+1	+2	+3
43. Separation from spouse (due to work, travel, etc.)	−3	−2	−1	0	+1	+2	+3
44. Engagement	−3	−2	−1	0	+1	+2	+3
45. Breaking up with boyfriend/girlfriend	−3	−2	−1	0	+1	+2	+3
46. Leaving home for the first time	−3	−2	−1	0	+1	+2	+3
47. Reconciliation with boyfriend/girlfriend	−3	−2	−1	0	+1	+2	+3
48. Others_____	−3	−2	−1	0	+1	+2	+3
49 _____	−3	−2	−1	0	+1	+2	+3
50. _____	−3	−2	−1	0	+1	+2	+3

LAB
14A

(Continued)

FIGURE 14A.1 *(Continued)*
The life experiences survey.

Section 2

51. Beginning a new school experience at a higher academic
    level (college, graduate school, professional school, etc.)   −3 −2 −1   0 +1 +2 +3

52. Changing to a new school at the same academic level
    undergraduate, graduate, etc.)   −3 −2 −1   0 +1 +2 +3

53. Academic probation   −3 −2 −1   0 +1 +2 +3

54. Being dismissed from dormitory or other residence   −3 −2 −1   0 +1 +2 +3

55. Failing an important exam   −3 −2 −1   0 +1 +2 +3

56. Changing a major   −3 −2 −1   0 +1 +2 +3

57. Failing a course   −3 −2 −1   0 +1 +2 +3

58. Dropping a course   −3 −2 −1   0 +1 +2 +3

59. Joining a fraternity/sorority   −3 −2 −1   0 +1 +2 +3

60. Financial problems concerning school (in danger of not
    having sufficient money to continue)   −3 −2 −1   0 +1 +2 +3

Total Negative Points: _____

Total Positive Points: _____

FIGURE 14A.1 *(Continued)*
The life experiences survey.

TYPE A PERSONALITY ASSESSMENT AND BEHAVIORAL OBJECTIVES FOR STRESS REDUCTION AND PERSONALITY CHANGE

Name: _____ Date: _____ Grade: _____

Instructor: _____ Course: _____ Section: _____

NECESSARY LAB EQUIPMENT   None.

OBJECTIVE   To obtain a general Type A personality rating and write behavioral objectives for stress reduction and personality change.

INSTRUCTIONS   Please answer "yes" or "no" for each of the items listed in the Type A Personality Assessment Form given in Figure 14B.1. For questions 7, 15, and 16, give yourself one point for each "yes" answer. For the rest of the questions, give yourself one point for each "no" answer. Your level of Type A behavior, based on your total number of points, is given below. After determining your Type A rating, prepare your behavioral objectives for stress reduction and personality change by answering the six questions at the end of this lab.

Level of Type A Behavior Results

Results	Points	
Questions 7, 15, 16:	_____	(1 point for each "yes" answer)
All other questions:	_____	(1 point for each "no" answer)
Total Score:	_____	

Score Interpretation:

Rating	Points
High	0–7
Medium	8–13
Low	14–21

Your level of Type A: _____

Yes	No	
____	____	1. Do you feel your job carries heavy responsibility?
____	____	2. Would you describe yourself as a hard-driving, ambitious type of person?
____	____	3. Do you usually try to get things done as quickly as possible?
____	____	4. Would family members and close friends describe you as hard-driving and ambitious?
____	____	5. Have people close to you ever asked you to slow down in your work?
____	____	6. Do you think you drive harder to accomplish things than most of your associates?
____	____	7. When you play games with people your own age, do you play just for the fun of it?
____	____	8. If there's competition in your job, do you enjoy this?
____	____	9. When you are driving and there is a car in your lane going far too slowly for you, do you mutter and complain? Would anyone riding with you know that you are annoyed?
____	____	10. If you make an appointment with someone, would you be there on time in almost all cases?
____	____	11. If you were kept waiting, would you resent it?
____	____	12. If you see someone doing a job rather slowly and you know you could do it faster and better yourself, does it make you restless to watch him or her?
____	____	13. Would you be tempted to step in and do it yourself?
____	____	14. Do you eat rapidly? Walk rapidly?
____	____	15. After you've finished eating, do you like to sit around the table and chat?
____	____	16. When you go out to a restaurant and find eight or ten people waiting ahead of you for a table, will you wait?
____	____	17. Do you really resent having to wait in line at the bank or post office?
____	____	18. Do you always feel anxious to get going and finish whatever you have to do?
____	____	19. Do you have the feeling that time is passing too rapidly for you to accomplish all the things you'd like to get done in one day?
____	____	20. Do you often feel a sense of time urgency or time pressure?
____	____	21. Do you hurry in doing most things?

Form revised from The Structured Interview from the forum on Type A Behavior, National Heart/Lung/Blood Institute. Ray M. Rosenman, MD, 1981. This form is reproduced with permission from Patton, R. W., et. al *Implementing Health/Fitness Programs.* Champaign, IL: Human Kinetics Publisher, Inc., 1986.

LAB 14B

FIGURE 14B.1
Type A personality assessment questionnaire.

LAB 14C STRESS VULNERABILITY QUESTIONNAIRE

Name: _____ Date: _____ Grade: _____

Instructor: _____ Course: _____ Section: _____

NECESSARY LAB EQUIPMENT None required.

OBJECTIVE Determine your stress vulnerability rating and identify areas to reduce your vulnerability to stress.

INSTRUCTIONS Carefully read each statement and circle the number that best describes your feelings or behavior. Please be completely honest with your answers.

Stress Vulnerability Questionnaire

Item	Strongly Agree	Mildly Agree	Mildly Disagree	Strongly Disagree
1. I try to incorporate as much physical activity* as possible in my daily schedule.	1	2	3	4
2. I exercise aerobically for 20 minutes or more at least three times per week.	1	2	3	4
3. I regularly sleep 7 to 8 hours per night.	1	2	3	4
4. I take my time eating at least one hot balanced meal a day.	1	2	3	4
5. I drink less than two cups of coffee (or equivalent) per day.	1	2	3	4
6. I am at recommended body weight.	1	2	3	4
7. I enjoy good health.	1	2	3	4
8 I do not use tobacco in any form.	1	2	3	4
9. I limit my alcohol intake to no more than one drink per day.	1	2	3	4
10. I do not use hard drugs (chemical dependency).	1	2	3	4
11. There is someone I love, trust, and can rely on for help if I have a problem or need to make an essential decision.	1	2	3	4
12. There is love in my family.	1	2	3	4
13. I routinely give and receive affection.	1	2	3	4
14. I have close personal relationships with other people that provide me with a sense of emotional security.	1	2	3	4

(Continued)

LAB
14C

*Walk instead of driving, avoid escalators and elevators, or walk to neighboring offices, homes, and stores.

FIGURE 14C.1
Stress vulnerability questionnaire.

15. There are people close by that I can turn to for guidance in time of stress.	1	2	3	4
16. I can speak openly about feelings, emotions, and problems with people that I trust.	1	2	3	4
17. Other people rely on me for help.	1	2	3	4
18. I am able to keep my feelings of anger and hostility under control.	1	2	3	4
19. I have a network of friends who enjoy the same social activities that I do.	1	2	3	4
20. I take time to do something fun at least once a week.	1	2	3	4
21. My religious beliefs provide guidance and strength to my life.	1	2	3	4
22. I often provide service to others.	1	2	3	4
23. I enjoy my job (major or school).	1	2	3	4
24. I am a competent worker.	1	2	3	4
25. I get along well with co-workers (or students).	1	2	3	4
26. My income is sufficient for my needs.	1	2	3	4
27. I manage time adequately.	1	2	3	4
28. I have learned to say "no" to additional commitments when I am already pressed for time.	1	2	3	4
29. I take daily quiet time for myself.	1	2	3	4
30. I practice stress management as needed.	1	2	3	4

Total Points: _____

Scoring:

0-30 points ....Excellent (great stress resistance)
31-40 points ....Good (little vulnerability to stress)
41-50 points ....Average (somewhat vulnerable to stress)
51-60 points ....Fair (vulnerable to stress)
≥61 points ....Poor (very vulnerable to stress)

LAB 14C

This questionnaire helps you identify areas where improvements can be made to help you cope with stress more effectively. As you take this test, you will notice that most of the items describe situations and behaviors that are within your control. To make yourself less vulnerable to stress, improve the behaviors which make you more vulnerable to stress. Start by modifying those behaviors that are easiest to change before undertaking the most difficult ones.

FIGURE 14C.1 *(Continued)*
Stress vulnerability questionnaire.

LAB 14D GOALS AND TIME MANAGEMENT SKILLS

Name: _____ Date: _____ Grade: _____

Instructor: _____ Course: _____ Section: _____

NECESSARY LAB EQUIPMENT None required.

OBJECTIVE To help you develop time management skills.

INSTRUCTIONS If you feel that you don't have enough hours during the day to get everything done, this lab is for you. Be sure to read the *time management* section in Chapter 14 and fill out all the forms provided with this lab.

In the spaces provided below, list your goals as indicated. You may want to keep this form and review it in years to come.

I. List three goals that you wish to accomplish in this life:

    1. _____

    2. _____

    3. _____

II. List three goals that you wish to see accomplished ten years from now:

    1. _____

    2. _____

    3. _____

III. List three goals that you wish to accomplish this year:

    1. _____

    2. _____

    3. _____

IV. List three goals that you wish to accomplish this month:

    1. _____

    2. _____

    3. _____

V. List three goals that you wish to accomplish this week:

    1. _____

    2. _____

    3. _____

Signature: _____ Date: _____

FIGURE 14D.1
Long- and short-range goals.

Keep a four to seven-day log, and record at half-hour intervals the activities you do (make additional copies of this form as needed). Record the activities as you go through your typical day, so you will remember them all. At the end of each day, decide when you wasted time. Using a highlighter, identify the time killers on this form and plan necessary changes for the next day.

6:00	
6:30	
7:00	
7:30	
8:00	
8:30	
9:00	
9:30	
10:00	
10:30	
11:00	
11:30	
12:00	
12:30	
1:00	
1:30	
2:00	
2:30	
3:00	
3:30	
4:00	
4:30	
5:00	
5:30	
6:00	
6:30	
7:00	
7:30	
8:00	
8:30	
9:00	
9:30	
10:00	
10:30	
11:00	
11:30	
12:00	

LAB 14D

FIGURE 14D.2
Finding your time killers.

Take a few minutes each Sunday night and write down the goals or tasks you wish to accomplish that week. As with your daily goals, rank them as top, medium, low, or "trash" priorities (Make as many copies of this form as needed). At the end of the week evaluate how well you accomplished your goals. Cross off the goals you accomplished and carry over to the next week those you did not get done.

Week: ____/____/199___ to ____/____/199___

Top Priority Goals
1. _____
2. _____
3. _____
4. _____

Medium Priority Goals
1. _____
2. _____
3. _____
4. _____

Low Priority Goals
1. _____
2. _____
3. _____
4. _____

Trash (do only after all other goals have been accomplished)
1. _____
2. _____
3. _____
4. _____

Take 10 minutes each morning and write down the goals or tasks you wish to accomplish that day. Rank them as top, medium, low, or "trash" priorities (Make as many copies of this form as needed). At the end of the day evaluate how well you accomplished your tasks for the day. Cross off the goals you accomplished and carry over to the next day those you did not get done.

Date: _____ Day of the Week: _____

Top Priority Goals
1. _____
2. _____
3. _____
4. _____

Medium Priority Goals
1. _____
2. _____
3. _____
4. _____

Low Priority Goals
1. _____
2. _____
3. _____
4. _____

Trash (do only after all other goals have been accomplished)
1. _____
2. _____
3. _____
4. _____

FIGURE 14D.3
Daily and weekly goals and priorities.

LAB 14D

On a weekly basis, go through the list of strategies given below and provide a "Yes" or "No" answer to each statement. If you are able to answer "Yes" to most questions, congratulations, you are becoming a good time manager.

Strategy　　　　　　　Date:																
1. I periodically evaluate my time killers																
2. I have written down my long-range goals																
3. I have written down my short-range goals																
4. I use a daily planner																
5. I conduct nightly audits																
6. I conduct weekly audits																
7. I delegate activities that others can do																
8. I have learned to say no to additional tasks when I am already in "overload"																
9. I plan activities to avoid boredom																
10. I plan ahead for distractions																
11. I work on one task at a time, until it's done																
12. I have removed distractions from my work																
13. I set aside "overtimes"																
14. I set aside special time for myself daily																
15. I reward myself for a job well done																

LAB 14D

FIGURE 14D.4
Time management evaluation.

LAB 14E STRESS MANAGEMENT TECHNIQUES

Name: _____ Date: _____ Grade: _____

Instructor: _____ Course: _____ Section: _____

NECESSARY LAB EQUIPMENT   None required.

OBJECTIVE   Students will participate in a stress management session.

INSTRUCTIONS   The class should be divided into groups of about five students per group. Each group should select and go through a minimum of two of the following stress management techniques outlined in Chapter 14:

1. Progressive Muscle Relaxation
2. Breathing Techniques for Relaxation
3. Autogenic Training
4. Meditation

A group leader is chosen who will lead the exercise according to the instructions provided for each relaxation technique in Chapter 14. Be sure that this experience is conducted in a comfortable room, as free of noise as possible. If trained personnel or a tape recording for progressive muscle relaxation exercises is available, the entire class may participate in this experience at once. Institutions that have biofeedback equipment may use it in this laboratory as well. Upon completion of this lab, answer the four questions given below.

I.   Indicate the two relaxation techniques used in your lab:

    A. _____

    B. _____

II. In your own words, relate your feelings as you were going through exercises A and B above:

    Exercise A: _____

    _____

    _____

    Exercise B: _____

    _____

    _____

III. Indicate how you felt mentally, emotionally, and physically after participating in this experience:

    _____

    _____

    _____

IV. Are there situations in your daily life where you feel that you would benefit as a result of practicing the selected stress management exercises? If so, indicate:

    _____

    _____

    _____

Behavioral Objectives for Stress Reduction and Personality Change

1. Do you currently perceive stress to be a problem in your life? _____ Yes _____ No

2. Do you experience any of the typical stress symptoms outlined in Figure 14.2? If so, list them.

   _____

   _____

3. Indicate any specific events in your life that trigger a stress response.

   _____

   _____

   _____

   _____

4. Write specific objectives to either avoid or help you manage the various stress-inducing events listed above, including one or more stress management techniques.

   _____

   _____

   _____

   _____

5. Are there any behavior patterns in your life that you would like to modify? List those that you would like to change.

   _____

   _____

   _____

   _____

LAB 14E

6. List specific steps that you will take to change undesirable behaviors.

   _____

   _____

   _____

   _____

LAB 15A   SMOKING CESSATION FORMS

Name: _____ Date: _____ Grade: _____

Instructor: _____ Course: _____ Section: _____

NECESSARY LAB EQUIPMENT   None required.

OBJECTIVE   To aid the participants in the development of a smoking cessation program either for themselves and/or friends and relatives.

INTRODUCTION   The forms given in Figures 15A.1 (Why-Do-You-Smoke Test), 15A.2 (Do You Want To Quit Test), and 15A.3 (Smoking vs Quitting Reasons) have been designed to help smokers identify reasons why they smoke and their readiness to initiate a smoking cessation program. These forms should be filled out prior to initiating a smoking cessation program. The interpretation of the results for Figures 15A.1 and 15A.2 are contained in Chapter 15. The daily cigarette smoking log given in Figure 15A.4 has been developed to assist smokers in getting to know their habit, helping them to cut down on cigarettes not really needed, and in finding positive substitutes when confronted with situations that trigger their desire to smoke.

	Always	Fre-quently	Occa-sionally	Seldom	Never
A. I smoke cigarettes in order to keep myself from slowing down.	5	4	3	2	1
B Handling a cigarette is part of the enjoyment of smoking it.	5	4	3	2	1
C. Smoking cigarettes is pleasant and relaxing.	5	4	3	2	1
D. I light up a cigarette when I feel angry about something.	5	4	3	2	1
E. When I have run out of cigarettes I find it almost unbearable until I can get them.	5	4	3	2	1
F. I smoke cigarettes automatically without even being aware of it.	5	4	3	2	1
G. I smoke cigarettes to stimulate me, to perk myself up.	5	4	3	2	1
H. Part of the enjoyment of smoking a cigarette comes from the steps I take to light up.	5	4	3	2	1
I. I find cigarettes pleasurable.	5	4	3	2	1
J. When I feel uncomfortable or upset about something, I light up a cigarette.	5	4	3	2	1
K. I am very much aware of the fact when I am not smoking a cigarette.	5	4	3	2	1
L I light up a cigarette without realizing I still have one burning in the ashtray.	5	4	3	2	1
M. I smoke cigarettes to give me a "lift."	5	4	3	2	1
N. When I smoke a cigarette, part of the enjoyment is watching the smoke as I exhale it.	5	4	3	2	1
O. I want a cigarette most when I am comfortable and relaxed.	5	4	3	2	1
P. When I feel "blue" or want to take my mind off cares and worries, I smoke cigarettes.	5	4	3	2	1
Q. I get a real gnawing hunger for a cigarette when I haven't smoked for a while.	5	4	3	2	1
R. I've found a cigarette in my mouth and didn't remember putting it there.	5	4	3	2	1

Scoring Your Test:

Enter the numbers you have circled on the test questions in the spaces provided below, putting the number you have circled to question A on line A, to question B on line B, etc. Add the three scores on each line to get a total for each factor. For example, the sum of your scores over lines A, G, and M gives you your score on "Stimulation," lines B, H, and N give the score on "Handling," etc. Scores can vary from 3 to 15. Any score 11 and above is high; any score 7 and below is low.

A _____ + G _____ + M _____ = _____ Stimulation
B _____ + H _____ + N _____ = _____ Handling
C _____ + I _____ + O _____ = _____ Pleasure Relaxation
D _____ + J _____ + P _____ = _____ Crutch: Tension Reduction
E _____ + K _____ + Q _____ = _____ Craving: Psychological Addiction
F _____ + L _____ + R _____ = _____ Habit

From *A Self-Test for Smokers*. U.S. Department of Health and Human Services, 1983.

*See Chapter 15 to interpret your test results

LAB 15A

FIGURE 15A.1
Why-Do-You-Smoke Test* (from *A Self-Test for Smokers*, U.S. Department of Health and Human Services, 1983).

	Strongly Agree	Mildly Agree	Mildly Disagree	Strongly Disagree
A. Cigarette smoking might give me a serious illness.	4	3	2	1
B. My cigarette smoking sets a bad example for others.	4	3	2	1
C. I find cigarette smoking to be a messy kind of habit.	4	3	2	1
D. Controlling my cigarette smoking is a challenge to me.	4	3	2	1
E. Smoking causes shortness of breath.	4	3	2	1
F If I quit smoking cigarettes it might influence others to stop.	4	3	2	1
G. Cigarettes cause damage to clothing and other personal property.	4	3	2	1
H. Quitting smoking would show that I have willpower.	4	3	2	1
I. My cigarette smoking will have a harmful effect on my health.	4	3	2	1
J. My cigarette smoking influences others close to me to take up or continue smoking.	4	3	2	1
K. If I quit smoking, my sense of taste or smell would improve.	4	3	2	1
L. I do not like the idea of feeling dependent on smoking.	4	3	2	1

Scoring Your Test:

Write the number you have circled after each statement on the test in the corresponding space to the right. Add the scores on each line to get your totals. For example, the sum of your scores A, E, I gives you your score for the health factor. Scores can vary from 3 to 12. Any score of 9 or over is high; and score 6 or under is low.

```
A _____ + E _____ + I _____ = _____   Health
B _____ + F _____ + J _____ = _____   Example
C _____ + G _____ + K _____ = _____   Aesthetics
D _____ + H _____ + L _____ = _____   Mastery
```

From *A Self-Test for Smokers*. U.S. Department of Health and Human Services, 1983.

*See Chapter 15 to interpret your test results

FIGURE 15A.2
Do You Want To Quit Test* (from *A Self-Test for Smokers*, U.S. Department of Health and Human Services, 1983).

Name:_____ Date:_____

Reasons for Smoking Cigarettes

1. _____
2. _____
3. _____
4. _____
5. _____
6. _____
7. _____
8. _____

Reasons for Quitting Cigarette Smoking

1. _____
2. _____
3. _____
4. _____
5. _____
6. _____
7. _____
8. _____

FIGURE 15A.3
Smoking versus quitting reasons.

LAB
15A

Today's Date: _____ Quit Date: _____ Decision Date: _____

Cigarettes to be Smoked Today: _____ Brand:_____

No.	Time	Activity	Rating[a]	Amount Smoked[b]	Remarks/Substitutes

1. _____

2. _____

3. _____

4. _____

5. _____

6. _____

7. _____

8. _____

9. _____

10. _____

11. _____

12. _____

13. _____

14. _____

15. _____

16. _____

17. _____

18. _____

19. _____

20. _____

Additional comments, list of friends and/or activities to avoid

_____

_____

_____

_____

_____

_____

[a]Rating: 1 = desperately needed, 2 = moderately needed, 3 = no real need

[b]Amount Smoked: entire cigarette, two-thirds, half, etc.

FIGURE 15A.3
Daily cigarette smoking log.

LAB
15A

ALCOHOL ABUSE: ARE YOU DRINKING TOO MUCH?*

Name: _____ Date: _____ Grade: _____

Instructor: _____ Course: _____ Section: _____

NECESSARY LAB EQUIPMENT None required.

OBJECTIVE To determine possible addiction to alcohol.

INTRODUCTION The following questionnaire is for your own personal information. Answer all questions on a separate sheet of paper and keep that sheet for yourself. Only turn in this page to your instructor as proof that you have read and completed the questionnaire.

ALCOHOL ABUSE: ARE YOU DRINKING TOO MUCH?*

1. When you are holding an empty glass at a party, do you always actively look for a refill instead of waiting to be offered one?
2. If given the chance, do you frequently pour out a more generous drink for yourself than seems to be the "going" amount for others?
3. Do you often have a drink or two when you are alone, either at home or in a bar?
4. Is your drinking ever the direct cause of a family quarrel, or do quarrels often seem to occur, if only by coincidence, when you have had a drink or two?
5. Do you feel that you must have a drink at a specific time every day — right after work, for instance?
6. When worried or under unusual stress, do you almost automatically take a stiff drink to "settle your nerves?"
7. Are you untruthful about how much you have had to drink when questioned on the subject?
8. Does drinking ever cause you to take time off work, or to miss scheduled meetings or appointments?
9. Do you feel physically deprived if you cannot have at least one drink every day?
10. Do you sometimes crave a drink in the morning?
11. Do you sometimes have "mornings after" when you cannot remember what happened the night before?

Evaluation

You should regard a "yes" answer to any one of the above questions as a warning sign. Do not increase your consumption of alcohol. Two "yes" answers suggest that you may already be becoming dependent on alcohol. Three or more "yes" answers indicate that you may have a serious problem, and you should get professional help. Also refer to Chapter 16 for general guidelines to cut down your drinking.

------

*Reproduced with permission from *Family Medical Guide* by The American Medical Association. New York: Random House, 1982.

LAB 16B ADDICTIVE BEHAVIOR QUESTIONNAIRE

Name: _____ Date: _____ Grade: _____

Instructor: _____ Course: _____ Section: _____

NECESSARY LAB EQUIPMENT None required.

OBJECTIVE To determine possible addiction to narcotics.

INTRODUCTION The following questionnaire is for your own personal information. Answer all questions on a separate sheet of paper and keep that sheet for yourself. Only turn in this page to your instructor as proof that you have read and completed the questionnaire.

COULD YOU BE AN ADDICT?*

Directions

The following test, designed by Dr. Lawrence J. Hatterer, is not a way to diagnose whether you are in the early, middle, or chronic stage of addictive disease. It is merely meant to help you understand addictive behavior better so you can recognize it in yourself or perhaps in people you know.

1. I am a person of excesses. I can't regulate what I do for pleasure, and often use a substance or indulge in an activity heavily, in order to get high.
2. I am an extremely self-involved person. People tell me that I am into myself too much.
3. I am compulsive. I must have what I want when I want it, regardless of the consequences.
4. I am excessively dependent on or independent of others.
5. I am preoccupied. I spend a lot of time thinking or fantasizing about a particular activity or substance. Also, I will work my day around doing it or go to pains to make sure it's available.
6. I deny that I do this and lie about it to others who ask me.
7. I have been involved in this behavior for at least one year.
8. I've told myself I could easily stop, even though I've shown no signs of slowing down.
9. Once I start indulging in this behavior or substance, I find I have trouble stopping.
10. One or more members of my family are also involved in some kind of excessive behavior or substance abuse.
11. I find I gravitate mostly toward people who have the same behavior or take the same substance as I.
12. I seem to be developing a tolerance of the behavior or substance. I have had a need to steadily increase the amounts I take or the time I spend doing it.
13. I have found that my excessive use of highs has, in fact, only made my problems worse.
14. If someone tries to keep me from obtaining the substance or practicing the activity, I get angry and reject or abuse them.
15. I experience withdrawal symptoms if I cannot indulge in the substance or activity.
16. This has gotten in the way of my functioning. I have missed something important — days at work, time with my friends, family, children — because of it.
17. The substance/activity is destroying my home life. I know I am hurting those closest to me.

---

*Reprinted with permission from *McCall's Magazine*, November 1986.

18. I have failed in many goals in life, lost money, given up many social and occupational contacts, all because of my excessive behavior.

19. I have tried to stop or cut down on my excesses but have been unsuccessful.

20. I have physically endangered myself or others in accidents that were a direct result of my excessive behavior.

Evaluation

If you answer "yes" to one half or more of the questions, you may have a problem with addictive disease and should seek immediate professional help. For a referral, contact your local mental health clinic (look in the Yellow Pages) or speak to your doctor.

LAB 16C   SELF-QUIZ ON HIV AND AIDS

Name: _____ Date: _____ Grade: _____

Instructor: _____ Course: _____ Section: _____

NECESSARY LAB EQUIPMENT   None required.

OBJECTIVE   To evaluate basic understanding of AIDS.

INSTRUCTION   Please answer all of the following questions.

	Yes	No
1. AIDS or Acquired Immunodeficiency Syndrome, is the end stage of infection caused by the Human Immunodeficiency Virus or HIV.	_____	_____
2. HIV is a chronic infectious disease that spreads among individuals who choose to engage in risky behavior such as unprotected sex or the sharing of hypodermic needles.	_____	_____
3. There is a cure for AIDS.	_____	_____
4. Abstaining from sex is the only 100 percent sure way to protect yourself from HIV infection.	_____	_____
5. Using drugs and alcohol can make you willing to have sex when you really don't plan to.	_____	_____
6. Condoms are 100 percent effective in protecting you against HIV infection.	_____	_____
7. Using drugs and alcohol makes a person less likely to use a condom and use it correctly.	_____	_____
8. If you're sexually active, latex condoms provide the best protection against HIV infection.	_____	_____
9. Using drugs and alcohol can make you more likely to have unplanned and unprotected sex.	_____	_____
10. Each year more and more teens are getting infected with HIV.	_____	_____
11. You can become HIV infected by donated blood.	_____	_____
12. You can tell by looking at someone if he/she is HIV infected.	_____	_____
13. The only means to determine whether someone has HIV is through an HIV antibody test.	_____	_____
14. HIV can completely destroy the immune system.	_____	_____
15. The HIV virus may live in the body 10 years or longer before AIDS symptoms may develop.	_____	_____
16. People infected with HIV have AIDS.	_____	_____
17. Once infected with HIV, a person never becomes uninfected.	_____	_____
18. HIV infection is preventable.	_____	_____

LAB 16C

Selected items on this questionnaire are adapted from *Test Your Survival Smarts: Self-Quiz on Drugs and AIDS*. National Institute on Drug Abuse, U.S. Department of Health & Human Services.

Answers:

1. Yes. AIDS is the term used to define the manifestation of opportunistic diseases and cancers that occur as a result of HIV infection (also referred to as HIV disease).

2. Yes. People do not get HIV because of who they are, but because of what they do. Almost all of the people who get HIV do so because they choose to engage in risky behaviors.

3. No. There is no cure for AIDS and there doesn't appear to be one in the foreseeable future.

4. Yes. Abstinence will protect you from HIV infection. But you may still get the disease by sharing hypodermic needles.

5. Yes. When you use alcohol or drugs, you can forget what you know about safe sex, and do things that you normally wouldn't do. If you're drunk or high, you might have sex even though you really don't plan to.

6. No. Only abstaining from sex gives you 100 percent protection, but condoms are very effective in protecting against HIV infection if they're used correctly.

7. Yes. Teens who are drunk or high are less likely to use condoms because, under the influence, they forget or feel that nothing "bad" can happen.

8. Yes. Proper use, however, is necessary to minimize the risk of infection.

9. Yes. Otherwise prudent people often act irrationally and engage in risky behaviors when they are under the influence of drugs and alcohol.

10. Yes. In the early 90s, the number of infected teens increased by 96% over a short span of two years. One reason for the increase may be that teens who are under the influence of drugs or alcohol often engage in risky sex. It is believed that about 20% of the AIDS patients today were infected as teenagers.

11. No. A myth regarding HIV is that it can be transmitted by donating blood. People cannot get HIV from giving blood. A brand new needle is used by health professionals every time blood is taken out. These needles are only used once and are destroyed and thrown away immediately after each individual has donated blood.

12. No. The symptoms of AIDS are often not noticeable until several years after a person has been infected with HIV. That's why, no matter who your partner is, it's important to always protect yourself against HIV and the risk of developing AIDS — either by abstaining from sex or by using condoms if you decide to have sex.

13. Yes. Not you, not a nurse, not even a doctor can tell; unless an HIV antibody test is done. Upon HIV infection, the immune system's line of defense against the virus is the formation of antibodies that bind to the virus. On the average it takes three months for the body to manufacture enough antibodies so as to show positive in an HIV antibody test. Sometimes it may take six months or longer.

14. Yes. The virus multiplies, attacks, and destroys white blood cells. These cells are part of the immune system and their function is to fight off infections and diseases in the body. As the number of white blood cells killed increases, the body's immune system gradually breaks down or may be completely destroyed.

15. Yes. Up to 10 years may go by before the person develops AIDS.

16. No. Being HIV positive does not necessarily mean that the person has AIDS. On the average, it takes 7 to 8 years following infection before the individual develops the symptoms that fit the case definition of AIDS. From that point on, the person may live another 2 to 3 years. In essence, from the point of infection, the individual may endure a chronic disease for 8 to 10 years.

17. Yes. There is no second chance. Everyone must protect him or herself against HIV infection.

18. Yes. The best prevention technique is abstaining from sex until the time comes for a mutually monogamous sexual relationship. That is, two people have sexual relationships only with each other. That one behavior, according to Dr. James Mason, director of the Centers for Disease Control in Atlanta, will almost completely remove you from any risk of HIV infection or developing any other sexually transmitted disease.

LAB 17A HEALTH PROTECTION PLAN FOR ENVIRONMENTAL HAZARDS, CRIME PREVENTION, AND PERSONAL SAFETY*

Name: _____ Date: _____ Grade: _____

Instructor: _____ Course: _____ Section: _____

NECESSARY LAB EQUIPMENT None required.

OBJECTIVE To educate regarding accident prevention and personal safety.

INTRODUCTION The questionnaire used in this lab has been developed to raise awareness of factors that help prevent accidents and increase personal safety. Answer each question carefully and read the respective information on "risk factors" and "awareness counts." Keep in mind that you control most actions in your life, and by following the recommendations given, you can further enhance your personal safety and well-being. After completing the questionnaire, briefly state changes that you need to implement in your life to minimize personal risk.

1. Personal Environment:

   _____

   _____

   _____

   _____

2. Crime Prevention:

   _____

   _____

   _____

   _____

3. Personal Safety:

   _____

   _____

   _____

   _____

*Questionnaire published by the Preventive Medicine Institute/Strang Clinic. New York, 1982. Reproduced with permission.

Personal Environment In addition to environmental

problems in the community at large there are also important problems
in our own immediate environment that affect our health, well-being, and comfort.
These are problems we can control and improve ourselves.
The following self-assessment relates to environmental hazards dealing
with water, wastes, noise and air pollution in our everyday lives.
All "no" answers are a cue to ACTION.

Concerning AIR POLLUTION, do you...?	YES	NO
...Know the optimal conditions for temperature, humidity and air movement in your home?	○	○
...Change the air filters once a year in your air conditioners or forced air heating systems?	○	○
...Are your work areas ventilated so that fumes and dusts do not accumulate?	○	○
...Do your throat or nasal passages feel moist and clear in the morning (not dry or stuffy)?	○	○
...Know what to do when the weather report says the quality of the air is unsatisfactory?	○	○
...Know what a "killer smog" is?	○	○
...If you smoke, do you avoid smoking in a bedroom or areas where children play?	○	○

RISK FACTORS:

- *Bronchitis, asthma, emphysema, and heart disease are all aggravated by air pollution.*
- *Chronic exposure to dusts of metal or wood are risk factors for cancer of the respiratory passages.*
- *Children of cigarette smokers have a higher than usual incidence of respiratory infections.*
- *Many so-called allergies of the sinuses and upper respiratory tract are really due to air pollution.*

AWARENESS COUNTS:

- **The optimal air comfort levels are 66-68°F temperature, 30-40% humidity, and air movement at 20-50 feet per minute. Lower humidity will lead to dryness of the respiratory passages, increase skin evaporation and make your home feel colder than it is.**
- **When the air quality is reported as "unsatisfactory" people with heart and lung disease should stay indoors.**
- **"Killer smog" refers to trapped air which cannot rise, with no available dispersing breeze, which accumulates industrial, auto and heating combustion products into a suffocating density. This may be fatal to those with cardiopulmonary disease, and uncomfortable for everyone.**

LAB 17A

Concerning WATER...?	YES	NO
...Have you checked your home drinking water in the last year for clarity, color and taste?	○	○
...If you shake up a glass of tap water does it remain clear (not foamy or frothy)?	○	○
...Do you have a screen filter on your water tap?	○	○
...Do you check restaurant water and ice for clarity and cleanliness?	○	○
...Do you know the common water-borne diseases?	○	○
...Do you know what kind of water purification tablets are best for traveling?	○	○
...Do you take care when traveling in developing countries or in unsettled areas to drink bottled water, or coffee, tea, or soup made with boiling water, and to avoid ice cubes?	○	○
...Do you think all wilderness water is safe?	○	○
...Do you know what source of water is almost always safe to drink?	○	○

Concerning WASTE…?	YES	NO
…Do you place ordinary kitchen waste in plastic bags for disposal?	○	○
…Do you know what kinds of wastes require special handling?	○	○
…Are your garbage cans free from bad odors?	○	○
…Is your sink or toilet bowl free from bad odors or back up of waste water in your drain?	○	○
…If you live in a home with a septic tank do you know its location?	○	○
…Do you know the last time the septic tank was cleaned?	○	○

RISK FACTORS: WATER AND WASTE

- *Diseases associated with water and waste include: typhoid fever, cholera, hepatitis, poliomyelitis, E. coli dysentery and amoebic dysentery.*
- *Very hard water containing large amounts of magnesium can cause diarrhea in children. It is difficult to wash with, and will cause deposits in water pipes.*
- *Chlorine is commonly used for water purification. An excess is harmful since it may be converted into chloroform, a toxic chemical.*
- *The presence of water supplies in proximity to industrial plants is a cause for concern since there are many instances of toxic chemicals leaking into local water supplies in this country.*

AWARENESS COUNTS: WATER

- All water taps should have screen filters to trap particulate material which may accidentally enter the water supply. These should be removed and cleaned regularly.
- Frothy water is due to detergents leaking into the water supply and this can cause intestinal upsets.
- Cloudy water may be due only to rusty pipes and while it may stain kitchen utensils it is not harmful; but turbid water with an odor may be due to seepage of sewage or industrial wastes into the water supply and this can be dangerous to health. Every state has a water supply agency that can give you information on the condition of your local water supply. However, if your water comes from a well, no one is checking it for purity. You must take the initiative and find out from the state agency how this can be done.
- The best type of water purification tablets is the iodine-releasing variety rather than the chlorine type. These are obtainable from your local pharmacy. Use these only if traveling in an area where bottled water is not available.
- Not all wilderness water is pure. It may come from springs which have toxic chemicals, or be contaminated by animal use upstream. If purified water is not available, the safest water to drink is rain water. (Make sure it is stored in a clean container.)

AWARENESS COUNTS: WASTE

- Plastic bags for disposal of ordinary wastes have the advantage of keeping your garbage containers, indoor and outdoor, clean and free of odors. This helps prevent fly, roach, and rodent infestation, and the accidental contamination of food.
- Aerosol cans, solvents, and fuels should not be placed in plastic bags, and should not be disposed of with household wastes because of the hazards of fire and explosion; your local waste disposal service should be contacted regarding special handling.
- Bad odors or backup of waste water into your sink, tub, or toilet is a serious matter since this is untreated sewage and poses a health hazard. There may be an obstruction in the sewage system; check with your plumber first. If you have a septic tank, it may have to be cleaned. The frequency of cleaning of septic tanks depends on size and use. Three to four years of regular use is an average duration of time before cleaning is necessary.
- It's important to know the location of your septic tank and also those of your neighbors in relationship to your well water supply. There should be a distance of 100 feet between the septic tank and well. Your board of health can give you additional information about specific conditions in your area.

LAB
17A

Concerning NOISE...?	YES	NO
...Do you know how to tell if you are in an environment which could damage your hearing?	○	○
...Do you know that permanent hearing loss can occur with a single exposure to a painfully loud noise?	○	○
...Are you aware of the other effects on your health that noise can have other than hearing loss?	○	○
...Do you know the accidents that can occur due to noise causing "warning concealment"?	○	○
...Are you aware of "slow reaction time" as a noise associated danger?	○	○
... Do you know what age group is especially susceptible to noise induced hearing loss?	○	○

RISK FACTORS:

NOISE

- *Noise hazards can lead not only to permanent hearing damage, but it has been established that noise can cause personality disorders, increase aggressive behavior and have an aggravating effect on headaches, hypertension, and peptic ulcers. It also lowers work efficiency and interferes with sleep patterns.*

AWARENESS COUNTS:

- *If you are in a noisy environment several hours a day where you have to raise your voice to be heard, you are in an area of potential danger for hearing loss. Noise that is painfully loud, such as pneumatic hammers or amplified rock music, has the greatest potential to damage hearing.*

- *The age group in which there is particular susceptibility to hearing loss is adolescence.*

- *It is particularly important to sleep in a quiet environment; use rugs, drapes, double windows, and finally ear plugs if necessary, to obliterate disturbing sound. (Cotton makes a poor plug unless saturated with wax or vaseline. Sponge plastic ear plugs are better.)*

- *Pleasant background music can sometimes be used to mask disturbing sounds. However, background noise can conceal safety warnings, or lead to slow reaction time and thus contribute to accidents.*

FOLLOW-THROUGH

For information on all environmental hazards, write to:
The U.S. Environmental Protection Agency
Office of Public Affairs (A-107) Washington, D.C. 20460

For information about noise hazards, write to:
The National Information Center for Quiet
P.O. Box 57171 Washington, D.C. 20037

LAB 17A

Crime Prevention *Through your own efforts, you can learn to reduce the opportunity and temptation for the criminal by accepting the responsibility to do everything possible for the protection of your personal well being and property. All "no" answers are a cue to ACTION.*

To protect yourself, do you…?	YES	NO
…Always us a peephole or chain lock to identify your visitor?	○	○
…Watch out for suspicious people or cars in your neighborhood?	○	○
…Make an effort to get better acquainted with your neighbors, especially if you live in a large apartment building?	○	○
…Avoid resisting the orders of a robber or purse snatcher?	○	○
…List only your last name and initials in the phone directory and on the mailbox?	○	○
…Always lock your doors during the day, even if you are at home?	○	○
…Leave lights on doors you will be using when you return after dark?	○	○
…Always have your key in your hand when you return home so you can open the door immediately?	○	○

RISK FACTORS:
PROTECTING YOURSELF

- *Women alone and the elderly are at highest risk at being victims of crime.*

- *People who are disabled are more vulnerable to crime.*

- *Certain areas of every large city are high crime areas and should be avoided if possible.*

AWARENESS COUNTS:

- **List only your last name and initial in the phone directory and on the mailbox, particularly if you are a woman living alone.**
- **Always have your key ready when you return home.**
- **Always ask a visitor to identify himself before you let him in.**
- **Use automatic timers to turn on lights, radio, etc.**
- **If a window or lock has been forced or broken while you were out, use a neighbor's phone to call the police and wait outside until they arrive.**
- **Be cautious of unidentified phone callers. Hang up immediately if the caller will not identify himself.**
- **When traveling about at night, try to have a companion with you.**
- **Remember to ask for identification *before* you let repairmen, meter readers, or any other stranger into your home.**

To protect yourself, do you…?	YES	NO
…Make specal plans for your home when you are away on vacation?	○	○
…Avoid leaving a key under the doormat or in any accessible area?	○	○
…Have you made sure that your door (s) have sturdy locks?	○	○
…Check all windows and doors regularly for security?	○	○
…Stop newspaper and milk deliveries when you go on vacation?	○	○
…Keep especially valuable items in a safety deposit box away from home?	○	○

RISK FACTORS:
PROTECTING YOUR HOME

- Those at higher risk of home crime are people who leave their homes unattended for long periods of time and those who are nighttime travellers.
- Most crime takes place under cover of darkness.
- Letting mail and newspapers accumulate at your door announces the vulnerability of your home.

AWARENESS COUNTS:

- **Keep your doors locked at all times.**
- **Have lights on an automatic timer while you are away.**
- **An alarm system is a useful crime deterrent.**
- **Make sure windows are secured.**
- **Make sure doorways and hallways are well lighted.**
- **Leave a radio on (a radio uses little electricity and gives the impression that your home is occupied).**

About Locks: Doors should be equipped with either a drop-bolt or dead-bolt lock. Do not use spring locks on any outside door. Spring locks work simply by closing the door and can be easily opened with a plastic card. Drop-bolt or dead-bolt locks can only be unlocked with a key.

FOLLOW-THROUGH

Check with your local police department about joining the Operation Identification Program. You are provided with a sticker to display on your home and your valuable property is engraved with a non-removable code number. The police have a registered list of this property and statistics show that burglars avoid such homes because marked items are difficult to dispose of. Many police departments have crime prevention units and will give you personal advice.

Many states make available the Federal Crime Insurance Program – it provides federal crime insurance against burglary and robbery losses – rates depend upon the crime rate in the area where your home is located. For more information write to:

Federal Crime Insurance, P.O. Box 11033
Washington, D.C. 20014 Toll Free (800) 638-8780

Review your homeowner's insurance coverage to make sure you have adequate coverage.

LAB
17A

Personal Safety

While not all accidents are preventable, many are. Failure to take simple precautionary measures increases the risk of an avoidable accident. See if you can identify safety problem areas. All "yes" answers are a cue to Action.

Concerning PERSONAL SAFETY,	YES	NO
...Have you had any accidents in the past years which could have been prevented?	○	○
...If yes, where did this occur? at home?	○	○
in your automobile?	○	○
at work?	○	○

To ensure your SAFETY AT HOME,	YES	NO
...Do you fail to go through your dwelling, room by room, deliberately looking for safety hazards once a year?	○	○
...Does your dwelling have fewer than two means of escape in the event of an emergency?	○	○

	YES	NO
...If you smoke, do you ever smoke in bed?	○	○
...Do you fail to keep a first aid kit, smoke alarm and fire extinguisher at home?	○	○
...Are there loose electrical wiring or fixtures around your home?	○	○
...Are carpets put down without non-skid backings?	○	○
...Are poisons and pills in areas within reach of pre-school children?	○	○

In the BATHROOM, do you fail to...	YES	NO
...Check the temperature of bath or shower water with your hand first?	○	○
...Make sure electrical appliances are never used near water?	○	○
...Use non-skid paste-ons or rubber mats for bathtub and shower surfaces?	○	○

In the KITCHEN, do you fail to...	YES	NO
...Store knives with points away from the hand, or in special holders?	○	○
...Keep curtains away from the cooking range?	○	○
...Keep electrical appliances away from water?	○	○
...Keep floors clean of grease and dirt?	○	○
...Are you currently exposed to any of the material listed below?	○	○
dust (such as wood, leather, heavy metals, dyestuff)?	○	○
petroleum products?	○	○
radiation?	○	○
solvents?	○	○
...If yes to any of the above...was your exposure usually indoors?	○	○

	YES	NO
...Did your exposure occur for an equivalent of at least one eight hour day per week for a period of five years?	○	○
...If yes to dust, chemicals or petroleum products, was your skin or clothing regularly contacted by these materials?	○	○

To ensure your SAFETY IN YOUR AUTOMOBILE, do you...?	YES	NO
...Neglect to <u>always</u> fasten your seat belts?	○	○
...Ever drink alcoholic beverages before driving?	○	○
...Drive even when you are sleepy?	○	○
...Drive more than <u>40%</u> of the time in the dark?	○	○
...Have you received more than <u>one</u> moving traffic violation this past year?	○	○
...Have you had more than <u>one</u> accident this past year?	○	○

RISK FACTORS: PERSONAL SAFETY

- *Accidents are the leading cause of death among those under 44 years old.*
- *Accidents are the fourth most common cause of death in this country ranking behind heart disease, cancer and stroke.*

AWARENESS COUNTS:

- It is especially important that potential problem areas at home, on the road, and at work be identified so that you can create a relatively accident free environment. Improving your accident-prone behavior is the only way to decrease your risk of accidents.
- Your home or apartment should be regularly checked for safety hazards: ■ Slippery stairways ■ Unfastened carpets ■ Faulty fixtures or outlets ■ Store poisons, firearms in safe place ■ Have safety guard rails on upper level windows ■ Place smoke detectors in strategic areas ■ Have emergency numbers posted by the phone ■ Fire strikes more than 1,500 homes every day.
- Automobile accidents take more lives each year than any other type of accident or illness. Many of these can be prevented: ■ Make sure your car is in safe running condition, especially brakes and tires ■ Wear seat belts at <u>all</u> times. ■ Never drive while drinking. ■ Never drive while sleepy. ■ Always lock your car.

To ensure your SAFETY AT WORK,	YES	NO	
...Does your place of work fail to have regular safety checks?	○	○	
...Does your place of work fail to have regular emergency drills such as fire drills?	○	○	
...Does your place of work fail to have a current fire emergency plan?	○	○	
...Does your place of work fail to have rules governing the use of machinery and protective equipment?	○	○	
...Have you ever worked at a job where you were exposed to: asbestos? ○○ chemicals? ○○ coal dust? ○○			

RISK FACTORS:

SAFETY AT WORK

- *13,000 accidental deaths per year occur on the job and over 2 million people are disabled or injured.*
- *Almost 30 billion dollars per year and about 25 million work days are lost due to accidents at work.*

AWARENESS COUNTS:

- Know where fire extinguishers are located.
- Is there a fire emergency plan in your office?
- Know the mandatory safety standards which apply to your business or industry.
- Use all protective clothing required.
- Know the names and hazards of <u>all</u> materials you are exposed to.

FOLLOW-THROUGH

For information regarding safety procedures and requirements <u>on the job</u> write to:
The U.S. Department of Labor, Washington, D.C. 20212
Or get in touch with the Department of Labor office in your region. Or write to:
The National Institute for Occupational Safety and Health, Post Office Building, Cincinnati, Ohio 45202
For information regarding the safety of consumer products, write to:
U.S. Consumer Product Safety Commission Office of Washington, D.C. 20207
For information regarding all kinds of accidents, write to:
The National Safety Council, 444 N. Michigan Avenue, Chicago, Illinois 60611

Preventive Medicine Institute /Strang Clinic 55 East 34 Street • New York, N.Y. 10016 • (212) 683-1000

LAB
17A

LAB 17B THE PREVENTION INDEX

Name: _____ Date: _____ Grade: _____

Instructor: _____ Course: _____ Section: _____

NECESSARY LAB EQUIPMENT None required.

OBJECTIVE To determine your personal prevention index based on the 21 most significant health promoting behaviors.

PREPARATION The Prevention Index is an annual measure of the effort Americans are making to prevent disease and accidents and to promote good health and longevity. Prior to completing this questionnaire, read the section on The Prevention Index contained in Chapter 17

Please carefully check "YES" or "NO" to each of the following questions.

Yes No

☐ ☐ 1 Do you have a blood pressure reading at least once a year?

☐ ☐ 2. Do you go to the dentist at least once a year for treatment or a checkup?

☐ ☐ 3. Avoid eating too much salt or sodium?

☐ ☐ 4. Avoid eating too much fat?

☐ ☐ 5. Eat enough fiber from whole grains, cereals, fruits, and vegetables?

☐ ☐ 6. Avoid eating too many high cholesterol foods, such as eggs, dairy products, and fatty meats?

☐ ☐ 7. Get enough vitamins and minerals in your diet?

☐ ☐ 8. Avoid getting too much sugar and sweet food?

☐ ☐ 9. Is your body weight within the recommended range for your sex, height, and bone structure?

☐ ☐ 10. Do you exercise strenuously (that is, so you breathe heavily and your heart and pulse rate are accelerated for a period lasting at least 20 minutes) three days or more a week?

☐ ☐ 11. Do you smoke cigarettes now?

☐ ☐ 12. Do you consciously take steps to control or reduce stress in your life?

☐ ☐ 13. Do you usually sleep a total of 7 to 8 hours during each 24-hour day? (if you usually sleep either more or less than this, please mark "no".)

☐ ☐ 14. Do you socialize with close friends, relatives or neighbors at least once a week?

☐ ☐ 15. In general, when you drink alcoholic beverages, do you consume less than 14 drinks per week and less than two on any single day? (Mark "yes" only if the answer to both parts of this question is "yes". If you never drink at all, also mark "yes". A "drink" means a drink with a shot of hard liquor, a can or bottle of beer, or a glass of wine.)

☐ ☐ 16. Do you wear a seat belt all the time when you are in the front seat of a car?

☐ ☐ 17. Do you drive at or below the speed limit all the time? (If you don't drive, please mark "yes".)

☐ ☐ 18. Do you ever drive after drinking? (If you don't drink, please mark "no".)

*The Prevention Index: A Louis Harris & Associates, Inc. survey conducted for Prevention Magazine.

LAB
17B

Yes No

☐   ☐   19. Do you have a smoke detector in your home?

☐   ☐   20. Does anyone in your household smoke in bed?

☐   ☐   21. Do you take any special steps or precautions to avoid accidents in and around your home?

Interpreting The Prevention Index (PI)

The correct answer for questions 11, 18, and 20 is "no." The correct answer for all other questions is "yes." Add up your total number of correct responses. Then, divide that number by 21 to obtain the percentage of the 21 Prevention Index behaviors that you practice.

$$PI = \frac{\text{Number of correct answers}}{21} =$$

RATINGS

Prevention Index	Category
90>	Excellent
70-89	Good
60-69	Average
<59	Poor

LAB 17C — SELF-EVALUATION AND BEHAVIORAL OBJECTIVES FOR THE FUTURE

Name: _____ Date: _____ Grade: _____

Instructor: _____ Course: _____ Section: _____

NECESSARY LAB EQUIPMENT None required, unless fitness tests are repeated.

OBJECTIVE To conduct a self-evaluation of the objectives achieved during this course and write behavioral objectives for the future.

LAB PREPARATION Read the section on self-evaluation and behavioral objectives for the future given in Chapter 17. If time allows and technicians are available, repeat the assessments for the health-related components of physical fitness.

PART A: Self-Evaluation

In this first part you will conduct a self-evaluation of the objectives that you accomplished in this course. To carry out this assignment, you will need to review the objectives written in previous laboratories. If you were able to repeat the various assessments, you can objectively indicate if your objectives were met. If you were unable to conduct the reassessments, subjectively determine how well you reached your objectives (only answer the "yes" or "no" questions under number 1 below).

1. Did you accomplish your objective for:

   Cardiovascular Endurance (see Lab 5A)   _____ Yes _____ No

   Pre-assessment Max. VO_2: _____ ml/kg/min   Fitness Classification: _____

   Post-assessment Max. VO_2: _____ ml/kg/min   Fitness Classification: _____

   Body Composition (see Labs 3A and 3B)   _____ Yes _____ No

   Pre-assessment Percent Body Fat: _____   Body Composition Classification: _____

   Post-assessment Percent Body Fat: _____   Body Composition Classification: _____

   Muscular Strength and Endurance (see Lab 7A)   _____ Yes _____ No

   Pre-assessment Percentile Rank: _____   Fitness Classification: _____

   Post-assessment Percentile Rank: _____   Fitness Classification: _____

   Muscular Flexibility (see Lab 9A)   _____ Yes _____ No

   Pre-assessment Percentile Rank: _____   Fitness Classification: _____

   Post-assessment Percentile Rank: _____   Fitness Classification: _____

2. Indicate nutritional and dietary changes that you were able to implement this semester (refer to Chapters 2 and 4 and Labs 2A, 2B, 4A, and 4B).

   _____

   _____

   _____

3. Did you implement your regular exercise program as outlined in Labs 4B, 6C, 8A, 10A, and Chapters 6, 8, and 10?

   _____

4. Indicate any lifestyle changes that you were able to make that will decrease your personal risk for cardiovascular disease and cancer. (Including stress management and smoking cessation. Refer also to Labs 12A, 13A, and 13C).

_____

_____

_____

5. Briefly evaluate this course and indicate whether it has had an effect on the quality of your life and your personal well-being.

_____

_____

_____

_____

PART B: Behavioral Objectives for the Future

Using the Wellness Compass, rate yourself for each component and plan objectives for the future according to the following instructions:

1. Color in red a number from five to one to indicate where you stood on each component at the beginning of the semester (five = poor rating, one = excellent or ideal rating).

2. Color in blue a second number from five to one to indicate where you stand on each component at the present time.

3. Select one or two components that you intend to work on in the next two months. Start with components where you feel you will have a high chance for success. Color in yellow the intended objective (number) to accomplish by the end of the two months. Once you achieve your objective, you may later color another number, also in yellow, to indicate your next objective.

Indicate below one or two general objectives that you will work on in the next couple of months and write specific behavioral objectives that you will use to accomplish each general objective (you may not need eight specific objectives, only write as many as you need).

General Objective: _____

Specific Objectives:

1. _____
2. _____
3. _____
4. _____
5. _____
6. _____
7. _____
8. _____

General Objective: _____

Specific Objectives:

1. _____
2. _____
3. _____
4. _____
5. _____
6. _____
7. _____
8. _____

LAB 17C

FIGURE 17A-1
The Wellness Compass.

Nutritive Value of Selected Foods

APPENDIX

A

Code	Food	Amount	Weight gm	Calories	Protein gm	Fat gm	Sat. Fat gm	Cholesterol mg	Carbohydrate gm	Calcium mg	Iron mg	Sodium mg	Vit A I.U.	Thiamin (Vit B₁) mg	Riboflavin (Vit B₂) mg	Niacin mg	Vit C mg
1.	Almond Joy, candy bar	1.5 oz.	42	227	2.5	12	10.2	0	28	3	1.2	0	0	0.00	0.00	0.0	0
2.	Almonds, shelled	1/4 c	36	213	6.6	19	1.4	0	9	83	1.7	2	0	0.09	0.33	1.3	0
3.	Apple, raw, unpared	1 med	150	80	0.3	1	0.0	0	20	10	0.4	1	120	0.04	0.03	0.1	6
4.	Apple juice, canned or bottled	1/2 c	124	59	0.1	0	0.0	0	15	8	0.7	1	0	0.01	0.03	0.1	1
5.	Apple Pie, McDonald's	1	307	260	2	15	10.0	6	30	0	0.48	240	0	0.06	0	0	12
6.	Applesauce, canned, sweetened	1/2 c	128	116	0.3	0	0.0	0	31	5	0.7	3	50	0.02	0.01	0.0	2
7.	Apricots, canned, heavy syrup liq.	3 halves; 1¼ tbsp liq.	85	73	0.5	0	0.0	0	19	9	0.3	1	1,480	0.02	0.02	0.3	3
8.	Apricots, dried, sulfured, uncooked	10 med halves	35	91	1.8	0	0.0	0	23	23	1.9	9	3,820	0.00	0.06	1.2	4
9.	Apricots, raw	3 (12 per lb)	114	55	1.1	0	0.0	0	14	18	0.5	1	2,890	0.06	0.04	0.6	11
10.	Arby Q, Arby's	1	190	389	18	15	5.5	29	48	84	6.1	1268	0	0.27	0.41	9.2	0
11.	Arby Sauce, Arby's	.5 oz.	14	15	0	0	0.0	0	3	0	0.2	113	0	0.00	0.00	0.0	0
12.	Asparagus, cooked green spears	4 med	60	12	1.3	0	0.0	0	2	13	0.4	1	540	0.10	0.11	0.8	16
13.	Avocado, raw	1/2 med	120	185	2.4	19	3.2	0	7	11	0.6	4	310	0.12	0.22	1.7	15
14.	Bacon, cooked, drained	2 slices	15	86	3.8	8	2.7	30	1	2	0.5	153	0	0.08	0.05	0.8	0
15.	Bacon, lettuce, tomato sandwich	1	130	327	11.6	19	4.7	21	31	84	2.5	661	426	0.42	0.28	4.1	12
16.	Bagel	1 3½ in.	68	180	7.0	1	0.2	0	35	20	2.1	124	0	0.26	0.20	2.4	0
17.	Banana, raw	1 sm (7¼")	140	81	1.0	0	0.0	0	21	8	0.7	1	180	0.05	0.06	0.7	10
18.	Banana, nut bread	1 slice	50	169	3.0	8	1.5	33	22	18	0.9	172	49	0.09	0.09	0.8	1
19.	BBQ Sauce, McDonald's	1.12 oz.	31.75	50	0	0.6	0.2	0	12	0.0	0.0	350	200	0.00	0.00	0	2.4
20.	Beans, green snap, cooked	1/2 c	65	16	1.0	0	0.0	0	3	32	0.4	4	340	0.05	0.06	0.3	8
21.	Beans, lentils	1/4 c	50	53	3.9	0	0.0	0	10	12	1.0	0	10	0.03	0.04	0.4	0
22.	Beans, lima (Fordhook), froz., cooked	1/2 c	85	84	6.0	0	0.0	0	17	40	2.1	1	240	0.15	0.08	1.1	15
23.	Beans, red kidney, cooked	1 c	185	218	14.4	1	0.0	0	40	70	4.4	6	10	0.20	0.11	1.3	0
24.	Beans, refried	1/2 c	145	148	9.0	1	0.2	0	25	71	2.6	614	0	0.07	0.08	0.7	9
25.	Bean sprouts, mung, raw	1/2 c	52	18	2.0	0	0.0	0	4	10	0.7	3	10	0.07	0.07	0.4	10
26.	Beef, chuck, cooked	3 oz.	85	212	25.0	12	7.8	80	0	11	3.1	43	20	0.05	0.19	3.8	0
27.	Beef, corned, canned	3 oz.	85	163	21.0	10	8.0	70	0	22	5.0	802	0	0.02	0.27	3.9	0
28.	Beef, ground, lean	3 oz.	85	186	23.3	10	5.0	81	0	10	3.0	57	20	0.08	0.20	5.1	0
29.	Beef, Lite Roast Deluxe, Arby's	1	182	294	18	10	3.5	42	33	156	3.0	826	200	0.27	0.52	8.4	8
30.	Beef, meatloaf	1 piece	111	246	20.0	15	6.1	125	6	37	2.4	434	181	0.08	0.23	4.1	1
31.	Beef N' Cheddar, Arby's	1	194	508	25	27	7.7	52	43	180	4.1	1166	0	0.42	0.67	9.8	1
32.	Beef, round steak, trimmed	3 oz.	85	222	24.3	13	6.0	77	0	10	3.0	60	20	0.07	0.20	4.8	0
33.	Beef, rump roast	3 oz.	85	177	24.7	9	4.0	80	0	10	3.1	61	10	0.06	0.19	4.4	0
34.	Beef, sirloin, cooked	3 oz.	85	329	19.6	27	13.0	77	0	9	2.5	48	50	0.05	0.15	4.0	0
35.	Beef, T-bone steak	3 oz.	85	403	16.7	37	15.6	66	0	7	2.2	40	23	0.07	0.14	3.5	0
36.	Beef, thin, sliced	3 oz.	85	105	18.5	3	1.4	36	0	11	1.8	1,409	0	0.07	0.16	4.5	0
37.	Beer	12 fl. oz.	360	151	1.1	0	1.1	0	14	18	0.0	25	0	0.01	0.11	2.2	0
38.	Beer, light	12 fl. oz.	354	96	0.7	0	0.0	0	4	17	0.1	10	0	0.03	0.10	1.3	0
39.	Beets, red, canned, drained	1/2 c	80	32	0.8	0	0.0	0	8	15	0.6	164	15	0.01	0.02	0.1	2
40.	Beet greens, cooked	1/2 c	73	13	1.3	0	0.0	0	2	72	1.4	55	3,700	0.05	0.11	0.2	11
41.	Biscuits, baking powder	1 med	35	114	2.5	6	1.1	0	18	60	0.8	272	0	0.06	0.06	0.7	0
42.	Blueberries, fresh cultivated	1/2 c	73	45	0.5	0	0.0	0	11	10	0.8	1	75	0.02	0.05	0.4	10

No.	Food	Amount	Weight (g)	Calories	Protein (g)	Fat (g)	Sat. Fat (g)	Chol. (mg)	Carb. (g)	Calcium (mg)	Iron (mg)	Sodium (mg)	Vit. A (IU)	Thiamin (mg)	Riboflavin (mg)	Niacin (mg)	Vit. C (mg)
43	Bologna	1 slice (1 oz.)	28	86	3.4	8	3.0	15	0	2	0.5	369	0	0.05	0.06	0.7	0
44	Bologna, turkey	2 slices	57	113	7.8	9	3.0	56	1	47	0.9	498	0	0.03	0.09	2.1	0
45	Bouillon, broth	1 cube	4	5	0.8	0	0.0	0	0	0	0.0	960	0	0.00	0.00	0.0	0
46	Brandy	1 oz.	28	69	0.0	0	0.0	0	11	0	0.0	1	0	0.00	0.00	0.0	0
47	Bread, Corn	1 slice	78	161	5.8	6	0.1	0	23	94	0.9	490	120	0.10	0.15	0.5	1
48	Bread, Cracked wheat	1 slice	25	65	2.3	1	0.2	0	12	16	0.7	106	0	0.10	0.10	0.8	0
49	Bread, French enriched	1 slice	35	102	3.2	1	0.2	0	19	15	0.8	203	0	0.12	0.08	0.9	0
50	Bread, Oatmeal	1 slice	25	65	2.1	1	0.2	0	12	15	0.7	124	0	0.27	0.07	0.9	0
51	Bread, Pita pocket	1 piece	60	165	6.2	1	0.1	0	33	49	1.5	339	0	0.11	0.13	2.3	0
52	Bread, Pumpernickel	1 slice	32	80	2.9	1	0.2	0	15	23	0.9	277	0	0.05	0.17	1.1	0
53	Bread, Rye (American)	1 slice	25	61	2.3	0	0.0	0	13	19	0.4	139	0	0.06	0.02	0.4	0
54	Bread, white enriched	1 slice	25	68	2.2	1	0.2	0	13	21	0.6	127	0	0.03	0.05	0.6	0
55	Bread, whole wheat	1 slice	25	61	2.6	1	0.6	0	12	25	0.8	132	0	0.13	0.03	0.7	0
56	Broccoli, cooked drained	1 sm stalk	140	36	4.3	1	0.0	0	6	123	1.1	14	3,500	0.10	0.28	1.1	126
57	Broccoli, raw	1 sm stalk	114	38	4.1	1	0.0	0	7	117	1.3	17	2,835	0.05	0.23	0.9	125
58	Brownies, with nuts	1	20	95	1.3	6	2.3	18	11	9	0.4	51	20	0.06	0.05	0.3	0
59	Brussels sprouts, froz., cooked, drained	1/2 c	78	28	3.2	0	0.0	0	5	25	0.8	8	405	0.07	0.11	0.5	63
60	Bulgur, wheat	1 c	135	227	8.4	1	0.0	0	47	27	1.8	809	0	0.15	0.04	3.2	0
61	Burrito, bean	1	166	307	12.5	10	3.6	14	45	173	2.4	983	283	0.34	0.22	2.3	5
62	Burrito, combination, Taco Bell	1	175	404	21.0	16	0.0	0	43	91	3.7	300	1,666	0.00	0.31	4.6	15
63	Butter	1 tsp	5	36	0.0	4	0.4	12	0	1	0.0	46	160	0.00	0.00	0.0	0
64	Buttermilk, cultured	1 c	245	88	8.8	0	1.3	5	12	296	0.1	319	10	0.10	0.44	0.2	2
65	Cabbage, boiled, drained wedge	1/2 c	85	16	0.9	0	0.0	0	3	36	0.3	10	100	0.02	0.02	0.1	21
66	Cabbage, raw chopped	1/2 c	45	11	0.6	0	0.0	0	3	22	0.2	9	60	0.03	0.03	0.2	21
67	Cake, Angel food, plain	1 piece	60	161	4.3	0	0.0	0	36	5	0.1	170	0	0.01	0.08	0.1	1
68	Cake, Carrot	1 piece	96	385	4.2	21	4.1	74	48	44	1.3	279	75	0.11	0.12	0.9	0
69	Cake, Cheesecake	1 piece (3½")	85	257	4.6	16	9.0	150	24	48	0.4	189	216	0.03	0.11	0.4	4
70	Cake, Chocolate, w/icing	1 piece	69	235	3.0	8	3.6	37	40	41	1.4	181	100	0.07	0.10	0.6	0
71	Cake, Coffee	1 piece	72	230	4.5	7	2.5	47	38	44	1.2	310	120	0.14	0.15	1.3	0
72	Cake, Devil's food, iced	1 piece	99	365	4.5	16	5.0	68	55	69	1.0	233	160	0.02	0.10	0.2	0
73	Cake, Pound	1 piece	30	120	2.0	5	1.0	32	15	20	0.5	98	200	0.05	0.06	0.5	0
74	Cake, White, choc. icing	1 piece	71	268	3.5	11	3.7	2	48	35	0.3	162	40	0.19	0.14	1.6	0
75	Candy, hard	1 oz.	28	109	0.0	0	0.0	0	28	6	0.5	9	0	0.00	0.00	0.6	0
76	Cantaloupe	1/4 melon 5" diam.	239	35	2.0	0	0.0	0	10	20	0.8	17	4,620	0.06	0.04	0.6	45
77	Caramel (candy, plain or choc.)	1 oz.	28	113	1.1	3	1.6	3	22	42	0.4	64	0	0.01	0.05	0.1	0
78	Carrots, cooked, drained	1/2 c	73	23	0.7	0	0.0	0	5	24	0.5	10	7,615	0.04	0.04	0.4	5
79	Carrots, raw	1 carrot 7½" long	81	30	0.8	0	0.0	0	7	27	0.5	34	7,930	0.04	0.04	0.4	6
80	Cashew, roasted, unsalted	2 oz.	57	326	9.2	27	5.4	0	16	23	2.3	10	0	0.24	0.10	1.0	0
81	Cauliflower, cooked, drained	1/2 c	63	14	1.5	0	0.0	0	3	13	0.5	6	40	0.06	0.05	0.4	35
82	Celery, green, raw, long	1 outer stalk 8"	40	7	0.4	0	0.0	0	2	16	0.1	50	110	0.01	0.01	0.1	4
83	Cereal, All-Bran	1/4 c	21	53	3.0	0	0.1	0	16	17	3.4	242	947	0.28	0.33	3.8	11
84	Cereal, Alpha Bits	1 c	28	111	2.2	1	0.0	0	25	8	1.8	219	1,875	0.40	0.40	5.0	0
85	Cereal, Bran	1/2 c	30	72	3.8	1	0.0	0	22	25	3.0	247	2,000	1.00	0.80	3.0	20
86	Cereal, Cheerios	1 c	23	89	3.4	1	1.2	0	16	38	3.6	246	949	0.32	0.32	4.0	12
87	Cereal, Corn Chex	1 c	28	111	2.0	0	0.1	0	25	3	1.8	271	75	0.40	0.07	5.0	15
88	Cereal, Corn Flakes	1 c	25	97	2.0	0	0.1	0	21	3	0.6	251	180	0.29	0.55	2.9	9
89	Cereal, Cream of Wheat	1 c	244	140	3.6	0	0.1	0	29	54	10.9	5	0	0.24	0.07	1.5	0
90	Cereal, Frosted Mini-Wheats	4 biscuits	31	111	3.2	1	0.1	0	26	10	2.0	9	2,050	0.40	0.50	5.5	16

Code	Food	Amount	Weight gm	Calories	Protein gm	Fat gm	Sat. Fat gm	Cholesterol mg	Carbohydrate gm	Calcium mg	Iron mg	Sodium mg	Vit A I.U.	Thiamin (Vit B₁) mg	Riboflavin (Vit B₂) mg	Niacin mg	Vit C mg
91.	Cereal, Fruit & Fibre w/dates	1 c	56	180	6.0	2	0.3	0	42	20	9.0	340	3,780	0.75	0.85	10.0	0
92.	Cereal, Granola, Nature Valley	1/2 c	57	252	5.8	10	7.0	0	38	36	1.9	116	41	0.20	0.10	0.4	0
93.	Cereal, Grape Nuts	1/2 c	57	202	6.6	0	0.0	0	47	22	2.5	394	3,815	0.80	0.80	10.0	0
94.	Cereal, Life	1 c	44	162	8.1	1	0.1	0	32	154	11.6	229	0	0.95	1.00	11.6	0
95.	Cereal, Nutri-Grain Wheat	1 c	44	158	3.8	1	0.1	0	37	12	1.2	299	2,915	0.60	0.70	7.7	23
96.	Cereal, Oatmeal, quick, cooked	1/2 c	120	66	2.4	1	0.2	0	12	11	0.7	262	0	0.10	0.03	0.1	0
97.	Cereal, Raisin Bran	1 c	49	160	4.0	1	0.2	0	40	25	24.0	293	2,500	0.51	0.57	6.7	0
98.	Cereal, Rice Krispies	3/4 c	22	85	1.4	0	0.0	0	19	3	1.4	255	971	0.30	0.30	3.8	11
99.	Cereal, Shredded Wheat	1 c	19	65	2.1	0	0.0	0	11	8	0.6	1	0	0.06	0.05	0.9	0
100.	Cereal, Special K	1 c	21	83	4.2	0	0.0	0	16	6	3.4	199	1,430	0.30	0.30	3.8	11
101.	Cereal, Sugar Corn Pops	1 c	28	108	1.4	0	0.0	0	26	1	1.8	103	1,875	0.40	0.40	5.0	15
102.	Cereal, Sugar Frosted Flakes	1 c	35	133	1.8	0	0.0	0	32	1	2.2	284	2,315	0.50	0.50	6.2	19
103.	Cereal, Sugar Smacks	1 c	37	141	2.7	1	0.1	0	32	4	2.4	100	2,500	0.49	0.57	6.7	20
104.	Cereal, Total	1 c	33	116	3.3	1	0.1	0	26	56	21.0	409	8,845	1.70	2.00	23.3	70
105.	Cereal, Wheat Chex	1 c	46	169	4.5	1	0.2	0	38	18	7.3	308	0	0.60	0.17	8.1	24
106.	Cereal, whole wheat, cooked	1/2 c	123	55	2.2	0	0.0	0	12	9	0.06	260	0	0.08	0.03	0.8	0
107.	Cereal, whole wheat flakes, ready-to-eat	1 c	30	106	3.1	1	0.0	0	24	12	2.0	310	1,410	0.35	0.42	3.5	11
108.	Cereal, 40% Bran Flakes	1 c	39	125	4.9	1	0.1	0	31	19	11.2	363	2,610	0.51	0.59	6.9	0
109.	Cereal, 100% Bran	1/2 c	33	89	4.2	2	0.3	0	24	23	4.1	229	0	0.80	0.90	10.4	31
110.	Champagne	4 oz.	113	87	0.2	0	0.1	0	0	6	0.4	7	0	0.00	0.01	0.1	0
111.	Cheese, American	1 oz. slice	28	100	6.0	8	5.6	27	0	188	0.1	307	343	0.01	0.10	0.0	0
112.	Cheese, Bleu	1 oz.	28	100	6.0	8	5.3	25	1	89	0.1	510	204	0.01	0.11	0.3	0
113.	Cheese, Cheddar	1 oz.	28	114	7.0	9	6.0	30	0	204	0.2	171	300	0.01	0.11	0.0	0
114.	Cheese, Cottage, 2%	1/2 c	113	103	15.5	2	1.4	10	4	78	0.2	459	79	0.03	0.21	0.2	0
115.	Cheese, Cottage, creamed	1/2 c	105	112	14.0	5	6.4	15	3	99	0.3	241	180	0.03	0.26	0.1	0
116.	Cheese, Creamed	1 oz.	28	99	6.0	8	3.0	31	1	167	0.3	71	320	0.02	0.14	0.0	0
117.	Cheese, Feta	1 oz.	28	75	4.5	6	4.2	25	1	140	0.2	316	180	0.04	0.23	0.3	0
118.	Cheese, Monterey jack	1 oz.	28	106	6.9	9	5.4	26	0	212	0.2	152	405	0.00	0.11	0.0	0
119.	Cheese, Mozzarella, skim	1 oz.	28	80	7.6	5	3.1	15	1	207	0.1	150	216	0.01	0.10	0.0	0
120.	Cheese, Parmesan	1 tbsp	5	23	2.1	2	1.0	4	0	69	0.1	93	45	0.00	0.02	0.0	0
121.	Cheese, Ricotta, part skim	1 oz.	28	39	3.2	2	1.4	9	1	77	0.1	35	160	0.01	0.05	0.2	0
122.	Cheese, Souffle	1 portion	110	240	10.9	19	9.5	189	7	221	1.1	400	880	0.06	0.26	0.0	0
123.	Cheese, Swiss	1 oz.	28	107	8.0	8	5.0	26	1	272	0.1	74	360	0.01	0.10	0.0	0
124.	Cheese puffs, Cheetos	1 oz.	28	158	2.2	10	4.8	5	14	17	0.4	344	130	0.01	0.03	0.2	0
125.	Cheeseburger, McDonald's	1	115	321	15.2	16	6.7	40	29	170	2.9	736	353	0.30	0.24	4.4	2
126.	Cherries	10	75	47	0.9	0	0.0	0	12	15	0.3	8	450	0.20	0.24	1.6	41
127.	Chicken, BK Broiler sandwich, Burger King	1 sandwich	168	379	24.0	18	3.0	53	31	48	2.3	764	350	0.42	0.22	9.2	5
128.	Chicken Breast Filet, Arby's	1	204	445	22	23.0	3.0	45	52	72	1.9	958	0	0.23	0.58	9.0	5
129.	Chicken breast, roast w/skin	1	98	193	29.2	8	2.1	83	0	14	1.0	69	91	0.07	0.12	12.5	0
130.	Chicken chow mein	1 c	250	255	31.0	11	3.6	75	10	58	2.5	718	250	0.08	0.23	4.3	10
131.	Chicken club sandwich, Wendy's	1	220	520	30	25	6.0	75	44	120	9.6	980	100	0.60	0.45	16.0	9
132.	Chicken Cordon Bleu, Arby's	1	225	518	30	27	5.3	92	52	204	2.1	1463	0	0.42	0.68	10.2	5
133.	Chicken, drumstick Kentucky Fried	1	54	136	14.0	8	2.2	73	2	20	0.9	320	30	0.04	0.12	2.7	0
134.	Chicken, drumstick, roasted	1	52	112	14.1	6	1.6	48	0	6	0.7	47	52	0.04	0.11	3.1	0

No.	Food	Amount	Weight (g)	Calories	Protein (g)	Fat (g)	Sat. Fat (g)	Cholesterol (mg)	Carbohydrate (g)	Calcium (mg)	Iron (mg)	Sodium (mg)	Vit. A (IU)	Thiamin (mg)	Riboflavin (mg)	Niacin (mg)	Vit. C (mg)
135.	Chicken McNuggets	6	111	329	19.5	21	5.2	64	15	11	1.3	521	92	0.16	0.14	7.7	2
136.	Chicken Nuggets, Wendy's	6 pc.	94	280	14	20	5.0	50	12	48	0.48	600	0	0.090	0.110	6.0	0
137.	Chicken, patty sandwich	1	157	436	24.8	23	6.1	68	34	44	1.9	2,732	47	0.13	0.26	9.2	4
138.	Chicken, wing, Kentucky Fried	1	45	151	11.0	10	2.9	70	4	0	0.6	300	0	0.03	0.07	0.0	0
139.	Chicken, roast, light meat without skin	3 oz.	85	141	27.0	3	0.4	45	0	10	1.2	54	51	0.03	0.09	9.9	0
140.	Chicken, roast, dark meat without skin	3 oz.	85	149	24.0	5	0.8	50	0	11	1.5	54	127	0.06	0.19	4.7	0
141.	Chicken, Roast Deluxe, Arby's	1	195	276	24	7	1.7	33	33	156	1.9	777	200	0.440	0.800	9.4	7
142.	Chicken Sandwich, breaded Wendy's	1	208	450	26	20	4.0	60	44	120	9.6	740	100	0.450	0.360	14.0	6
143.	Chicken Sandwich, Grilled, Wendy's	1	177	290	24	7	1.0	60	35	120	2.4	670	100	0.375	0.270	10.0	6
144.	Chicken Sandwich, McChicken	1	187	415	19	19	9.0	50	39	180	1.8	830	100	0.900	0.180	9.0	2.4
145.	Chili con carne	1 c	255	339	19.1	16	5.8	28	31	82	4.3	1,354	150	0.08	0.18	3.3	8
146.	Chocolate fudge	1 oz.	28	115	0.6	3	2.1	1	22	22	0.3	54	0	0.01	0.03	0.1	0
147.	Chocolate, milk	1 oz.	28	147	2.0	9	3.6	5	21	65	0.3	27	80	0.02	0.10	0.1	0
148.	Chocolate, milk w/almonds	1 oz.	28	150	2.9	10	4.4	5	16	61	0.6	23	30	0.03	0.13	0.3	0
149.	Clam, canned, drained	3 oz.	85	83	13.0	2	0.2	50	15	46	3.5	750	93	0.01	0.09	0.9	9
150.	Cocoa, hot, with whole milk	1 c	250	218	9.1	9	6.1	33	26	298	0.8	123	318	0.10	0.44	0.4	2
151.	Cocoa, plain, dry	1 tbsp	5	14	0.9	1	0.0	0	3	7	0.6	0	0	0.01	0.02	0.1	0
152.	Coconut, shredded, packed	1/2 c	65	225	2.3	23	20.0	0	6	8	1.1	165	0	0.03	0.01	0.3	2
153.	Cod, batter fried	3.5 oz.	100	199	19.6	10	3.9	55	8	80	0.5	100	2	0.02	0.02	1.8	0
154.	Cod, cooked	3 oz.	85	144	24.3	4	1.5	60	0	27	0.9	63	150	0.06	0.09	2.7	0
155.	Cod, poached	3.5 oz.	100	94	20.9	1	0.3	60	0	29	0.5	110	2	0.08	0.08	3.0	0
156.	Coffee	3/4 cup	180	1	0.0	1	0.0	0	0	1	0.2	2	2	0.00	0.00	0.1	0
157.	Coleslaw	1 c	120	173	1.6	17	1.0	5	6	53	0.5	144	190	0.06	0.06	0.4	35
158.	Collards, leaves without stems, cooked, drained	1/2 c	95	32	3.4	1	2.0	0	5	178	0.8	28	7,410	0.01	0.19	1.2	72
159.	Cookies, Chocolate chip homemade	2 2¼" diam.	20	103	1.0	6	1.7	14	12	7	0.4	70	20	0.02	0.02	0.2	0
160.	Cookies, Fig bars	4 bars	56	210	2.0	4	1.0	27	42	40	1.4	180	31	0.08	0.07	0.7	0
161.	Cookies, Oatmeal raisin	2 2" diam.	26	122	1.5	5	1.3	1	18	9	0.6	74	20	0.04	0.04	0.5	0
162.	Cookies, Peanut butter, homemade	2 cookies	24	123	2.0	7	2.0	11	14	10	0.5	71	12	0.03	0.03	0.9	0
163.	Cookies, sandwich, all	4 cookies	40	195	2.0	8	2.0	0	29	12	1.4	189	0	0.90	0.07	0.8	0
164.	Cookies, Shortbread	4 cookies	32	155	2.0	8	2.9	27	20	13	0.8	123	40	0.10	0.09	0.9	0
165.	Cookies, Vanilla	5 1¾" diam.	20	93	1.0	3	0.8	10	15	8	0.1	50	25	0.00	0.01	0.0	0
166.	Cookies, Vanilla wafers	10 wafers	40	185	2.0	7	1.8	25	29	16	0.8	150	70	0.07	0.10	1.0	0
167.	Corn, boiled on cob	1 ear 5" long	140	70	2.5	1	0.0	0	16	2	0.5	1	310	0.09	0.08	1.1	7
168.	Corn, canned, drained	1/2 c	83	70	2.2	1	0.0	0	16	4	0.4	195	290	0.03	0.04	0.8	4
169.	Corn chips	1 oz.	28	155	2.0	9	1.8	0	16	35	0.5	233	110	0.04	0.05	0.4	1
170.	Cornmeal, degermed, yellow, enriched, cooked	1/2 c	120	60	1.3	0	0.0	0	13	1	0.5	264	70	0.07	0.05	0.6	0
171.	Crab, canned	1 c	135	135	23.0	3	0.5	135	1	61	1.1	1,350	70	0.11	0.11	2.6	0
172.	Crackers, Cheese	10 crackers	10	50	1.0	3	0.9	6	5	11	0.4	112	25	0.05	0.04	0.4	0
173.	Crackers, Graham	2 squares	14	55	1.1	1	0.3	0	10	6	0.2	95	0	0.01	0.03	0.2	0
174.	Crackers, Ritz	1 cracker	3	15	0.2	1	0.2	0	2	3	0.1	30	0	0.01	0.01	0.1	0
175.	Crackers, Ryewafers, whole grain	2 crackers	14	55	1.0	1	0.3	0	10	7	0.5	115	0	0.06	0.03	0.5	0
176.	Crackers, Saltines	4 squares	11	48	1.0	1	0.3	0	8	2	0.1	123	0	0.00	0.00	0.1	0
177.	Crackers, Soda	1	3	13	0.3	0	0.1	0	2	1	0.1	39	0	0.02	0.01	0.1	0

Code	Food	Amount	Weight gm	Calories	Protein gm	Fat gm	Sat. Fat gm	Cholesterol mg	Carbohydrate gm	Calcium mg	Iron mg	Sodium mg	Vit A I.U.	Thiamin (Vit B₁) mg	Riboflavin (Vit B₂) mg	Niacin mg	Vit C mg
178.	Crackers, Triscuits	1	5	23	0.4	1	0.3	0	3	1	0.0	0	0	0.00	0.00	0.0	0
179.	Crackers, Wheat Thins	1	2	9	0.2	0	0.1	0	1	1	0.1	17	0	0.01	0.01	0.1	0
180.	Cranberry juice	1 c	253	145	0.1	0	0.0	0	36	8	0.4	5	5	0.02	0.02	0.1	90
181.	Cream, light coffee or table	1 tbsp	15	20	0.5	2	0.5	5	1	16	0.0	7	70	0.00	0.02	0.0	0
182.	Cream, heavy whipping	1 tbsp	15	53	0.3	6	1.3	12	1	11	0.0	5	230	0.00	0.02	0.0	0
183.	Croissant		57	235	4.7	12	4.0	13	27	20	2.1	452	50	0.17	0.13	1.3	0
184.	Croissants (Sara Lee)	1 roll	18	59	1.6	2	0.3	0	8	22	0.6	105	0	0.14	0.09	0.8	0
185.	Croissan'wich, egg, cheese	1 sandwich	110	315	13.0	20	7.0	222	19	112	1.8	607	500	0.22	0.37	1.4	0
	Burger King																
186.	Cucumbers, raw pared	9 sm slices	28	4	0.3	0	0.0	0	1	7	0.3	2	70	0.01	0.01	0.1	3
187.	Danish, Apple, McDonald's	1	115	390	6	17	11.0	25	51	0	0.96	370	0	0.30	0.18	2.0	15
188.	Danish, Cinnamon Raisin	1	110	440	6	21	13.0	34	58	48	0.12	430	0	0.30	0.27	3.0	3.6
189.	Dates hydrated	5	46	110	0.9	0	0.0	0	29	24	1.2	1	20	0.04	0.04	0.9	0
190.	Doughnut, plain	1	42	164	1.9	8	2.0	19	22	17	0.6	210	30	0.07	0.07	0.5	0
191.	Doughnut, yeast raised	1	27	235	4.0	13	5.2	21	26	17	1.4	222	2	0.28	0.12	1.8	0
192.	Dressing, Bleu cheese	1 tbsp	15	77	0.7	8	1.9	4	1	12	0.0	8	32	0.00	0.02	0.0	0
193.	Dressing, French	1 tbsp	16	83	0.1	9	1.4	0	1	2	0.1	184	0	0.00	0.00	0.0	0
194.	Dressing, French, low cal	1 tbsp.	15	24	0.0	0	0.2	0	2	6	0.1	306	0	0.00	0.00	0.0	0
195.	Dressing, Italian	1 tbsp.	15	69	0.1	9	1.3	0	2	1	0.0	73	29	0.00	0.00	0.0	0
196.	Dressing, Italian, low cal	1 tbsp.	15	10	0.0	1	0.0	0	1	1	0.0	136	1	0.00	0.00	0.0	0
197.	Dressing, Ranch style	1 tbsp.	15	54	0.4	6	0.9	6	1	15	0.0	65	36	0.01	0.02	0.0	0
198.	Dressing, Thousand island	1 tbsp.	15	60	0.2	6	1.0	4	2	2	0.1	110	75	0.00	0.01	0.0	1
199.	Dressing, Thousand island, low cal	1 tbsp.	15	25	0.1	2	0.2	2	3	2	0.1	153	70	0.00	0.00	0.0	0
200.	Eggs, hard cooked	1 large	50	72	6.0	5	1.8	250	1	24	1.0	113	520	0.05	0.13	0.0	0
201.	Egg, fried with butter		46	95	5.4	6	2.4	278	1	28	0.9	162	320	0.04	0.13	0.0	0
202.	Egg McMuffin	1	138	327	18.5	15	5.9	259	31	226	2.9	885	591	0.47	0.44	3.8	1
203.	Egg salad sandwich	1	111	325	10.0	19	3.9	215	28	95	2.5	461	242	0.29	0.29	2.1	0
204.	Egg, scrambled, with milk, butter	1 egg	64	95	6.0	7	3.0	282	1	54	0.9	176	510	0.04	0.18	0.0	0
205.	Eggs, white	1 large	33	17	3.6	0	0.0	0	0	3	0.0	48	0	0.00	0.09	0.0	0
206.	Eggs, yolk, raw	1 yolk	17	63	2.8	6	1.7	248	0	26	1.0	8	390	0.04	0.07	0.0	0
207.	Enchilada, beef	1	200	487	21.8	23	8.8	63	26	425	2.9	262	595	0.02	0.27	3.5	5
208.	Enchilada, cheese	1	230	632	25.3	34	17.6	82	31	876	2.6	596	1,672	0.13	0.40	1.2	15
209.	Figs, dried	1 large	21	60	1.0	0	0.0	0	15	26	0.6	1	20	0.16	0.17	3.9	0
210.	Filet of Fish, McDonald's	1	131	402	15.0	23	7.9	43	34	105	1.8	709	152	0.28	0.28	3.9	4
211.	Fish sandwich, Wendy's	1	182	460	16	25	5.0	55	42	120	1.8	780	0	0.60	0.45	4.0	1.2
212.	Fish, sticks	2	56	140	12.0	6	1.6	52	8	22	0.6	106	40	0.06	0.10	1.2	3
213.	Flounder	3 oz.	85	171	25.5	7	1.0	60	0	21	1.2	201	0	0.06	0.06	2.1	3
214.	Flour, all purpose enriched	1 c	125	455	13.0	1	0.0	0	95	20	3.6	3	0	0.55	0.33	4.4	0
215.	Flour, whole wheat	1 c	120	400	16.0	2	0.0	0	85	49	4.0	4	0	0.66	0.14	5.2	0
216.	Frankfurter, cooked	1	57	176	7.0	16	5.6	45	1	4	1.1	627	0	0.09	0.11	1.5	0
217.	Frankfurter, turkey, cooked	1	45	102	6.4	8	2.7	39	1	58	0.8	454	60	0.04	0.08	1.7	0
218.	French Dip, Arby's	1	154	368	22	15	5.6	43	35	60	2.8	1018	285	0.20	0.50	8.4	0
219.	French toast	1 piece	65	123	4.9	4	1.1	73	15	79	1.1	189	285	0.15	0.17	1.1	0
220.	Fries, Curly, Arby's	1	99	337	4	18	7.4	0	43	24	0.96	167	370	0.06	0.07	2.0	5
221.	Fruit cocktail	1 c	245	91	1.0	0	0.0	0	24	22	1.0	12	370	0.05	0.02	1.2	5
222.	Fruit cocktail, juice pack	1 c	248	115	1.1	0	0.0	0	29	20	0.5	10	380	0.03	0.04	1.0	7
223.	Grapefruit, raw white	1/2 med	301	56	1.0	0	0.0	0	15	22	0.5	1	10	0.05	0.03	0.3	52

#	Food	Portion														
224.	Grapefruit, juice unsweetened canned	1/2 c	124	50	0.6	0	0.0	0	12	11	0.2	2	10	0.05	0.03	0.3	46
225.	Grapes, seedless, European	10 grapes	50	34	0.3	0	0.0	0	9	6	0.2	2	50	0.03	0.03	0.2	2
226.	Grape juice, unsweetened bottled	1/2 c	127	84	0.3	0	0.0	0	21	14	0.4	3	0	0.05	0.03	0.3	0
227.	Gravy, beef, homemade	1 tbsp	17	19	0.3	2	1.0	1	1	1	0.1	49	0	0.01	0.01	0.2	0
228.	Haddock, fried (dipped in egg, milk, bread crumbs)	3 oz.	85	141	17.0	5	1.0	54	5	33	0.9	150	0	0.06	0.06	2.7	3
229.	Halibut, broiled with butter or margarine	3 oz.	85	144	21.0	6	2.1	55	0	15	0.6	114	570	0.06	0.06	7.2	1
230.	Ham (cured pork)	3 oz.	85	318	20.0	26	9.4	77	0	9	2.6	48	0	0.43	0.20	3.8	0
231.	Ham, lunch meat	1 slice	28	37	5.5	1	0.5	13	.3	2	0.2	405	0	0.26	0.06	1.4	7
232.	Hamburger, Big Classic, Wendy's	1	251	480	27	23	7.0	75	44	180	4.2	850	300	0.45	0.27	7.0	12
233.	Hamburger, Big Mac	1	204	581	25.1	36	12.0	85	40	207	5.0	999	388	0.49	0.39	7.3	3
234.	Hamburger bun	1 bun	40	129	3.7	2	1.0	0	23	61	1.3	271	2	0.22	0.15	1.8	3
235.	Hamburger, Jr. Bacon	1	170	440	22	25	8.0	65	33	240	3.0	870	300	0.45	0.27	6.0	0
236.	Hamburger, McDonald's	1	99	257	13.0	9	3.7	26	30	63	3.0	526	231	0.23	0.23	5.1	9
237.	Hamburger, McLean Deluxe	1	206	320	22	10	5.0	60	35	180	2.4	670	500	0.375	0.36	7.0	2
238.	Hamburger, McLean Deluxe	1	219	370	24	14	8.0	75	35	240	2.4	890	750	0.375	0.36	7.0	6
239.	Hamburger, Quarter pounder	1 burger	160	427	24.6	24	9.1	80	29	98	4.3	718	115	0.35	0.32	7.2	6
240.	Hamburger, Quarter pounder, with cheese	1 burger	186	525	29.6	32	12.8	107	31	255	4.8	1,195	640	0.37	0.41	7.1	6
241.	Hamburger, Wendy's	1	219	440	26	23	7.0	75	36	120	3.6	850	300	0.375	0.18	7.0	3
242.	Ham N' Cheese, Arby's	1	169	355	25	14	5.1	55	35	204	1.8	1400	0	0.83	0.40	7.8	3
243.	Honey	1 tbsp	21	64	0.0	0	0.0	0	17	1	0.1	1	0	0.00	0.01	0.1	0
244.	Honeydew melon	1 slice (1/10 melon)	129	45	0.6	0	0.0	0	12	8	0.1	13	25	0.10	0.02	0.8	32
245.	Horsey Sauce, Arby's	.5 oz.	14	55	0	5	2.0	0	3	24	0.00	105	0	0.00	0.00	0.0	0
246.	Hotcakes w/Margarine & Syrup, McDonald's	1	174	440	8	12	5.0	8	74	120	1.2	685	200	0.30	0.36	3.0	0
247.	Hotdog bun	1 bun	40	115	3.3	2	1.0	0	20	54	1.2	241	2	0.20	0.13	1.6	0
248.	Ice cream, vanilla	1/2 c	67	135	3.0	7	4.4	27	14	97	0.1	42	295	0.03	0.14	0.1	1
249.	Ice cream cone	1 small	115	185	4.3	5	2.2	24	30	183	0.1	109	218	0.06	0.36	0.4	1
250.	Ice cream cone, Dairy Queen	medium	142	230	6.0	7	4.6	15	35	200	0.0	150	300	0.09	0.26	0.0	1
251.	Ice cream, hot fudge sundae	1	164	357	7.0	11	5.4	27	58	215	0.6	170	233	0.07	0.31	1.1	1
252.	Ice milk, vanilla	1/2 c	61	100	3.0	3	1.8	13	15	102	0.1	45	140	0.04	0.15	0.1	1
253.	Instant breakfast, whole milk	1 c	281	280	15.0	8	5.1	33	34	301	8.0	286	2,057	0.39	0.46	5.2	29
254.	Instant breakfast, skim milk	1 c	282	216	15.4	0	0.0	4	35	312	8.0	292	1,635	0.39	0.41	5.2	29
255.	Jams or preserves	1 tbsp	7	18	0.0	0	0.0	0	5	1	0.1	3	1	0.00	0.00	0.0	0
256.	Jelly	1 tbsp	18	49	0.0	0	0.0	0	13	4	0.3	3	0	0.01	0.01	0.0	0
257.	Kale, fresh cooked, drained	1/2 c	55	22	2.5	0	0.0	0	3	103	0.9	24	4,565	0.06	0.10	0.9	51
258.	Kiwi fruit, raw	1 med	76	46	1.0	0	0.0	0	11	20	0.3	4	65	0.02	0.04	0.4	75
259.	Kool Aid, with sugar	1 c	240	100	0.0	0	0.0	0	25	0	0.0	0	0	0.00	0.00	0.0	6
260.	Lamb leg, roast, trimmed	3 oz.	85	237	22.0	16	7.3	60	0	9	1.4	53	0	0.13	0.23	4.7	0
261.	Lamb loin chop, broiled, lean	3 oz.	84	183	25.0	8	3.4	78	0	16	1.7	70	7	0.10	0.23	5.7	0
262.	Lasagna, homemade	1 piece	220	357	23.6	18	8.3	50	27	413	2.8	703	1,008	0.19	0.30	3.3	6
263.	Lemon juice, fresh	1 tbsp	15	4	0.1	0	0.0	0	1	1	0.0	0	0	0.00	0.00	0.0	7
264.	Lemonade (concentrate)	12 oz.	340	137	0.2	0	0.1	0	36	11	0.6	11	73	0.02	0.07	0.1	13
265.	Lentils, cooked	1/2 c	100	106	8.0	0	0.0	0	19	25	2.1	7	20	0.07	0.06	0.6	0
266.	Lettuce, crisp head	1 c sm chunks	75	10	0.7	0	0.0	0	2	15	0.4	5	250	0.05	0.05	0.2	5
267.	Lettuce, cos or romaine	1 c chopped	55	10	0.7	0	0.0	0	2	37	0.8		1,050	0.08	0.04	0.2	10
268.	Liver, beef, fried	1 slice 3 oz.	85	195	22.0	9	2.5	345	5	5	7.5	156	45,390	0.22	3.56	14.0	23
269.	Liverwurst, fresh	1 slice 1 oz.	28	87	5.0	7	3.5	50	3	3	1.5	0	1,800	0.06	0.37	1.6	0
270.	Lobster	1 c	145	138	27.0	2	1.0	293	0	94	1.2	305	0	0.15	0.10	0.0	0

Code	Food	Amount	Weight gm	Calories	Protein gm	Fat gm	Sat. Fat gm	Cholesterol mg	Carbohydrate gm	Calcium mg	Iron mg	Sodium mg	Vit A I.U.	Thiamin (Vit B$_1$) mg	Riboflavin (Vit B$_2$) mg	Niacin mg	Vit C mg
271.	M&M's, Chocolate, plain	1 oz.	28	140	1.9	6	3.3	0	19	47	0.5	24	30	0.01	0.07	0.2	0
272.	M&M's, Chocolate, w/peanuts	1 oz.	28	145	3.2	7	3.2	0	17	36	0.4	17	15	0.02	0.05	0.9	0
273.	Macaroni, enriched, cooked	1/2 c	70	78	2.4	0	0.0	0	16	6	0.7	1	0	0.10	0.06	0.8	0
274.	Macaroni and cheese	1/2 c	100	215	8.2	11	4.0	21	20	181	0.9	543	430	0.10	0.20	0.9	0
275.	Margarine	1 tsp	5	34	0.0	4	0.7	2	0	1	0.0	46	160	0.00	0.00	0.0	0
276.	Mars bar	1 bar	50	240	4.0	11	4.8	0	30	85	0.6	85	1	0.02	0.16	0.5	*
277.	Matzo	1 piece	30	117	3.0	0	0.0	0	25	*	*	0	*	*	*	*	*
278.	Mayonnaise	1 tsp	5	36	0.0	4	0.7	3	0	1	0.0	28	13	0.00	0.00	0.0	0
279.	Milk, chocolate, 2%	1 c	250	180	8.0	5	3.1	17	26	284	0.6	151	143	0.09	0.41	0.3	2
280.	Milk, evaporated whole	1/2 c	126	172	9.0	10	5.8	40	13	329	0.2	149	405	0.05	0.43	0.2	2
281.	Milk, lowfat (2% fat)	1 c	246	145	10	5	3.1	5	15	352	0.1	150	200	0.10	0.52	0.2	2
282.	Milk shake, chocolate	1 (10 fluid oz.)	340	433	11.5	13	7.8	45	70	383	1.1	328	312	0.20	0.83	0.5	0
283.	Milk shake, medium Frosty	16 oz.	324	460	13	13	7.0	55	76	480	0.96	260	500	0.15	1.08	0.8	0
284.	Milk shake, strawberry	1 (10 fluid oz.)	340	383	11.4	10	6.0	37	64	384	0.4	281	418	0.14	0.61	0.5	4
285.	Milk shake, vanilla, McDonald's	1	289	323	10	8	5.1	29	52	346	0.2	250	346	0.12	0.66	0.6	3
286.	Milk, skim	1 c	245	88	9.0	0	0.3	5	12	296	0.1	126	10	0.09	0.44	0.2	2
287.	Milk, whole (3.5% fat)	1 c	244	159	9.0	9	5.1	34	12	288	0.1	120	350	0.07	0.40	0.2	2
288.	Milky Way bar	1 bar	60	260	3.2	9	5.4	14	43	86	0.5	140	125	0.03	0.15	0.2	1
289.	Molasses, medium	1 tbsp	20	50	0.0	0	0.0	0	13	33	0.9	3	0	0.01	0.01	0.0	0
290.	Muffin, apple bran, fat free	1	75	180	5	0	0.0	0	40	48	0.72	200	0	0.15	0.18	2.0	0
291.	Muffin, blueberry	1	45	135	3.0	5	1.5	19	20	54	0.9	198	40	0.10	0.11	0.9	1
292.	Muffin, bran	1	45	125	3.0	6	1.4	24	19	60	1.4	189	230	0.11	0.13	1.3	3
293.	Muffin, cornmeal	1	45	145	3.0	5	1.5	23	21	66	0.9	169	80	0.11	0.11	0.9	0
294.	Muffin, English, plain	1	57	140	4.5	1	0.3	0	26	96	1.7	378	0	0.26	0.18	2.1	0
295.	Muffin, English w/butter	1	63	186	5.0	5	2.3	15	30	117	1.5	310	164	0.28	0.49	2.6	1
296.	Mushrooms, fresh cultivated	1/2 c sliced	35	12	1.0	0	0.0	0	2	4	0.5	4	0	0.04	0.12	2.4	1
297.	Mustard greens, cooked drained	1/2 c	70	16	1.7	0	0.0	0	3	96	1.2	13	4,060	0.05	0.10	0.4	33
298.	Noodles, egg, enriched cooked	1/2 c	80	100	3.3	1	0.0	0	19	8	0.7	2	55	0.11	0.07	1.0	0
299.	Nuts, Brazil	1 oz. (6–8 nuts)	28	185	4.1	19	4.8	0	3	53	1.0	0	0	0.27	0.03	0.5	0
300.	Nuts, Pecans	1 oz.	28	195	2.6	20	1.4	0	4	21	0.7	0	40	0.24	0.04	0.3	1
301.	Nuts, Walnuts	1 oz. (14 halves)	28	185	4.2	18	1.0	0	5	28	0.9	1	10	0.09	0.04	0.3	1
302.	Oil, Corn	1 tbsp.	15	125	0.0	14	1.8	0	0	0	0.0	0	0	0.00	0.00	0.0	0
303.	Oil, Olive	1 tbsp.	15	125	0.0	14	1.9	0	0	0	0.0	0	0	0.00	0.00	0.0	0
304.	Oil, Safflower	1 tbsp.	15	125	0.0	14	1.3	0	0	0	0.0	0	0	0.00	0.00	0.0	0
305.	Oil, Soybean	1 tsp.	5	44	0.0	5	2.0	0	0	0	0.0	0	0	0.00	0.00	0.0	0
306.	Okra, cooked, drained	1/2 c	80	23	1.6	0	0.0	0	5	74	0.4	2	390	0.11	0.15	0.7	16
307.	Olives, black, ripe	10 extra large	55	61	0.5	7	1.0	0	1	40	0.8	385	30	0.00	0.00	0.0	0
308.	Onions, mature, cooked, drained	1/2 c sliced	105	31	1.3	0	0.0	0	7	25	0.4	8	40	0.03	0.03	0.2	0
310.	Onion rings, fried	3	30	122	1.6	8	2.3	0	11	9	0.5	113	68	0.08	0.04	1.1	0
311.	Onion rings (Brazier) Dairy Queen	1 serving	85	360	6.0	17	6.0	15	33	20	0.4	125	125	0.09	0.00	0.4	2
312.	Orange juice, froz. reconstituted	1/2 c	125	61	0.9	0	0.0	0	15	13	0.1	1	270	0.12	0.02	0.5	60
313.	Orange, raw (medium skin)	1 med	180	64	1.3	0	0.0	0	16	54	0.5	1	260	0.13	0.05	0.5	66

(Column headings are not printed on this page; they appear on a preceding page of the appendix. The numeric columns are, in order: Weight (g), Calories, Protein (g), Fat (g), Saturated fat (g), Cholesterol (mg), Carbohydrate (g), Calcium (mg), Iron (mg), Sodium (mg), Vitamin A, Thiamin (mg), Riboflavin (mg), Niacin (mg), Vitamin C (mg).)

No.	Food	Measure	Wt (g)	Cal	Prot	Fat	Sat Fat	Chol	Carb	Ca	Fe	Na	Vit A	Thia	Ribo	Niac	Vit C
314.	Oysters, Eastern, breaded, fried	1 oyster	45	90	5.0	5	1.4	35	5	49	3.0	70	220	0.07	0.10	1.3	0
315.	Oysters, raw, Eastern	1/2 c (6-9 med)	120	79	10.0	2	1.3	60	4	113	6.6	145	370	0.17	0.22	3.0	0
316.	Pancakes	6" diam x 1/2" thick	73	169	5.2	5	1.0	36	25	74	0.9	310	90	0.12	0.16	0.9	0
317.	Pancakes, buckwheat	4 in. diam.	27	55	2.0	5	0.9	20	6	59	0.4	125	17	0.04	0.05	0.2	0
318.	Pancakes w/butter, syrup	1 large	100	250	4.0	5	1.9	24	47	31	1.1	535	160	0.13	0.18	1.1	2
319.	Papaya, raw	1/2 med	227	60	0.9	0	0.0	0	15	72	0.5	5	2,660	0.06	0.06	0.5	85
320.	Parsnips, cooked	1 large 9" long	160	106	2.4	1	0.0	0	24	4	1.0	13	50	0.11	0.13	0.2	16
321.	Peaches, canned, heavy syrup	1 half 2⅛ tbsp liq.	96	75	0.4	0	0.0	0	19	5	0.3	2	410	0.01	0.02	0.6	3
322.	Peaches, canned, juice pack	1 half	77	34	0.5	0	0.0	0	9	14	0.2	3	147	0.01	0.01	0.5	3
323.	Peaches, raw, peeled	1 2¾" diam.	175	58	0.9	0	0.0	0	15	18	0.8	2	2,030	0.03	0.08	1.5	11
324.	Peanut butter	2 tbsp	32	188	8.0	16	1.0	0	6	87	0.6	194	1	0.04	0.04	4.8	0
325.	Peanut butter, jam sandwich	1	100	340	11.4	14	2.6	0	45	21	2.3	414	0	0.32	0.22	5.3	0
326.	Peanuts, roasted	1 oz.	28	166	7.0	14	1.0	0	5	5	0.6	119	0	0.09	0.04	4.9	0
327.	Pears, canned, heavy syrup	1 half 2¼ tbsp liq.	103	78	0.2	0	0.0	0	20	7	0.2	1	0	0.01	0.02	0.1	1
328.	Pears, canned, juice pack	1 half	77	38	0.3	0	0.0	0	10	13	0.2	3	3	0.01	0.01	0.2	1
329.	Pears, raw	1 pear	180	100	1.1	1	0.0	0	25	22	0.5	3	3	0.03	0.07	0.2	7
330.	Peas, canned, drained	1/2 c	85	75	4.0	0	0.0	0	14	15	1.6	200	30	0.08	0.05	0.7	7
331.	Peas, frozen, cooked drained	1/2 c	80	55	4.1	0	0.0	0	10	15	1.5	92	585	0.22	0.07	0.7	7
332.	Peppers, sweet, raw	1 pepper 3¼" x 3" diam.	200	36	2.0	0	0.0	0	8	35	1.1	21	480	0.13	0.13	1.4	210
333.	Pickles, dill	1 large 4" long	135	15	0.9	0	0.0	0	3	4	1.4	1,928	690	0.00	0.03	0.8	8
334.	Pickles, sweet	1 large 3" long	35	51	0.2	0	0.0	0	13	9	0.4	0	140	0.00	0.01	0.0	2
335.	Pie, Apple	1 piece (3½")	118	302	2.6	13	3.5	120	45	12	0.4	355	30	0.02	0.02	0.0	1
336.	Pie, Apple, fried	1 pie	85	255	2.2	14	5.8	14	32	26	0.9	326	40	0.09	0.06	0.5	1
337.	Pie, Blueberry	1 piece (3½")	158	380	4.0	17	4.0	137	55	17	2.1	423	15	0.17	0.14	1.0	6
338.	Pie, Cherry	1 piece (3½")	118	308	3.1	13	5.0	13	45	11	0.4	355	140	0.02	0.02	1.7	1
339.	Pie, Cherry, fried	1 pie	85	250	2.0	14	5.8	137	32	160	0.7	371	40	0.06	0.06	0.5	1
340.	Pie, Chocolate cream	1 piece (1/6 pie)	175	311	7.4	13	4.5	15	42	25	1.1	427	95	0.15	0.30	0.6	1
341.	Pie, Lemon meringue	1 piece (1/6 pie)	140	355	4.7	14	3.5	137	53	35	1.4	395	170	0.10	0.14	1.1	4
342.	Pie, Pecan	1 piece (1/6 pie)	138	583	6.3	24	3.9	13	92	58	1.9	304	330	0.22	0.17	0.8	0
343.	Pie, Pumpkin	1 (3½")	114	241	4.6	13	3.0	70	28	14	0.6	244	2,810	0.03	0.11	1.1	9
344.	Pineapple, canned, heavy syrup	1/2 c	128	95	0.4	0	0.0	0	25	17	0.4	2	65	0.10	0.03	0.6	12
345.	Pineapple, canned, juice pack	1/2 c	125	75	0.5	0	0.0	0	20	13	0.3	1	24	0.12	0.24	0.3	13
346.	Pineapple, raw	1/2 c diced	78	41	0.3	0	0.0	0	11	11	0.4	1	55	0.07	0.03	0.3	1
347.	Pizza, Cheese, Thin 'n Crispy, Pizza Hut	1/2 10" pie	*	450	25.0	15	7.0	125	54	450	4.5	1,200	750	0.30	0.51	5.0	1
348.	Pizza, Cheese, Thick 'n Chewy, Pizza Hut	1/2 10" pie	*	560	34.0	14	6.0	110	71	500	5.4	1,100	1,000	0.68	0.68	7.0	4
349.	Plums, Japanese and hybrid, raw	1 plum 2⅛" diam.	70	32	0.3	0	0.0	0	8	8	0.3	1	160	0.02	0.02	0.3	4
350.	Popcorn, cooked, oil	1 c	11	55	0.9	3	0.5	0	6	6	0.3	86	20	0.01	0.02	0.1	0
351.	Popcorn, popped, plain, large kernel	1 c	6	12	0.8	0	0.0	0	5	3	0.2	0	0	0.00	0.01	0.1	0
352.	Pork roast, trimmed	2 slices 3 oz.	85	179	24.0	8	2.2	65	0	11	3.1	863	0	0.55	0.22	4.3	0
353.	Pork, sausage, cooked	1 sm link	17	72	2.8	6	2.1	13	0	0	0.3	221	0	0.00	0.00	0.0	0
354.	Potato, au gratin	1 c	245	228	5.6	10	6.3	12	32	203	0.8	1,076	380	0.05	0.20	2.3	8
355.	Potato, baked in skin	1 potato 2⅓ x 4¼"	202	145	1.1	0	0.0	0	33	14	1.1	6	0	0.15	0.07	2.7	31
356.	Potato chips	10 chips	20	114	2.1	8	2.1	0	10	8	0.4	150	0	0.04	0.01	1.0	3
357.	Potato, French fried long	10 strips 3½-4"	78	214	3.4	10	1.7	0	28	12	1.0	5	0	0.10	0.06	2.4	16
358.	Potato, Hashbrowns, McDonald's	1 patty	55	144	1.4	9	3.0	4	15	5	0.4	325	6	0.06	0.01	0.8	4

Code	Food	Amount	Weight gm	Calories	Protein gm	Fat gm	Sat. Fat gm	Cholesterol mg	Carbohydrate gm	Calcium mg	Iron mg	Sodium mg	Vit A I.U.	Thiamin (Vit B₁) mg	Riboflavin (Vit B₂) mg	Niacin mg	Vit C mg
359.	Potato, mashed, milk added	1/2 c	105	69	2.2	1	0.4	8	14	25	0.4	316	20	0.09	0.06	1.1	11
360.	Potato salad w/eggs, mayo	1/2 c	125	179	3.4	10	7.8	85	14	24	0.8	662	262	0.10	0.08	1.1	12
361.	Potato, hash brown	1/2 c	78	170	2.5	9	3.5	0	22	12	1.2	27	0	0.09	0.02	1.9	5
362.	Pretzel, thin, twists	1 oz.	28	113	2.8	1	0.3	0	23	8	0.6	456	0	0.09	0.07	1.2	0
363.	Prunes, dried "softenized" without pits	5 prunes	61	137	1.1	0	0.0	0	36	26	0.1	4	860	0.05	0.09	0.9	2
364.	Prune juice, canned or bottled	1/2 c	128	99	0.5	0	0.0	0	24	18	5.3	3	0	0.02	0.02	0.5	3
365.	Pudding, Chocolate, canned	5 oz.	142	205	3	11	9.5	1	30	74	1.2	285	155	0.04	0.17	0.6	0
366.	Pudding, Tapioca, canned	5 oz.	142	160	3	5	4.8	1	28	119	0.3	252	5	0.03	0.14	0.4	0
367.	Pudding, Vanilla, canned	5 oz.	142	220	2	10	9.5	1	33	79	0.2	305	5	0.03	0.12	0.6	0
368.	Quiche, Lorraine	1 piece	242	825	18	66	31.9	392	40	290	1.9	898	2,250	0.15	0.44	1.7	1
369.	Raisins, unbleached, seedless	1 oz.	28	82	0.7	0	0.0	0	22	18	1.0	8	10	0.03	0.02	0.1	0
370.	Raspberries, fresh	1 c	123	60	1.1	1	0.0	0	14	27	0.7	0	80	0.04	0.11	1.1	31
371.	Raspberries, frozen	1 c	250	255	1.7	1	0.0	0	62	38	1.6	3	75	0.05	0.11	1.5	41
372.	Rice, brown, cooked	1/2 c	96	116	2.5	1	0.0	0	25	12	0.5	275	0	0.09	0.02	1.3	0
373.	Rice, white enriched, cooked	1/2 c	103	113	2.1	0	0.0	0	25	11	0.9	384	0	0.12	0.01	1.1	0
374.	Rice, wild, cooked	1/2 c	100	92	3.6	0	0.0	0	19	5	1.1	2	0	0.11	0.16	1.6	0
375.	Roast Beef, Regular, Arby's	1	155	383	22	18	7.0	43	35	72	3.20	936	0	0.28	0.50	11.0	0
376.	Roast Beef Sub, Arby's	1	305	623	38	32	11.5	73	47	492	5.20	1847	500	0.56	0.76	14.2	9
377.	Roll, hard, white	1 roll	50	155	5	2	0.0	0	30	24	1.4	313	0	0.20	0.12	1.7	0
378.	Rueben sandwich	1	237	488	28.7	28	10.4	85	30	364	5.3	1,685	461	0.25	0.44	3.9	12
379.	Salad, Caesar side, Wendy's	1	130	160	10	6	1.0	10	18	96	1.20	700	1250	0.231	0.27	2.0	24
380.	Salad, Chef, Burger King	1 serving	273	178	17.0	9	4.0	103	7	128	1.6	568	4,750	0.35	0.26	3.6	15
381.	Salad, Chef, McDonald's	1	265	170	17	9	4.0	111	8	180	0.96	400	5000	0.30	0.27	4.0	21
382.	Salad, Chicken, Burger King	1 serving	258	142	20	4	1.0	49	8	32	1.3	443	4,600	0.14	0.17	8.5	20
383.	Salad, Chicken w/celery	1/2 c	78	266	10.5	25	4.1	48	1	16	0.7	199	153	0.03	0.08	3.3	1
384.	Salad, Deluxe Garden, Wendy's	1	271	110	7	5	1.0	0	9	240	0.96	380	3000	0.15	0.36	1.2	36
385.	Salad, Garden, Arby's	1	330	117	7	5	2.7	12	11	192	1.10	134	4900	0.17	0.20	1.2	52
386.	Salad, Grilled Chicken, Wendy's	1	338	200	25	8	1.0	55	9	240	1.80	690	3000	0.225	0.36	8.0	36
387.	Salad, Tuna	1 c	205	375	33	19	3.3	80	19	31	2.5	877	53	0.06	0.14	13.3	6
388.	Salami, dry	1 oz.	28	128	7.0	11	1.6	24	0	4	1.0	349	0	0.10	0.07	1.5	0
389.	Salmon, broiled with butter or margarine	3 oz.	85	156	23.0	6	2.2	53	0	0	0.9	99	150	0.15	0.06	8.4	0
390.	Salmon, canned Chinook	3 oz.	85	179	16.6	12	0.8	30	0	131	0.7	105	197	0.03	0.01	6.2	0
391.	Sardines, canned drained	1 oz.	28	58	7.0	3	1.0	20	0	124	0.8	233	60	0.01	0.06	1.5	0
392.	Sauerkraut, canned	1/2 c	118	21	1.2	0	0.0	0	5	43	0.6	878	60	0.04	0.05	0.3	17
393.	Sausage Biscuit w/Egg. McDonald's	1	175	505	19	33	20.0	260	33	120	2.4	1210	300	0.45	0.36	4.0	0
394.	Sausage McMuffin, McDonald's	1	135	345	15	20	11.0	57	27	240	1.8	770	200	0.525	0.27	5.0	0
395.	Sausage McMuffin, w/Egg	1	159	430	21	25	14.0	270	27	300	2.4	920	500	0.525	0.45	5.0	0
396.	Sausage, smoked link, pork	1	68	265	15	22	7.7	46	1	20	.79	1020	0	1.04	.29	5.0	14
397.	Scallops, breaded, cooked	6 pieces	90	195	15	10	2.5	70	10	39	2.0	298	105	0.11	0.11	1.6	0
398.	Sherbet	1/2 c	97	135	1.1	2	1.3	7	29	52	0.2	44	92	0.02	0.04	0.1	2
399.	Shrimp, boiled	3 oz.	85	99	18.0	1	0.1	128	7	99	2.7	0	60	0.00	0.03	1.5	0
400.	Shrimp, fried	7 medium	85	200	16.0	10	2.5	168	11	61	2.0	384	130	0.06	0.09	2.8	0
401.	Snickers bar	1 bar	61	290	6.6	4	5.4	0	37	70	0.5	170	25	0.03	0.11	1.8	0
402.	Soda pop, cola	12 oz.	369	144	0.0	0	0.0	0	37	27	0.1	30	0	0.00	0.00	0.0	0
403.	Soda pop, diet	12 oz.	340	2	0.1	0	0.0	0	0	13	0.1	31	0	0.00	0.00	0.0	0
404.	Soda pop, Ginger ale	12 oz.	366	113	0.0	0	0.0	0	29	0	0.0	45	0	0.00	0.00	0.0	0

No.	Food	Amount	Wt (g)	Cal	Protein (g)	Fat (g)	Sat. fat (g)	Chol (mg)	Carb (g)	Ca (mg)	Fe (mg)	Na (mg)	Vit. A (IU)	Thiamin (mg)	Riboflavin (mg)	Niacin (mg)	Vit. C (mg)
405.	Soda pop, Lemon-lime	12 oz.	340	138	0.0	0	0.0	0	35	8	0.2	38	0	0.00	0.00	0.0	0
406.	Soda pop, Root beer	12 oz.	340	140	0.0	0	0.0	0	36	17	0.2	45	0	0.00	0.00	0.0	0
407.	Soup, Chicken, cream	1 c	248	191	7.5	12	4.6	27	15	180	0.7	1,046	710	0.07	0.26	0.9	1
408.	Soup, Chicken noodle	1 c	241	75	4.0	2	0.7	7	9	17	0.8	900	711	0.05	0.06	1.4	0
409.	Soup, Clam chowder, Manhattan	1 c	244	78	4.2	2	0.4	2	12	34	1.9	1,808	460	0.06	0.05	1.3	3
410.	Soup, Clam chowder, north east	1 c	248	163	9.5	7	3.0	22	16	187	1.5	992	160	0.07	0.24	1.0	4
411.	Soup, Cream of mushroom condensed, prepared with equal volume of milk	1 c	245	216	7.0	14	5.4	15	16	191	0.5	955	250	0.05	0.34	0.7	1
412.	Soup, Minestrone	1 c	241	80	4.3	3	0.5	2	11	34	0.9	911	1,170	0.05	0.04	0.9	1
413.	Soup, Split pea, condensed, prepared with equal volume of water	1 c	245	145	9.0	3	1.1	0	21	29	1.5	941	440	0.25	0.15	1.5	1
414.	Soup, Tomato, condensed, prepared with equal volume of water	1 c	245	88	2.0	3	0.5	0	16	15	0.7	970	1,000	0.05	0.05	1.2	12
415.	Soup, Tomato with milk	1 c	248	160	6.0	6	2.9	17	22	159	1.8	932	850	0.13	0.25	1.5	68
416.	Soup, vegetable beef, condensed, prepared with equal volume of water	1 c	245	78	5.0	2	0.0	0	10	12	0.7	1,046	2,700	0.05	0.05	1.0	0
417.	Soup, Vegetarian vegetable	1 c	250	70	2.1	2	0.3	0	12	21	1.1	823	1,505	0.05	0.05	0.9	1
418.	Sour cream	1 tbsp	14	30	0.4	3	1.8	6	1	16	0.0	8	135	0.01	0.02	0.0	0
419.	Sour cream, imitation	1 tbsp.	14	29	0.3	3	2.5	0	1	0	0.0	14	0	0.00	0.00	0.0	0
420.	Spaghetti, in tomato sauce with cheese	1 c	250	260	8.8	9	2.0	10	37	80	2.3	955	1,080	0.25	0.18	2.3	13
421.	Spaghetti, plain, cooked	1 c	140	155	5.0	1	0.1	0	32	11	1.7	1	0	0.20	0.11	1.5	0
422.	Spaghetti, whole wheat, cooked	1 c	125	151	6.6	1	0.1	0	32	19	1.1	16	0	0.21	0.09	1.5	0
423.	Spaghetti, with meatballs and tomato sauce	1 c	248	332	18.6	11.7	3.0	75	39	124	3.7	1,009	1,590	0.25	0.30	4.0	22
424.	Spareribs, cooked	3 oz.	85	377	17.8	33	12.0	73	0	8	2.2	31	0	0.37	0.18	2.9	0
425.	Spinach, canned, drained	1/2 c	103	25	2.3	1	0.0	0	4	121	2.6	242	8,200	0.02	0.12	0.3	15
426.	Spinach, froz., cooked, drained	1/2 c	103	24	3.1	0	0.0	0	4	116	2.2	54	8,100	0.07	0.16	0.4	20
427.	Spinach, raw, chopped	1 c	55	14	1.8	0	0.0	0	2	51	1.7	39	4,460	0.06	0.11	0.3	28
428.	Squash, summer, cooked	1/2 c	90	13	0.8	0	0.0	0	3	23	0.4	1	350	0.05	0.07	0.7	9
429.	Squash, winter, baked mashed	1/2 c	103	70	1.9	0	0.0	0	18	41	1.0	8	6,560	0.05	0.14	0.7	8
430.	Strawberries, frozen, sweetened	1 c	250	245	1.4	0	0.0	0	66	28	1.5	8	31	0.04	0.13	1.0	106
431.	Strawberries, raw	1 c	149	55	1.0	1	0.0	0	13	31	1.5	1	90	0.04	0.10	0.9	88
432.	Stuffing, bread, prepared	1/2 c	70	250	4.6	15	3.1	0	25	46	1.1	627	455	0.09	0.10	1.3	0
433.	Sundae, choc. Dairy Queen	medium	184	300	6.0	7	4.9	79	53	200	1.1	175	300	0.06	0.26	0.0	0
434.	Sugar, brown granulated	1 tsp	5	17	0.0	0	0.0	0	5	4	0.1	0	0	0.00	0.00	0.1	0
435.	Sugar, white granulated	1 tsp	4	15	0.0	0	0.0	0	4	0	0.0	0	0	0.00	0.00	0.0	0
436.	Super Roast Beef, Arby's	1	254	552	24	28	7.6	43	54	108	4.3	1174	150	0.39	0.61	12.4	9
437.	Sweet N' Sour Sauce, McDonald's	1.12 oz.	31.75	60	0	0.2	0.1	0	14	46	0.0	190	300	0.10	0.08	0.8	25
438.	Sweet potato, baked	1 potato 5" long	146	161	2.4	1	0.0	0	37	33	1.0	14	0	0.00	0.00	0.0	0
439.	Syrup (maple)	1 tbsp	20	50	0.0	0	0.0	0	13								
440.	Taco Salad, Wendy's	1	510	640	34	30	12.0	80	70	540	5.4	960	1750	0.225	0.45	3.0	27
441.	Taco shell	1 shell	10	60	1.1	3	0.3	0	9	26	0.3	62	36	0.00	0.01	0.3	0
442.	Taco, Taco Bell	1	83	186	15.0	8	0.0	0	14	120	2.4	79	120	0.09	0.16	2.9	0
443.	Tangerine	1 med 2⅜" diam.	116	39	0.7	0	0.0	0	10	34	0.3	2	360	0.05	0.02	0.1	27
444.	Tartar sauce	1 tbsp.	14	74	0.2	8	1.2	4	1	3	0.1	182	54	0.00	0.00	0.0	0
445.	Tea, brewed	1/4 c	180	0	0.0	0	0.0	0	0	0	0.0	0	0	0.00	0.00	0.0	0

Code	Food	Amount	Weight gm	Calories	Protein gm	Fat gm	Sat. Fat gm	Cholesterol mg	Carbohydrate gm	Calcium mg	Iron mg	Sodium mg	Vit A I.U.	Thiamin (Vit B_1) mg	Riboflavin (Vit B_2) mg	Niacin mg	Vit C mg
446.	Tomato juice, canned	1 c	244	42	1.9	0	0.1	0	10	22	1.4	881	1,357	0.12	0.08	1.6	45
447.	Tomato sauce (catsup)	1 tbsp	15	16	0.3	0	0.0	0	4	3	0.1	156	105	0.01	0.01	0.2	2
448.	Tomato, canned	1/2 c	121	26	1.2	0	0.0	0	5	7	0.6	157	1,085	0.06	0.04	0.9	21
449.	Tomato, raw	1 tomato 3½ oz.	100	20	1.0	0	0.0	0	4	12	0.5	3	820	0.05	0.04	0.6	21
450.	Tortilla chips	1 oz.	28	139	2.2	8	1.1	0	17	82	1.0	140	7	0.01	0.02	0.2	0
451.	Tortilla, corn, lime	1 6" diam.	30	63	1.5	3	0.0	0	14	60	0.9	134	6	0.04	0.02	0.3	0
452.	Tortilla, flour	1	35	105	2.6	3	0.4	0	19	21	0.5			0.13	0.08	1.2	0
453.	Tostada	1	148	206	9.2	18	3.0	14	25	167	1.8	200	445	0.06	0.13	0.8	6
454.	Trout, broiled w/butter, lemon	3 oz.	85	175	21.0	9	4.1	71	0	26	1.0	122	300	0.07	0.07	2.3	1
455.	Tuna, canned, oil pack, drained	3 oz.	85	167	25.0	7	1.7	60	0	7	1.6	0	70	0.04	0.10	10.1	0
456.	Tuna, canned, water pack, solids and liquid	3½ oz.	99	126	27.7	1	0.0	55	0	16	1.6	161	0	0.00	0.10	13.2	0
457.	Turkey, Lite Roast Deluxe, Arby'	1	195	260	20	6	1.6	33	33	156	2.30	1262	200	0.29	0.43	15.4	12
458.	Turkey, roast (light and dark mixed)	3 oz.	85	162	27.0	5	1.5	73	0	7	1.5	111	0	0.04	0.15	6.5	0
459.	Turnip, cooked, drained	1/2 c cubed	78	18	0.6	0	0.0	0	4	27	0.3	27	0	0.03	0.04	0.3	17
460.	Turnip greens, cooked drained	1/2 c	73	19	2.1	0	0.0	0	3	98	1.3	14	5,695	0.04	0.08	0.4	16
461.	Veal, cooked loin	3 oz.	85	199	22.0	11	4.0	90	0	9	2.7	55	0	0.06	0.21	4.6	0
462.	Veal cutlet, braised, broiled	3 oz.	85	185	23.0	9	4.0	109	0	9	0.8	56	5	0.06	0.21	4.6	0
463.	Vegetables, mixed, cooked	1 c	182	116	5.8	0	0.0	0	24	46	2.4	348	4,505	0.02	0.13	2.0	15
464.	Waffles	1 waffle	75	205	6.9	8	2.7	59	27	179	1.2	515	49	0.14	0.23	0.9	0
465.	Watermelon	1 c diced	160	42	0.8	0	0.0	0	10	11	0.8	2	940	0.05	0.05	0.3	11
466.	Wheat germ, plain toasted	1 tbsp	6	23	1.8	1	0.0	0	3	3	0.5		10	0.11	0.05	0.3	0
467.	Whiskey, gin, rum, vodka 90 proof	1/2 11 oz (jigger)	42	110	0	0	0.0	0	0	0	0.0	0	0	0.00	0.00	0.0	0
468.	Whopper, Burger King	1 sandwich	270	614	27.0	36	12.0	90	45	64	4.9	865	550	0.34	0.41	6.1	12
469.	Whopper with cheese, Burger King	1 sandwich	294	706	32.0	44	16.0	115	47	176	4.9	1,177	950	0.34	0.48	6.1	12
470.	Whopper, double, Burger King	1 sandwich	351	844	46.0	53	19.0	169	45	72	7.2	933	550	0.35	0.56	9.4	12
471.	Wine, dry table 12% alc.	3½ fl. oz.	102	87	0.1	0	0.0	0	4	9	0.4	5	0	0.00	0.01	0.1	0
472.	Wine, red dry 18.8% alc.	2 fl. oz.	59	81	0.1	0	0.0	0	5	5	0.0	4	0	0.01	0.02	0.2	0
473.	Yeast, brewers	1 tbsp	8	23	3.1	0	0.0	0	3	17	1.4	10		1.25	0.34	3.0	0
474.	Yogurt, fruit	1 c	227	231	9.9	2	1.6	10	43	345	0.2	125	104	0.08	0.40	0.2	2
475.	Yogurt, Nonfat, TCBY	4 fl. oz.	113	110	4	4	0	0	23	96	0.1	45	0	0.03	0.144	0	0
476.	Yogurt, plain low fat	1 8-oz. container	226	113	7.7	4	2.3	15	12	271	0.1	115	150	0.09	0.41	0.2	2
477.	Yogurt, Regular, TCBY	4 fl. oz.	113	120	4	3	2.0	13	23	180	0.48	60	0	0.06	0.18	0	0
478.	Yogurt, Sugar Free, TCBY	4 fl. oz.	113	80	4	0	0	0	18	96	0	40	200	0.06	0.18	0	0
479.	Yogurt, Vanilla Lowfat, McDonald's	3 oz.	85	105	4	1	0.3	3	22	120	0	80	100	0.03	0.18	0.4	0

"0" represents both less than 1 and 0

Sources:

Nutritive Value of American Foods in Common Units. *Agriculture Handbook No. 456.* U.S. Dept. of Agriculture. Washington, D.C. 1988.

Young, E. A., E. H. Brennan, and C. L. Irving. Guest Eds. Perspectives on Fast Foods. *Public Health Currents,* 19(1), 1979, Published by Ross Laboratories, Columbus, OH.

Dennison, D. *The Dine System: the Nutrition Plan For Better Health.* C. V. Mosby Company St. Louis, Missouri, 1982.

Pennington, S. A. T. and H. N. Church. *Food Values of Portions Commonly Used.* Harper and Row Publishers, New York, 1985.

Kullman, D. A. *ABC Milligram Cholesterol Diet Guide.* Merit Publications, Inc. North Miami Beach, Florida 1978.

Food Processor nutrient analysis software by Esha Corporation, P.O. Box 13028, Salem, Oregon, 97309. With permission.

The recommended quality and quantity of exercise for developing and maintaining cardiorespiratory and muscular fitness in healthy adults*

AMERICAN COLLEGE of SPORTS MEDICINE

POSITION STAND

The Recommended Quantity and Quality of Exercise for Developing and Maintaining Cardiorespiratory and Muscular Fitness in Healthy Adults

This Position Stand replaces the 1978 ACSM position paper, "The Recommended Quantity and Quality of Exercise for Developing and Maintaining Fitness in Healthy Adults."

Increasing numbers of persons are becoming involved in endurance training and other forms of physical activity, and, thus, the need for guidelines for exercise prescription is apparent. Based on the existing evidence concerning exercise prescription for healthy adults and the need for guidelines, the American College of Sports Medicine (ACSM) makes the following recommendations for the quantity and quality of training for developing and maintaining cardiorespiratory fitness, body composition, and muscular strength and endurance in the healthy adult:

1. Frequency of training: 3–5 $d \cdot wk^{-1}$.
2. Intensity of training: 60–90% of maximum heart rate (HR_{max}), or 50–85% of maximum oxygen uptake ($\dot{V}O_{2max}$) or HR_{max} reserve.[1]
3. Duration of training: 20–60 min of continuous aerobic activity. Duration is dependent on the intensity of the activity; thus, lower intensity activity should be conducted over a longer period of time. Because of the importance of "total fitness" and the fact that it is more readily attained in longer duration programs, and because of the potential hazards and compliance problems associated with high intensity activity, lower to moderate intensity activity of longer duration is recommended for the nonathletic adult.
4. Mode of activity: any activity that uses large muscle groups, can be maintained continuously, and is rhythmical and aerobic in nature, e.g., walking-hiking, running-jogging, cycling-bicycling, cross-country skiing, dancing, rope skipping, rowing, stair climbing, swimming, skating, and various endurance game activities.
5. Resistance training: Strength training of a moderate intensity, sufficient to develop and maintain fat-free weight (FFW), should be an integral part of an adult fitness program. One set of 8–12 repetitions of eight to ten exercises that condition the major muscle groups at least 2 $d \cdot wk^{-1}$ is the recommended minimum.

RATIONALE AND RESEARCH BACKGROUND

Introduction

The questions "How much exercise is enough," and "What type of exercise is best for developing and maintaining fitness?" are frequently asked. It is recognized that the term "physical fitness" is composed of a variety of characteristics included in the broad categories of cardiovascular-respiratory fitness, body composition, muscular strength and endurance, and flexibility. In this context fitness is defined as the ability to perform moderate to vigorous levels of physical activity without undue fatigue and the capability of maintaining such ability throughout life (167). It is also recognized that the adaptive response to training is complex and includes peripheral, central, structural, and functional factors (5,172). Although many such variables and their adaptive response to training have been documented, the lack of sufficient in-depth and comparative data relative to frequency, intensity, and duration of training makes them inadequate to use as comparative models. Thus, in respect to the above questions, fitness is limited mainly to changes in $\dot{V}O_{2max}$, muscular strength and endurance, and body composition, which includes total body mass, fat weight (FW), and FFW. Further, the rationale and research background used for this position stand will be divided into programs for cardiorespiratory fitness and weight control and programs for muscular strength and endurance.

Fitness versus health benefits of exercise. Since the original position statement was published in 1978, an important distinction has been made between physical activity as it relates to health versus fitness. It has been pointed out that the quantity and quality of ex-

---

[1] Maximum heart rate reserve is calculated from the difference between resting and maximum heart rate. To estimate training intensity, a percentage of this value is added to the resting heart rate and is expressed as a percentage of HR_{max} reserve (85).

ercise needed to attain health-related benefits may differ from what is recommended for fitness benefits. It is now clear that lower levels of physical activity than recommended by this position statement may reduce the risk for certain chronic degenerative diseases and yet may not be of sufficient quantity or quality to improve $\dot{V}O_{2max}$ (71,72,98,167). ACSM recognizes the potential health benefits of regular exercise performed more frequently and for a longer duration, but at lower intensities than prescribed in this position statement (13A,71,100,120,160). ACSM will address the issue concerning the proper amount of physical activity necessary to derive health benefits in another statement.

Need for standardization of procedures and reporting results. Despite an abundance of information available concerning the training of the human organism, the lack of standardization of testing protocols and procedures, of methodology in relation to training procedures and experimental design, and of a preciseness in the documentation and reporting of the quantity and quality of training prescribed make interpretation difficult (123,133,139,164,167). Interpretation and comparison of results are also dependent on the initial level of fitness (42,43,58,114,148,151,156), length of time of the training experiment (17,45,125,128,139, 145,150), and specificity of the testing and training (5,43,130,139,145A,172). For example, data from training studies using subjects with varied levels of $\dot{V}O_{2max}$, total body mass, and FW have found changes to occur in relation to their initial values (14,33,109, 112,113,148,151); i.e., the lower the initial $\dot{V}O_{2max}$ the larger the percentage of improvement found, and the higher the FW the greater the reduction. Also, data evaluating trainability with age, comparison of the different magnitudes and quantities of effort, and comparison of the trainability of men and women may have been influenced by the initial fitness levels.

In view of the fact that improvement in the fitness variables discussed in this position statement continues over many months of training (27,86,139,145,150), it is reasonable to believe that short-term studies conducted over a few weeks have certain limitations. Middle-aged sedentary and older participants may take several weeks to adapt to the initial rigors of training, and thus need a longer adaptation period to get the full benefit from a program. For example, Seals et al. (150) exercise trained 60–69-yr-olds for 12 months. Their subjects showed a 12% improvement in $\dot{V}O_{2max}$ after 6 months of moderate intensity walking training. A further 18% increase in $\dot{V}O_{2max}$ occurred during the next 6 months of training when jogging was introduced. How long a training experiment should be conducted is difficult to determine, but 15–20 wk may be a good minimum standard. Although it is difficult to control exercise training experiments for more than 1 yr, there is a need to study this effect. As stated earlier, lower

doses of exercise may improve $\dot{V}O_{2max}$ and control or maintain body composition, but at a slower rate.

Although most of the information concerning training described in this position statement has been conducted on men, the available evidence indicates that women tend to adapt to endurance training in the same manner as men (19,38,46,47,49,62,65,68,90,92,122, 166).

Exercise Prescription for Cardiorespiratory Fitness and Weight Control

Exercise prescription is based upon the frequency, intensity, and duration of training, the mode of activity (aerobic in nature, e.g., listed under No. 4 above), and the initial level of fitness. In evaluating these factors, the following observations have been derived from studies conducted for up to 6–12 months with endurance training programs.

Improvement in $\dot{V}O_{2max}$ is directly related to frequency (3,6,50,75–77,125,126,152,154,164), intensity (3,6,26,29,58,61,75–77,80,85,93,118,152,164), and duration (3,29,60,61,70,75–77,101,109,118,152,162, 164,168) of training. Depending upon the quantity and quality of training, improvement in $\dot{V}O_{2max}$ ranges from 5 to 30% (8,29,30,48,59,61,65,67,69,75–77,82,84,96, 99,101,102,111,115,119,123,127,139,141,143,149, 150,152,153,158,164,168,173). These studies show that a minimum increase in $\dot{V}O_{2max}$ of 15% is generally attained in programs that meet the above stated guidelines. Although changes in $\dot{V}O_{2max}$ greater than 30% have been shown, they are usually associated with large total body mass and FW loss, in cardiac patients, or in persons with a very low initial level of fitness. Also, as a result of leg fatigue or a lack of motivation, persons with low initial fitness may have spuriously low initial $\dot{V}O_{2max}$ values. Klissouras (94A) and Bouchard (16A) have shown that human variation in the trainability of $\dot{V}O_{2max}$ is important and related to current phenotype level. That is, there is a genetically determined pretraining status of the trait and capacity to adapt to physical training. Thus, physiological results should be interpreted with respect to both genetic variation and the quality and quantity of training performed.

Intensity-duration. Intensity and duration of training are interrelated, with total amount of work accomplished being an important factor in improvement in fitness (12,20,27,48,90,92,123,127,128,136,149,151,164). Although more comprehensive inquiry is necessary, present evidence suggests that, when exercise is performed above the minimum intensity threshold, the total amount of work accomplished is an important factor in fitness development (19,27,126,127,149,151) and maintenance (134). That is, improvement will be similar for activities performed at a lower intensity-longer duration compared to higher intensity-shorter duration if the total energy costs of the activities are equal. Higher intensity exercise is associated with greater cardiovascular risk (156A), orthopedic injury (124,139) and lower compliance to training than lower intensity exercise (36,105,124,146). Therefore, programs emphasizing low to moderate intensity training with longer duration are recommended for most adults.

The minimal training intensity threshold for improvement in $\dot{V}O_{2max}$ is approximately 60% of the HR_{max} (50% of $\dot{V}O_{2max}$ or HR_{max} reserve) (80,85). The 50% of HR_{max} reserve represents a heart rate of approximately 130–135 beats·min^{-1} for young persons. As a result of the age-related change in maximum heart rate, the absolute heart rate to achieve this threshold is inversely related to age and can be as low as 105–115 beats·min^{-1} for older persons (35,65,150). Patients who are taking beta-adrenergic blocking drugs may have significantly lower heart rate values (171). Initial level of fitness is another important consideration in prescribing exercise (26,90,104,148,151). The person with a low fitness level can achieve a significant training effect with a sustained training heart rate as low as 40–50% of HR_{max} reserve, while persons with higher fitness levels require a higher training stimulus (35,58,152,164).

Classification of exercise intensity. The classification of exercise intensity and its standardization for exercise prescription based on a 20–60 min training session has been confusing, misinterpreted, and often taken out of context. The most quoted exercise classification system is based on the energy expenditure (kcal·min^{-1}·kg^{-1}) of industrial tasks (40,89). The original data for this classification system were published by Christensen (24) in 1953 and were based on the energy expenditure of working in the steel mill for an 8-h day. The classification of industrial and leisure-time tasks by using absolute values of energy expenditure have been valuable for use in the occupational and nutritional setting. Although this classification system has broad application in medicine and, in particular, making recommendations for weight control and job placement, it has little or no meaning for preventive and rehabilitation exercise training programs. To extrapolate absolute values of energy expenditure for completing an industrial task based on an 8-h work day to 20–60 min regimens of exercise training does not make sense. For example, walking and jogging/running can be accomplished at a wide range of speeds; thus, the relative intensity becomes important under these conditions. Because the endurance training regimens recommended by ACSM for nonathletic adults are geared for 60 min or less of physical activity, the system of classification of exercise training intensity shown in Table 1 is recommended (139). The use of a realistic time period for training and an individual's relative exercise intensity makes this system amenable to young,

TABLE 1. Classification of intensity of exercise based on 20–60 min of endurance training.

Relative Intensity (%)		Rating of Perceived Exertion	Classification of Intensity
HR_{max}*	$\dot{V}O_{2max}$* or HR_{max} reserve		
<35%	<30%	<10	Very light
35–59%	30–49%	10–11	Light
60–79%	50–74%	12–13	Moderate (somewhat hard)
80–89%	75–84%	14–16	Heavy
≥90%	≥85%	>16	Very heavy

Table from Pollock, M. L. and J. H. Wilmore. *Exercise in Health and Disease: Evaluation and Prescription for Prevention and Rehabilitation*, 2nd Ed. Philadelphia: W.B. Saunders, 1990. Published with permission.
* HR_{max} = maximum heart rate; $\dot{V}O_{2max}$ = maximum oxygen uptake.

middle-aged, and elderly participants, as well as patients with a limited exercise capacity (3,137,139).

Table 1 also describes the relationship between relative intensity based on percent HR_{max}, percentage of HR_{max} reserve or percentage of $\dot{V}O_{2max}$, and the rating of perceived exertion (RPE) (15,16,137). The use of heart rate as an estimate of intensity of training is the common standard (3,139).

The use of RPE has become a valid tool in the monitoring of intensity in exercise training programs (11,37,137,139). It is generally considered an adjunct to heart rate in monitoring relative exercise intensity, but once the relationship between heart rate and RPE is known, RPE can be used in place of heart rate (23,139). This would not be the case in certain patient populations where a more precise knowledge of heart rate may be critical to the safety of the program.

Frequency. The amount of improvement in $\dot{V}O_{2max}$ tends to plateau when frequency of training is increased above 3 d·wk^{-1} (50,123,139). The value of the added improvement found with training more than 5 d·wk^{-1} is small to not apparent in regard to improvement in $\dot{V}O_{2max}$ (75–77,106,123). Training of less than 2 d·wk^{-1} does not generally show a meaningful change in $\dot{V}O_{2max}$ (29,50,118,123,152,164).

Mode. If frequency, intensity, and duration of training are similar (total kcal expenditure), the training adaptations appear to be independent of the mode of aerobic activity (101A,118,130). Therefore, a variety of endurance activities, e.g., those listed above, may be used to derive the same training effect.

Endurance activities that require running and jumping are considered high impact types of activity and generally cause significantly more debilitating injuries to beginning as well as long-term exercisers than do low impact and non-weight bearing type activities (13,93, 117,124,127,135,140,142). This is particularly evident in the elderly (139). Beginning joggers have increased foot, leg, and knee injuries when training is performed more than 3 d·wk^{-1} and longer than 30 min duration per exercise session (135). High intensity interval training (run-walk) compared to continuous jogging training was also associated with a higher incidence of injury (124,136). Thus, caution should be taken when recommending the type of activity and exercise prescription for the beginning exerciser. Orthopedic injuries as related to overuse increase linearly in runners/joggers when performing these activities (13,140). Thus, there is a need for more inquiry into the effect that different types of activities and the quantity and quality of training has on injuries over short-term and long-term participation.

An activity such as weight training should not be considered as a means of training for developing $\dot{V}O_{2max}$, but it has significant value for increasing muscular strength and endurance and FFW (32,54,107, 110,165). Studies evaluating circuit weight training (weight training conducted almost continuously with moderate weights, using 10–15 repetitions per exercise session with 15–30 s rest between bouts of activity) show an average improvement in $\dot{V}O_{2max}$ of 6% (1,51–54,83,94,108,170). Thus, circuit weight training is not recommended as the only activity used in exercise programs for developing $\dot{V}O_{2max}$.

Age. Age in itself does not appear to be a deterrent to endurance training. Although some earlier studies showed a lower training effect with middle-aged or elderly participants (9,34,79,157,168), more recent studies show the relative change in $\dot{V}O_{2max}$ to be similar to younger age groups (7,8,65,132,150,161,163). Although more investigation is necessary concerning the rate of improvement in $\dot{V}O_{2max}$ with training at various ages, at present it appears that elderly participants need longer periods of time to adapt (34,132,150). Earlier studies showing moderate to no improvement in $\dot{V}O_{2max}$ were conducted over a short time span (9), or exercise was conducted at a moderate to low intensity (34), thus making the interpretation of the results difficult.

Although $\dot{V}O_{2max}$ decreases with age and total body mass and FW increase with age, evidence suggests that this trend can be altered with endurance training (22,27,86–88,139). A 9% reduction in $\dot{V}O_{2max}$ per decade for sedentary adults after age 25 has been shown (31,73), but for active individuals the reduction may be less than 5% per decade (21,31,39,73). Ten or more yr follow-up studies where participants continued training at a similar level showed maintenance of cardiorespiratory fitness (4,87,88,138). A cross-sectional study of older competitive runners showed progressively lower values in $\dot{V}O_{2max}$ from the fourth to seventh decades of life, but also showed less training in the older groups (129). More recent 10-yr follow-up data on these same athletes (50–82 yr of age) showed $\dot{V}O_{2max}$ to be unchanged when training quantity and quality remained unchanged (138). Thus, lifestyle plays a significant role in the maintenance of fitness. More inquiry into the relationship of long-term training (quantity and qual-

ity), for both competitors and noncompetitors, and physiological function with increasing age is necessary before more definitive statements can be made.

Maintenance of training effect. In order to maintain the training effect, exercise must be continued on a regular basis (18,25,28,47,97,111,144,147). A significant reduction in cardiorespiratory fitness occurs after 2 wk of detraining (25,144), with participants returning to near pretraining levels of fitness after 10 wk (47) to 8 months of detraining (97). A loss of 50% of their initial improvement in $\dot{V}O_{2max}$ has been shown after 4–12 wk of detraining (47,91,144). Those individuals who have undergone years of continuous training maintain some benefits for longer periods of detraining than subjects from short-term training studies (25). While stopping training shows dramatic reductions in $\dot{V}O_{2max}$, reduced training shows modest to no reductions for periods of 5–15 wk (18,75–77,144). Hickson et al., in a series of experiments where frequency (75), duration (76), or intensity (77) of training were manipulated, found that, if intensity of training remained unchanged, $\dot{V}O_{2max}$ was maintained for up to 15 wk when frequency and duration of training were reduced by as much as ⅔. When frequency and duration of training remained constant and intensity of training was reduced by ⅓ or ⅔, $\dot{V}O_{2max}$ was significantly reduced. Similar findings were found in regards to reduced strength training exercise. When strength training exercise was reduced from 3 or 2 d·wk⁻¹ to at least 1 d·wk⁻¹, strength was maintained for 12 wk of reduced training (62). Thus, it appears that missing an exercise session periodically or reducing training for up to 15 wk will not adversely effect $\dot{V}O_{2max}$ or muscular strength and endurance as long as training intensity is maintained.

Even though many new studies have given added insight into the proper amount of exercise, investigation is necessary to evaluate the rate of increase and decrease of fitness when varying training loads and reduction in training in relation to level of fitness, age, and length of time in training. Also, more information is needed to better identify the minimal level of exercise necessary to maintain fitness.

Weight control and body composition. Although there is variability in human response to body composition change with exercise, total body mass and FW are generally reduced with endurance training programs (133,139,171A), while FFW remains constant (123,133,139,169) or increases slightly (116,174). For example, Wilmore (171A) reported the results of 32 studies that met the criteria for developing cardiorespiratory fitness that are outlined in this position stand and found an average loss in total body mass of 1.5 kg and percent fat of 2.2%. Weight loss programs using dietary manipulation that result in a more dramatic decrease in total body mass show reductions in both FW and FFW (2,78,174). When these programs are conducted in conjunction with exercise training, FFW loss is more modest than in programs using diet alone (78,121). Programs that are conducted at least 3 d·wk^{-1} (123,125,126,128,169), of at least 20 min duration (109,123,169), and of sufficient intensity to expend approximately 300 kcal per exercise session (75 kg person)^2 are suggested as a threshold level for total body mass and FW loss (27,64,77,123,133,139). An expenditure of 200 kcal per session has also been shown to be useful in weight reduction if the exercise frequency is at least 4 d·wk^{-1} (155). If the primary purpose of the training program is for weight loss, then regimens of greater frequency and duration of training and low to moderate intensity are recommended (2,139). Programs with less participation generally show little or no change in body composition (44,57,93,123,133,159,162,169). Significant increases in $\dot{V}O_{2max}$ have been shown with 10–15 min of high intensity training (6,79,109,118,123,152,153); thus, if total body mass and FW reduction are not considerations, then shorter duration, higher intensity programs may be recommended for healthy individuals at low risk for cardiovascular disease and orthopedic injury.

Exercise Prescription for Muscular Strength and Endurance

The addition of resistance/strength training to the position statement results from the need for a well-rounded program that exercises all the major muscle groups of the body. Thus, the inclusion of resistance training in adult fitness programs should be effective in the development and maintenance of FFW. The effect of exercise training is specific to the area of the body being trained (5,43,145A,172). For example, training the legs will have little or no effect on the arms, shoulders, and trunk muscles. A 10-yr follow-up of master runners who continued their training regimen, but did no upper body exercise, showed maintenance of $\dot{V}O_{2max}$ and a 2-kg reduction in FFW (138). Their leg circumference remained unchanged, but arm circumference was significantly lower. These data indicate a loss of muscle mass in the untrained areas. Three of the athletes who practiced weight training exercise for the upper body and trunk muscles maintained their FFW. A comprehensive review by Sale (145A) carefully documents available information on specificity of training.

Specificity of training was further addressed by Graves et al. (63). Using a bilateral knee extension exercise, they trained four groups: group A, first ½ of the range of motion; group B, second ½ of the range of motion; group AB, full range of motion; and a control group that did not train. The results clearly showed that

the training result was specific to the range of motion trained, with group AB getting the best full range effect. Thus, resistance training should be performed through a full range of motion for maximum benefit (63,95).

Muscular strength and endurance are developed by the overload principle, i.e., by increasing more than normal the resistance to movement or frequency and duration of activity (32,41,43,74,145). Muscular strength is best developed by using heavy weights (that require maximum or nearly maximum tension development) with few repetitions, and muscular endurance is best developed by using lighter weights with a greater number of repetitions (10,41,43,145). To some extent, both muscular strength and endurance are developed under each condition, but each system favors a more specific type of development (43,145). Thus, to elicit improvement in both muscular strength and endurance, most experts recommend 8–12 repetitions per bout of exercise.

Any magnitude of overload will result in strength development, but higher intensity effort at or near maximal effort will give a significantly greater effect (43,74,101B,103,145,172). The intensity of resistance training can be manipulated by varying the weight load, repetitions, rest interval between exercises, and number of sets completed (43). Caution is advised for training that emphasizes lengthening (eccentric) contractions, compared to shortening (concentric) or isometric contractions, as the potential for skeletal muscle soreness and injury is accentuated (3A,84A).

Muscular strength and endurance can be developed by means of static (isometric) or dynamic (isotonic or isokinetic) exercises. Although each type of training has its favorable and weak points, for healthy adults, dynamic resistance exercises are recommended. Resistance training for the average participant should be rhythmical, performed at a moderate to slow speed, move through a full range of motion, and not impede normal forced breathing. Heavy resistance exercise can cause a dramatic acute increase in both systolic and diastolic blood pressure (100A,101C).

The expected improvement in strength from resistance training is difficult to assess because increases in strength are affected by the participants' initial level of strength and their potential for improvement (43,66,74,114,172). For example, Mueller and Rohmert (114) found increases in strength ranging from 2 to 9% per week depending on initial strength levels. Although the literature reflects a wide range of improvement in strength with resistance training programs, the average improvement for sedentary young and middle-aged men and women for up to 6 months of training is 25–30%. Fleck and Kraemer (43), in a review of 13 studies representing various forms of isotonic training, showed an average improvement in bench press strength of 23.3% when subjects were tested on the

---

^{2} Haskell and Haskell et al. (71,72) have suggested the use of 4 kcal·kg^{-1} of body weight of energy expenditure per day for a minimum standard for use in exercise programs.

equipment with which they were trained and 16.5% when tested on special isotonic or isokinetic ergometers (six studies). Fleck and Kraemer (43) also reported an average increase in leg strength of 26.6% when subjects were tested with the equipment that they trained on (six studies) and 21.2% when tested with special isotonic or isokinetic ergometers (five studies). Results of improvement in strength resulting from isometric training have been of the same magnitude as found with isotonic training (17,43,62,63).

In light of the information reported above, the following guidelines for resistance training are recommended for the average healthy adult. A minimum of 8–10 exercises involving the major muscle groups should be performed a minimum of two times per week. A minimum of one set of 8–12 repetitions to near fatigue should be completed. These minimal standards for resistance training are based on two factors. First, the time it takes to complete a comprehensive, well-rounded exercise program is important. Programs lasting more than 60 min per session are associated with higher dropout rates (124). Second, although greater frequencies of training (17,43,56) and additional sets or combinations of sets and repetitions elicit larger strength gains (10,32,43,74,145,172), the magnitude of difference is usually small. For example, Braith et al. (17) compared training 2 $d \cdot wk^{-1}$ with 3 $d \cdot wk^{-1}$ for 18 wk. The subjects performed one set of 7–10 repetitions to fatigue. The 2 $d \cdot wk^{-1}$ group showed a 21% increase in strength compared to 28% in the 3 $d \cdot wk^{-1}$ group. In other words, 75% of what could be attained in a 3 $d \cdot wk^{-1}$ program was attained in 2 $d \cdot wk^{-1}$. Also, the 21% improvement in strength found by the 2 $d \cdot wk^{-1}$ regimen is 70–80% of the improvement reported by other programs using additional frequencies of training and combinations of sets and repetitions (43). Graves et al. (62,63), Gettman et al. (55), Hurley et al. (83) and Braith et al. (17) found that programs using one set to fatigue showed a greater than 25% increase in strength. Although resistance training equipment may provide a better graduated and quantitative stimulus for overload than traditional calisthenic exercises, calisthenics and other resistance types of exercise can still be effective in improving and maintaining strength.

SUMMARY

The combination of frequency, intensity, and duration of chronic exercise has been found to be effective for producing a training effect. The interaction of these factors provide the overload stimulus. In general, the lower the stimulus the lower the training effect, and the greater the stimulus the greater the effect. As a result of specificity of training and the need for maintaining muscular strength and endurance, and flexibility of the major muscle groups, a well-rounded training program including resistance training and flexibility exercises is recommended. Although age in itself is not a limiting factor to exercise training, a more gradual approach in applying the prescription at older ages seems prudent. It has also been shown that endurance training of fewer than 2 $d \cdot wk^{-1}$, at less than 50% of maximum oxygen uptake and for less than 10 $min \cdot d^{-1}$, is inadequate for developing and maintaining fitness for healthy adults.

In the interpretation of this position statement, it must be recognized that the recommendations should be used in the context of participants' needs, goals, and initial abilities. In this regard, a sliding scale as to the amount of time allotted and intensity of effort should be carefully gauged for both the cardiorespiratory and muscular strength and endurance components of the program. An appropriate warm-up and cool-down, which would include flexibility exercises, is also recommended. The important factor is to design a program for the individual to provide the proper amount of physical activity to attain maximal benefit at the lowest risk. Emphasis should be placed on factors that result in permanent lifestyle change and encourage a lifetime of physical activity.

REFERENCES

1. ALLEN, T. E., R. J. BYRD, and D. P. SMITH. Hemodynamic consequences of circuit weight training. *Res. Q.* 43:299–306, 1976.
2. AMERICAN COLLEGE OF SPORTS MEDICINE. Proper and improper weight loss programs. *Med. Sci. Sports Exerc.* 15:ix–xiii, 1983.
3. AMERICAN COLLEGE OF SPORTS MEDICINE. *Guidelines for Graded Exercise Testing and Exercise Prescription*, 3rd Ed. Philadelphia: Lea and Febiger, 1986.
3A. ARMSTRONG, R. B. Mechanisms of exercise-induced delayed onset muscular soreness: a brief review. *Med. Sci. Sports Exerc.* 16:529–538, 1984.
4. ÅSTRAND, P. O. Exercise physiology of the mature athlete. In: *Sports Medicine for the Mature Athlete*, J. R. Sutton and R. M. Brock (Eds.). Indianapolis, IN: Benchmark Press, Inc., 1986, pp. 3–16.
5. ÅSTRAND, P. O. and K. RODAHL. *Textbook of Work Physiology*, 3rd Ed. New York: McGraw-Hill, 1986, pp. 412–485.
6. ATOMI, Y., K. ITO, H. IWASASKI, and M. MIYASHITA. Effects of intensity and frequency of training on aerobic work capacity of young females. *J. Sports Med.* 18:3–9, 1978.
7. BADENHOP, D. T., P. A. CLEARY, S. F. SCHAAL, E. L. FOX, and R. L. BARTELS. Physiological adjustments to higher- or lower-intensity exercise in elders. *Med. Sci. Sports Exerc.* 15:496–502, 1983.
8. BARRY, A. J., J. W. DALY, E. D. R. PRUETT, et al. The effects of physical conditioning on older individuals. I. Work capacity, circulatory-respiratory function, and work electrocardiogram. *J. Gerontol.* 21:182–191, 1966.
9. BENESTAD, A. M. Trainability of old men. *Acta Med. Scand.* 178:321–327, 1965.
10. BERGER, R. A. Effect of varied weight training programs on strength. *Res. Q.* 33:168–181, 1962.

11. BIRK, T. J. and C. A. BIRK. Use of ratings of perceived exertion for exercise prescription. *Sports Med.* 4:1–8, 1987.

12. BLAIR, S. N., J. V. CHANDLER, D. B. ELLISOR, and J. LANGLEY. Improving physical fitness by exercise training programs. *South. Med. J.* 73:1594–1596, 1980.

13. BLAIR, S. N., H. W. KOHL, and N. N. GOODYEAR. Rates and risks for running and exercise injuries: studies in three populations. *Res. Q. Exerc. Sports* 58:221–228, 1987.

13A.BLAIR, S. N., H. W. KOHL, III, R. S. PAFFENBARGER, D. G. CLARK, K. H. COOPER, and L. H. GIBBONS. Physical fitness and all-cause mortality. A prospective study of healthy men and women. *J.A.M.A.* 262:2395–2401, 1989.

14. BOILEAU, R. A., E. R. BUSKIRK, D. H. HORSTMAN, J. MENDEZ, and W. NICHOLAS. Body composition changes in obese and lean men during physical conditioning. *Med. Sci. Sports* 3:183–189, 1971.

15. BORG, G. A. V. Psychophysical bases of perceived exertion. *Med. Sci. Sports Exerc.* 14:377–381, 1982.

16. BORG, G. and D. OTTOSON (Eds.). *The Perception of Exertion in Physical Work.* London, England: The MacMillan Press, Ltd., 1986, pp. 4–7.

16A.BOUCHARD, C. Gene-environment interaction in human adaptability. In: *The Academy Papers*, R. B. Malina and H. M. Eckert (Eds.). Champaign, IL: Human Kinetics Publishers, 1988, pp. 56–66.

17. BRAITH, R. W., J. E. GRAVES, M. L. POLLOCK, S. L. LEGGETT, D. M. CARPENTER, and A. B. COLVIN. Comparison of two versus three days per week of variable resistance training during 10 and 18 week programs. *Int. J. Sports Med.* 10:450–454, 1989.

18. BRYNTESON, P. and W. E. SINNING. The effects of training frequencies on the retention of cardiovascular fitness. *Med. Sci. Sports* 5:29–33, 1973.

19. BURKE, E. J. Physiological effects of similar training programs in males and females. *Res. Q.* 48:510–517, 1977.

20. BURKE, E. J. and B. D. FRANKS. Changes in $\dot{V}O_{2max}$ resulting from bicycle training at different intensities holding total mechanical work constant. *Res. Q.* 46:31–37, 1975.

21. BUSKIRK, E. R. and J. L. HODGSON. Age and aerobic power: the rate of change in men and women. *Fed. Proc.* 46:1824–1829, 1987.

22. CARTER, J. E. L. and W. H. PHILLIPS. Structural changes in exercising middle-aged males during a 2-year period. *J. Appl. Physiol.* 27:787–794, 1969.

23. CHOW, J. R. and J. H. WILMORE. The regulation of exercise intensity by ratings of perceived exertion. *J. Cardiac Rehabil.* 4:382–387, 1984.

24. CHRISTENSEN, E. H. Physiological evaluation of work in the Nykroppa iron works. In: *Ergonomics Society Symposium on Fatigue*, W. F. Floyd and A. T. Welford (Eds.). London, England: Lewis, 1953, pp. 93–108.

25. COYLE, E. F., W. H. MARTIN, D. R. SINACORE, M. J. JOYNER, J. M. HAGBERG, and J. O. HOLLOSZY. Time course of loss of adaptation after stopping prolonged intense endurance training. *J. Appl. Physiol.* 57:1857–1864, 1984.

26. CREWS, T. R. and J. A. ROBERTS. Effects of interaction of frequency and intensity of training. *Res. Q.* 47:48–55, 1976.

27. CURETON, T. K. *The Physiological Effects of Exercise Programs upon Adults.* Springfield, IL: Charles C. Thomas Co., 1969, pp. 3–6, 33–77.

28. CURETON, T. K. and E. E. PHILLIPS. Physical fitness changes in middle-aged men attributable to equal eight-week periods of training, non-training and retraining. *J. Sports Med. Phys. Fitness* 4:1–7, 1964.

29. DAVIES, C. T. M. and A. V. KNIBBS. The training stimulus, the effects of intensity, duration and frequency of effort on maximum aerobic power output. *Int. Z. Angew. Physiol.* 29:299–305, 1971.

30. DAVIS, J. A., M. H. FRANK, B. J. WHIPP, and K. WASSERMAN. Anaerobic threshold alterations caused by endurance training in middle-aged men. *J. Appl. Physiol.* 46:1039–1049, 1979.

31. DEHN, M. M. and R. A. BRUCE. Longitudinal variations in maximal oxygen intake with age and activity. *J. Appl. Physiol.* 33:805–807, 1972.

32. DELORME, T. L. Restoration of muscle power by heavy resistance exercise. *J. Bone Joint Surg.* 27:645–667, 1945.

33. DEMPSEY, J. A. Anthropometrical observations on obese and nonobese young men undergoing a program of vigorous physical exercise. *Res. Q.* 35:275–287, 1964.

34. DEVRIES, H. A. Physiological effects of an exercise training regimen upon men aged 52 to 88. *J. Gerontol.* 24:325–336, 1970.

35. DEVRIES, H. A. Exercise intensity threshold for improvement of cardiovascular-respiratory function in older men. *Geriatrics* 26:94–101, 1971.

36. DISHMAN, R. K., J. SALLIS, and D. ORENSTEIN. The determinants of physical activity and exercise. *Public Health Rep.* 100:158–180, 1985.

37. DISHMAN, R. K., R. W. PATTON, J. SMITH, R. WEINBERG, and A. JACKSON. Using perceived exertion to prescribe and monitor exercise training heart rate. *Int. J. Sports Med.* 8:208–213, 1987.

38. DRINKWATER, B. L. Physiological responses of women to exercise. In: *Exercise and Sports Sciences Reviews*, Vol. 1, J. H. Wilmore (Ed.). New York: Academic Press, 1973, pp. 126–154.

39. DRINKWATER, B. L., S. M. HORVATH, and C. L. WELLS. Aerobic power of females, ages 10 to 68. *J. Gerontol.* 30:385–394, 1975.

40. DURNIN, J. V. G. A. and R. PASSMORE. *Energy, Work and Leisure.* London, England: Heinemann Educational Books, Ltd., 1967, pp. 47–82.

41. EDSTROM, L. and L. GRIMBY. Effect of exercise on the motor unit. *Muscle Nerve* 9:104–126, 1986.

42. EKBLOM, B., P. O. ÅSTRAND, B. SALTIN, J. STENBERG, and B. WALLSTROM. Effect of training on circulatory response to exercise. *J. Appl. Physiol.* 24:518–528, 1968.

43. FLECK, S. J. and W. J. KRAEMER. *Designing Resistance Training Programs.* Champaign, IL: Human Kinetics Books, 1987, pp. 15–46, 161–162.

44. FLINT, M. M., B. L. DRINKWATER, and S. M. HORVATH. Effects of training on women's response to submaximal exercise. *Med. Sci. Sports* 6:89–94, 1974.

45. FOX, E. L., R. L. BARTELS, C. E. BILLINGS, R. O'BRIEN, R. BASON, and D. K. MATHEWS. Frequency and duration of interval training programs and changes in aerobic power. *J. Appl. Physiol.* 38:481–484, 1975.

46. FRANKLIN, B., E. BUSKIRK, J. HODGSON, H. GAHAGAN, J. KOLLIAS, and J. MENDEZ. Effects of physical conditioning on cardiorespiratory function, body composition and serum lipids in relatively normal weight and obese middle-age women. *Int. J. Obes.* 3:97–109, 1979.

47. FRINGER, M. N. and A. G. STULL. Changes in cardiorespiratory parameters during periods of training and detraining in young female adults. *Med. Sci. Sports* 6:20–25, 1974.

48. GAESSER, G. A. and R. G. RICH. Effects of high- and low-intensity exercise training on aerobic capacity and blood lipids. *Med. Sci. Sports Exerc.* 16:269–274, 1984.

49. GETCHELL, L. H. and J. C. MOORE. Physical training: comparative responses of middle-aged adults. *Arch. Phys. Med. Rehabil.* 56:250–254, 1975.

50. GETTMAN, L. R., M. L. POLLOCK, J. L. DURSTINE, A. WARD, J. AYRES, and A. C. LINNERUD. Physiological responses of men to 1,3, and 5 day per week training programs. *Res. Q.* 47:638–646, 1976.

51. GETTMAN, L. R., J. J. AYRES, M. L. POLLOCK, and A. JACKSON. The effect of circuit weight training on strength, cardiorespiratory function, and body composition of adult men. *Med. Sci. Sports* 10:171–176, 1978.

52. GETTMAN, L. R., J. AYRES, M. L. POLLOCK, J. L. DURSTINE, and W. GRANTHAM. Physiological effects of circuit strength training and jogging. *Arch. Phys. Med. Rehabil.* 60:115–120, 1979.

53. GETTMAN, L. R., L. A. CULTER, and T. STRATHMAN. Physiologic changes after 20 weeks of isotonic vs. isokinetic circuit training. *J. Sports Med. Phys. Fitness* 20:265–274, 1980.

54. GETTMAN, L. R. and M. L. POLLOCK. Circuit weight training: a critical review of its physiological benefits. *Phys. Sports Med.* 9:44–60, 1981.

55. GETTMAN, L. R., P. WARD, and R. D. HAGMAN. A comparison of combined running and weight training with circuit weight

training. *Med. Sci. Sports Exerc.* 14:229–234, 1982.

56. GILLAM, G. M. Effects of frequency of weight training on muscle strength enhancement. *J. Sports Med.* 21:432–436, 1981.

57. GIRANDOLA, R. N. Body composition changes in women: effects of high and low exercise intensity. *Arch. Phys. Med. Rehabil.* 57:297–300, 1976.

58. GLEDHILL, N. and R. B. EYNON. The intensity of training. In: *Training Scientific Basis and Application*, A. W. Taylor and M. L. Howell (Eds.). Springfield, IL: Charles C Thomas Co., 1972, pp. 97–102.

59. GOLDING, L. Effects of physical training upon total serum cholesterol levels. *Res. Q.* 32:499–505, 1961.

60. GOODE, R. C., A. VIRGIN, T. T. ROMET, et al. Effects of a short period of physical activity in adolescent boys and girls. *Can. J. Appl. Sports Sci.* 1:241–250, 1976.

61. GOSSARD, D., W. L. HASKELL, B. TAYLOR, et al. Effects of low- and high-intensity home-based exercise training on functional capacity in healthy middle-age men. *Am. J. Cardiol.* 57:446–449, 1986.

62. GRAVES, J. E., M. L. POLLOCK, S. H. LEGGETT, R. W. BRAITH, D. M. CARPENTER, and L. E. BISHOP. Effect of reduced training frequency on muscular strength. *Int. J. Sports Med.* 9:316–319, 1988.

63. GRAVES, J. E., M. L. POLLOCK, A. E. JONES, A. B. COLVIN, and S. H. LEGGETT. Specificity of limited range of motion variable resistance training. *Med. Sci. Sports Exerc.* 21:84–89, 1989.

64. GWINUP, G. Effect of exercise alone on the weight of obese women. *Arch. Int. Med.* 135:676–680, 1975.

65. HAGBERG, J. M., J. E. GRAVES, M. LIMACHER, et al. Cardiovascular responses of 70–79 year old men and women to exercise training. *J. Appl. Physiol.* 66:2589–2594,1989.

66. HAKKINEN, K. Factors influencing trainability of muscular strength during short term and prolonged training. *Natl. Strength Cond. Assoc. J.* 7:32–34, 1985.

67. HANSON, J. S., B. S. TABAKIN, A. M. LEVY, and W. NEDDE. Long-term physical training and cardiovascular dynamics in middle-aged men. *Circulation* 38:783–799, 1968.

68. HANSON, J. S. and W. H. NEDDE. Long-term physical training effect in sedentary females. *J. Appl. Physiol.* 37:112–116, 1974.

69. HARTLEY, L. H., G. GRIMBY, A. KILBOM, et al. Physical training in sedentary middle-aged and older men. *Scand. J. Clin. Lab. Invest.* 24:335–344, 1969.

70. HARTUNG, G. H., M. H. SMOLENSKY, R. B. HARRIST, and R. RUNGE. Effects of varied durations of training on improvement in cardiorespiratory endurance. *J. Hum. Ergol.* 6:61–68, 1977.

71. HASKELL, W. L. Physical activity and health: need to define the required stimulus. *Am. J. Cardiol.* 55:4D–9D, 1985.

72. HASKELL, W. L., H. J. MONTOYE, and D. ORENSTEIN. Physical activity and exercise to achieve health-related physical fitness components. *Public Health Rep.* 100:202–212, 1985.

73. HEATH, G. W., J. M. HAGBERG, A. A. EHSANI, and J. O. HOLLOSZY. A physiological comparison of young and older endurance athletes. *J. Appl. Physiol.* 51:634–640, 1981.

74. HETTINGER, T. *Physiology of Strength*. Springfield, IL: C. C Thomas Publisher, 1961, pp. 18–40.

75. HICKSON, R. C. and M. A. ROSENKOETTER. Reduced training frequencies and maintenance of increased aerobic power. *Med. Sci. Sports Exerc.* 13:13–16, 1981.

76. HICKSON, R. C., C. KANAKIS, J. R. DAVIS, A. M. MOORE, and S. RICH. Reduced training duration effects on aerobic power, endurance, and cardiac growth. *J. Appl. Physiol.* 53:225–229, 1982.

77. HICKSON, R. C., C. FOSTER, M. L. POLLOCK, T. M. GALASSI, and S. RICH. Reduced training intensities and loss of aerobic power, endurance, and cardiac growth. *J. Appl. Physiol.* 58:492–499, 1985.

78. HILL, J. O., P. B. SPARLING, T. W. SHIELDS, and P. A. HELLER. Effects of exercise and food restriction on body composition and metabolic rate in obese women. *Am. J. Clin. Nutr.* 46:622–630, 1987.

79. HOLLMANN, W. *Changes in the Capacity for Maximal and Continuous Effort in Relation to Age. Int. Res. Sports Phys. Ed.*, E. Jokl and E. Simon (Eds.). Springfield, IL: Charles C Thomas Co., 1964, pp. 369–371.

80. HOLLMANN, W. and H. VENRATH. Die Beinflussung von Herzgrösse, maximaler O₂–Aufnahme und Ausdauergrenze durch ein Ausdauertraining mittlerer und hoher Intensität. *Der Sportarzt* 9:189–193, 1963.

81. No reference 81 due to renumbering in proof.

82. HUIBREGTSE, W. H., H. H. HARTLEY, L. R. JONES, W. D. DOOLITTLE, and T. L. CRIBLEZ. Improvement of aerobic work capacity following non-strenuous exercise. *Arch. Environ. Health* 27:12–15, 1973.

83. HURLEY, B. F., D. R. SEALS, A. A. EHSANI, et al. Effects of high-intensity strength training on cardiovascular function. *Med. Sci. Sports Exerc.* 16:483–488, 1984.

84. ISMAIL, A. H., D. CORRIGAN, and D. F. MCLEOD. Effect of an eight-month exercise program on selected physiological, biochemical, and audiological variables in adult men. *Br. J. Sports Med.* 7:230–240, 1973.

84A. JONES, D. A., D. J. NEWMAN, J. M. ROUND, and S. E. L. TOLFREE. Experimental human muscle damage: morphological changes in relation to other indices of damage. *J. Physiol. (Lond.)* 375:435–438, 1986.

85. KARVONEN, M., K. KENTALA, and O. MUSTALA. The effects of training heart rate: a longitudinal study. *Ann. Med. Exp. Biol. Fenn* 35:307–315, 1957.

86. KASCH, F. W., W. H. PHILLIPS, J. E. L. CARTER, and J. L. BOYER. Cardiovascular changes in middle-aged men during two years of training. *J. Appl. Physiol.* 314:53–57, 1972.

87. KASCH, F. W. and J. P. WALLACE. Physiological variables during 10 years of endurance exercise. *Med. Sci. Sports* 8:5–8, 1976.

88. KASCH, F. W., J. P. WALLACE, and S. P. VAN CAMP. Effects of 18 years of endurance exercise on physical work capacity of older men. *J. Cardiopulmonary Rehabil.* 5:308–312, 1985.

89. KATCH, F. I. and W. D. MCARDLE. *Nutrition, Weight Control and Exercise*, 3rd Ed. Philadelphia: Lea and Febiger, 1988, pp. 110–112.

90. KEARNEY, J. T., A. G. STULL, J. L. EWING, and J. W. STREIN. Cardiorespiratory responses of sedentary college women as a function of training intensity. *J. Appl. Physiol.* 41:822–825, 1976.

91. KENDRICK, Z. B., M. L. POLLOCK, T. N. HICKMAN, and H. S. MILLER. Effects of training and detraining on cardiovascular efficiency. *Am. Corr. Ther. J.* 25:79–83, 1971.

92. KILBOM, A. Physical training in women. *Scand. J. Clin. Lab. Invest.* 119 (Suppl.):1–34, 1971.

93. KILBOM, A., L. HARTLEY, B. SALTIN, J. BJURE, G. GRIMBY, and I. ASTRAND. Physical training in sedentary middle-aged and older men. *Scand. J. Clin. Lab. Invest.* 24:315–322, 1969.

94. KIMURA, Y., H. ITOW, and S. YAMAZAKIE. The effects of circuit weight training on VO₂max and body composition of trained and untrained college men. *J. Physiol. Soc. Jpn.* 43:593–596, 1981.

94A. KLISSOURAS, V., F. PIRNAY, and J. PETIT. Adaptation to maximal effort: genetics and age. *J. Appl. Physiol.* 35:288–293, 1973.

95. KNAPIK, J. J., R. H. MAUDSLEY, and N. V. RAMMOS. Angular specificity and test mode specificity of isometric and isokinetic strength training. *J. Orthop. Sports Phys. Ther.* 5:58–65, 1983.

96. KNEHR, C. A., D. B. DILL, and W. NEUFELD. Training and its effect on man at rest and at work. *Am. J. Physiol.* 136:148–156, 1942.

97. KNUTTGEN, H. G., L. O. NORDESJO, B. OLLANDER, and B. SALTIN. Physical conditioning through interval training with young male adults. *Med. Sci. Sports* 5:220–226, 1973.

98. LAPORTE, R. E., L. L. ADAMS, D. D. SAVAGE, G. BRENES, S. DEARWATER, and T. COOK. The spectrum of physical activity, cardiovascular disease and health: an epidemiologic perspective. *Am. J. Epidemiol.* 120:507–517, 1984.

99. LEON, A. S., J. CONRAD, D. B. HUNNINGHAKE, and R. SERFASS. Effects of a vigorous walking program on body composition, and carbohydrate and lipid metabolism of obese young men. *Am. J. Clin. Nutr.* 32:1776–1787, 1979.

100. LEON, A. S., J. CONNETT, D. R. JACOBS, and R. RAURAMAA. Leisure-time physical activity levels and risk of coronary heart disease and death: the multiple risk of coronary heart disease and death: the multiple risk factor intervention trial. *J.A.M.A.* 258:2388–2395, 1987.

100A. LEWIS, S. F., W. F. TAYLOR, R. M. GRAHAM, W. A. PETTINGER,

J. E. SHUTTE, and C. G. BLOMQVIST. Cardiovascular responses to exercise as functions of absolute and relative work load. *J. Appl. Physiol.* 54:1314–1323, 1983.

101. LIANG, M. T., J. F. ALEXANDER, H. L. TAYLOR, R. C. SERFRASS, A. S. LEON, and G. A. STULL. Aerobic training threshold, intensity duration, and frequency of exercise. *Scand. J. Sports Sci.* 4:5–8, 1982.

101A. LIEBER, D. C., R. L. LIEBER, and W. C. ADAMS. Effects of run-training and swim-training at similar absolute intensities on treadmill $\dot{V}O_{2max}$. *Med. Sci. Sports Exerc.* 21:655–661, 1989.

101B. MACDOUGALL, J. D., G. R. WARD, D. G. SALE, and J. R. SUTTON. Biochemical adaptation of human skeletal muscle to heavy resistance training and immobilization. *J. Appl. Physiol.* 43:700–703, 1977.

101C. MACDOUGALL, J. D., D. TUXEN, D. G. SALE, J. R. MOROZ, and J. R. SUTTON. Arterial blood pressure response to heavy resistance training. *J. Appl. Physiol.* 58:785–790, 1985.

102. MANN, G. V., L. H. GARRETT, A. FARHI, et al. Exercise to prevent coronary heart disease. *Am. J. Med.* 46:12–27, 1969.

103. MARCINIK, E. J., J. A. HODGDON, U. MITTLEMAN, and J. J. O'BRIEN. Aerobic/calisthenic and aerobic/circuit weight training programs for Navy men: a comparative study. *Med. Sci. Sports Exerc.* 17:482–487, 1985.

104. MARIGOLD, E. A. The effect of training at predetermined heart rate levels for sedentary college women. *Med. Sci. Sports* 6:14–19, 1974.

105. MARTIN, J. E. and P. M. DUBBERT. Adherence to exercise. In: *Exercise and Sports Sciences Reviews*, Vol. 13, R. L. Terjung (Ed.). New York: MacMillan Publishing Co., 1985, pp. 137–167.

106. MARTIN, W. H., J. MONTGOMERY, P. G. SNELL, et al. Cardiovascular adaptations to intense swim training in sedentary middle-aged men and women. *Circulation* 75:323–330, 1987.

107. MAYHEW, J. L. and P. M. GROSS. Body composition changes in young women with high resistance weight training. *Res. Q.* 45:433–439, 1974.

108. MESSIER, J. P. and M. DILL. Alterations in strength and maximal oxygen uptake consequent to Nautilus circuit weight training. *Res. Q. Exerc. Sport* 56:345–351, 1985.

109. MILESIS, C. A., M. L. POLLOCK, M. D. BAH, J. J. AYRES, A. WARD, and A. C. Linnerud. Effects of different durations of training on cardiorespiratory function, body composition and serum lipids. *Res Q.* 47:716–725, 1976.

110. MISNER, J. E., R. A. BOILEAU, B. H. MASSEY, and J. H. MAYHEW. Alterations in body composition of adult men during selected physical training programs. *J. Am. Geriatr. Soc.* 22:33–38, 1974.

111. MIYASHITA, M., S. HAGA, and T. MITZUTA. Training and detraining effects on aerobic power in middle-aged and older men. *J. Sports Med.* 18:131–137, 1978.

112. MOODY, D. L., J. KOLLIAS, and E. R. BUSKIRK. The effect of a moderate exercise program on body weight and skinfold thickness in overweight college women. *Med. Sci. Sports* 1:75–80, 1969.

113. MOODY, D. L., J. H. WILMORE, R. N. GIRANDOLA, and J. P. ROYCE. The effects of a jogging program on the body composition of normal and obese high school girls. *Med. Sci. Sports* 4:210–213, 1972.

114. MUELLER, E. A. and W. ROHMERT. Die geschwindigkeit der muskelkraft zunahme bein isometrischen training. *Int. Z. Angew. Physiol.* 19:403–419, 1963.

115. NAUGHTON, J. and F. NAGLE. Peak oxygen intake during physical fitness program for middle-aged men. *J.A.M.A.* 191:899–901, 1965.

116. O'HARA, W., C. ALLEN, and R. J. SHEPHARD. Loss of body weight and fat during exercise in a cold chamber. *Eur. J. Appl. Physiol.* 37:205–218, 1977.

117. OJA, P., P. TERASLINNA, T. PARTANEN, and R. KARAVA. Feasibility of an 18 months' physical training program for middle-aged men and its effect on physical fitness. *Am. J. Public Health* 64:459–465, 1975.

118. OLREE, H. D., B. CORBIN, J. PENROD, and C. SMITH. Methods of achieving and maintaining physical fitness for prolonged space flight. Final Progress Rep. to NASA, Grant No. NGR-04-002-004, 1969.

119. OSCAI, L. B., T. WILLIAMS, and B. HERTIG. Effects of exercise on blood volume. *J. Appl. Physiol.* 24:622–624, 1968.

120. PAFFENBARGER, R. S., R. T. HYDE, A. L. WING, and C. HSIEH. Physical activity and all-cause mortality, and longevity of college alumni. *N. Engl. J. Med.* 314:605–613, 1986.

121. PAVLOU, K. N., W. P. STEFFEE, R. H. LEARMAN, and B. A. BURROWS. Effects of dieting and exercise on lean body mass, oxygen uptake, and strength. *Med. Sci. Sports Exerc.* 17:466–471, 1985.

122. PELS, A. E., M. L. POLLOCK, T. E. DOHMEIER, K. A. LEMBERGER, and B. F. OEHRLEIN. Effects of leg press training on cycling, leg press, and running peak cardiorespiratory measures. *Med. Sci. Sports Exerc.* 19:66–70, 1987.

123. POLLOCK, M. L. The quantification of endurance training programs. In: *Exercise and Sport Sciences Reviews*, J. H. Wilmore (Ed.). New York: Academic Press, 1973, pp. 155–188.

124. POLLOCK, M. L. Prescribing exercise for fitness and adherence. In: *Exercise Adherence: Its Impact on Public Health*, R. K. Dishman (Ed.). Champaign, IL: Human Kinetics Books, 1988, pp. 259–277

125. POLLOCK, M. L., T. K. CURETON, and L. GRENINGER. Effects of frequency of training on working capacity, cardiovascular function, and body composition of adult men. *Med. Sci. Sports* 1:70–74, 1969.

126. POLLOCK, M. L., J. TIFFANY, L. GETTMAN, R. JANEWAY, and H. LOFLAND. Effects of frequency of training on serum lipids, cardiovascular function, and body composition. In: *Exercise and Fitness*, B. D. Franks (Ed.). Chicago: Athletic Institute, 1969, pp. 161–178.

127. POLLOCK, M. L., H. MILLER, R. JANEWAY, A. C. LINNERUD, B. ROBERTSON, and R. VALENTINO. Effects of walking on body composition and cardiovascular function of middle-aged men. *J. Appl. Physiol.* 30:126–130, 1971.

128. POLLOCK, M. L., J. BROIDA, Z. KENDRICK, H. S. MILLER, R. JANEWAY, and A. C. LINNERUD. Effects of training two days per week at different intensities on middle-aged men. *Med. Sci. Sports* 4:192–197, 1972.

129. POLLOCK, M. L., H. S. MILLER, JR., and J. WILMORE. Physiological characteristics of champion American track athletes 40 to 70 years of age. *J. Gerontol.* 29:645–649, 1974.

130. POLLOCK, M. L., J. DIMMICK, H. S. MILLER, Z. KENDRICK, and A. C. LINNERUD. Effects of mode of training on cardiovascular function and body composition of middle-aged men. *Med. Sci. Sports* 7:139–145, 1975.

131. No reference 131 due to renumbering in proof.

132. POLLOCK, M. L., G. A. DAWSON, H. S. MILLER, JR., et al. Physiologic response of men 49 to 65 years of age to endurance training. *J. Am. Geriatr. Soc.* 24:97–104, 1976.

133. POLLOCK, M. L. and A. JACKSON. Body composition: measurement and changes resulting from physical training. Proceedings National College Physical Education Association for Men and Women, January, 1977, pp. 125–137.

134. POLLOCK, M. L., J. AYRES, and A. WARD. Cardiorespiratory fitness: response to differing intensities and durations of training. *Arch. Phys. Med. Rehabil.* 58:467–473, 1977.

135. POLLOCK, M. L., R. GETTMAN, C. A. MILESIS, M. D. BAH, J. L. DURSTINE, and R. B. JOHNSON. Effects of frequency and duration of training on attrition and incidence of injury. *Med. Sci. Sports* 9:31–36, 1977.

136. POLLOCK, M. L., L. R. GETTMAN, P. B. RAVEN, J. AYRES, M. BAH, and A. WARD. Physiological comparison of the effects of aerobic and anaerobic training. In: *Physical Fitness Programs for Law Enforcement Officers: A Manual for Police Administrators*, C. S. Price, M. L. Pollock, L. R. Gettman, and D. A. Kent (Eds.). Washington, D. C.: U. S. Government Printing Office, No. 027-000-00671-0, 1978, pp. 89–96.

137. POLLOCK, M. L., A. S. JACKSON, and C. FOSTER. The use of the perception scale for exercise prescription. In: *The Perception of Exertion in Physical Work*, G. Borg and D. Ottoson (Eds.). London, England: The MacMillan Press, Ltd., 1986, pp. 161–176.

138. POLLOCK, M. L., C. FOSTER, D. KNAPP, J. S. ROD, and D. H. SCHMIDT. Effect of age and training on aerobic capacity and

body composition of master athletes. *J. Appl. Physiol.* 62:725–731, 1987.

139. POLLOCK, M. L. and J. H. WILMORE. *Exercise in Health and Disease: Evaluation and Prescription for Prevention and Rehabilitation,* 2nd Ed. Philadelphia: W. B. Saunders, Co., 1990.

140. POWELL, K. E., H. W. KOHL, C. J. CASPERSEN, and S. N. BLAIR. An epidemiological perspective of the causes of running injuries. *Phys. Sportsmed.* 14:100–114, 1986.

141. RIBISL, P. M. Effects of training upon the maximal oxygen uptake of middle-aged men. *Int. Z. Angew. Physiol.* 26:272–278, 1969.

142. RICHIE, D. H., S. F. KELSO, and P. A. BELLUCCI. Aerobic dance injuries: a retrospective study of instructors and participants. *Phys. Sportsmed.* 13:130–140, 1985.

143. ROBINSON, S. and P. M. HARMON. Lactic acid mechanism and certain properties of blood in relation to training. *Am. J. Physiol.* 132:757–769, 1941.

144. ROSKAMM, H. Optimum patterns of exercise for healthy adults. *Can. Med. Assoc. J.* 96:895–899, 1967.

145. SALE, D. G. Influence of exercise and training on motor unit activation. In: *Exercise and Sport Sciences Reviews,* K. B. Pandolf (Ed.). New York: MacMillan Publishing Co., 1987, pp. 95–152.

145A.SALE, D. G. Neural adaptation to resistance training. *Med. Sci. Sports Exerc.* 20:S135–S145, 1988.

146. SALLIS, J. F., W. L. HASKELL, S. P. FORTMAN, K. M. VRANIZAN, C. B. TAYLOR, and D. S. SOLOMAN. Predictors of adoption and maintenance of physical activity in a community sample. *Prev. Med.* 15:131–141, 1986.

147. SALTIN, B., G. BLOMQVIST, J. MITCHELL, R. L. JOHNSON, K. WILDENTHAL, and C. B. CHAPMAN. Response to exercise after bed rest and after training. *Circulation* 37, 38(Suppl. 7):1–78, 1968.

148. SALTIN, B., L. HARTLEY, A. KILBOM, and I. ÅSTRAND. Physical training in sedentary middle-aged and older men. *Scand. J. Clin. Lab. Invest.* 24:323–334, 1969.

149. SANTIGO, M. C., J. F. ALEXANDER, G. A. STULL, R. C. SERFRASS, A. M. HAYDAY, and A. S. LEON. Physiological responses of sedentary women to a 20-week conditioning program of walking or jogging. *Scand. J. Sports Sci.* 9:33–39, 1987.

150. SEALS, D. R., J. M. HAGBERG, B. F. HURLEY, A. A. EHSANI, and J. O. HOLLOSZY. Endurance training in older men and women. I. Cardiovascular responses to exercise. *J. Appl. Physiol.* 57:1024–1029, 1984.

151. SHARKEY, B. J. Intensity and duration of training and the development of cardiorespiratory endurance. *Med. Sci. Sports* 2:197–202, 1970.

152. SHEPHARD, R. J. Intensity, duration, and frequency of exercise as determinants of the response to a training regime. *Int. Z. Angew. Physiol.* 26:272–278, 1969.

153. SHEPHARD, R. J. Future research on the quantifying of endurance training. *J. Hum. Ergol.* 3:163–181, 1975.

154. SIDNEY, K. H., R. B. EYNON, and D. A. CUNNINGHAM. Effect of frequency of training of exercise upon physical working performance and selected variables representative of cardiorespiratory fitness. In: *Training Scientific Basis and Application,* A. W. Taylor (Ed.). Springfield, IL: Charles C Thomas Co., 1972, pp. 144–188.

155. SIDNEY, K. H., R. J. SHEPHARD, and J. HARRISON. Endurance training and body composition of the elderly. *Am. J. Clin. Nutr.* 30:326–333, 1977.

156. SIEGEL, W., G. BLOMQVIST, and J. H. MITCHELL. Effects of a quantitated physical training program on middle-aged sedentary males. *Circulation* 41:19–29, 1970.

156A.SISCOVICK, D. S., N. S. WEISS, R. H. FLETCHER, and T. LASKY. The incidence of primary cardiac arrest during vigorous exer-

cise. *N. Engl. J. Med.* 311:874–877, 1984.

157. SKINNER, J. The cardiovascular system with aging and exercise. In: *Physical Activity and Aging,* D. Brunner and E. Jokl (Eds.). Baltimore: University Park Press, 1970, pp. 100–108.

158. SKINNER, J., J. HOLLOSZY, and T. CURETON. Effects of a program of endurance exercise on physical work capacity and anthropometric measurements of fifteen middle-aged men. *Am. J. Cardiol.* 14:747–752, 1964.

159. SMITH, D. P. and F. W. STRANSKY. The effect of training and detraining on the body composition and cardiovascular response of young women to exercise. *J. Sports Med.* 16:112–120, 1976.

160. SMITH, E. L., W. REDDAN, and P. E. SMITH. Physical activity and calcium modalities for bone mineral increase in aged women. *Med. Sci. Sports Exerc.* 13:60–64, 1981.

161. SUOMINEN, H., E. HEIKKINEN, and T. TARKATTI. Effect of eight weeks physical training on muscle and connective tissue of the m. vastus lateralis in 69-year-old men and women. *J. Gerontol.* 32:33–37, 1977.

162. TERJUNG, R. L., K. M. BALDWIN, J. COOKSEY, B. SAMSON, and R. A. SUTTER. Cardiovascular adaptation to twelve minutes of mild daily exercise in middle-aged sedentary men. *J. Am. Geriatr. Soc.* 21:164–168, 1973.

163. THOMAS, S. G., D. A. CUNNINGHAM, P. A. RECHNITZER, A. P. DONNER, and J. H. HOWARD. Determinants of the training response in elderly men. *Med. Sci. Sports Exerc.* 17:667–672, 1985.

164. WENGER, H. A. and G. J. BELL. The interactions of intensity, frequency, and duration of exercise training in altering cardiorespiratory fitness. *Sports Med.* 3:346–356, 1986.

165. WILMORE, J. H. Alterations in strength, body composition, and anthropometric measurements consequent to a 10-week weight training program. *Med. Sci. Sports* 6:133–138, 1974.

166. WILMORE, J. Inferiority of female athletes: myth or reality. *J. Sports Med.* 3:1–6, 1974.

167. WILMORE, J. H. Design issues and alternatives in assessing physical fitness among apparently healthy adults in a health examination survey of the general population. In: *Assessing Physical Fitness and Activity in General Population Studies,* T. F. Drury (Ed.). Washington, D.C.: U.S. Public Health Service, National Center for Health Statistics, 1988 (in press).

168. WILMORE, J. H., J. ROYCE, R. N. GIRANDOLA, F. I. KATCH, and V. L. KATCH. Physiological alternatives resulting from a 10-week jogging program. *Med. Sci. Sports* 2:7–14, 1970.

169. WILMORE, J. H., J. ROYCE, R. N. GIRANDOLA, F. I. KATCH, and V. L. KATCH. Body composition changes with a 10-week jogging program. *Med. Sci. Sports* 2:113–117, 1970.

170. WILMORE, J., R. B. PARR, P. A. VODAK, et al. Strength, endurance, BMR, and body composition changes with circuit weight training. *Med. Sci. Sports* 8:58–60, 1976.

171. WILMORE, J. H., G. A. EWY, A. R. MORTAN, et al. The effect of beta-adrenergic blockade on submaximal and maximal exercise performance. *J. Cardiac Rehabil.* 3:30–36, 1983.

171A.WILMORE, J. H. Body composition in sport and exercise: directions for future research. *Med. Sci. Sports Exerc.* 15:21–31, 1983.

172. WILMORE, J. H. and D. L. COSTILL. *Training for Sport and Activity. The Physiological Basis of the Conditioning Process,* 3rd Ed. Dubuque, IA: Wm. C. Brown, 1988, pp. 113–212.

173. WOOD, P. D., W. L. HASKELL, S. N. BLAIR, et al. Increased exercise level and plasma lipoprotein concentrations: a one-year, randomized, controlled study in sedentary, middle-aged men. *Metabolism* 32:31–39, 1983.

174. ZUTI, W. B. and L. A. GOLDING. Comparing diet and exercise as weight reduction tools. *Phys. Sports Med.* 4:49–53, 1976.

GLOSSARY

A

Accommodating resistance Strength-training program that requires the use of special equipment with mechanical devices that provide a variable resistance, with the intent of overloading the muscle group maximally through the entire range of motion.

Acquired immunodeficiency syndrome (AIDS) Virus (HIV) that destroys the immune system.

Addiction Compulsive and uncontrollable behavior(s) or use of substance(s), most frequently drugs.

Adenosine triphosphate (ATP) A high-energy chemical compound used for immediate energy by the body.

Adipose tissue Fat cells.

Aerobic exercise Exercise that requires oxygen to produce the necessary energy (ATP) to carry out the activity.

AIDS See acquired immunodeficiency syndrome.

Alcohol (drinking alcohol) Known as ethyl alcohol, a depressant drug that affects the brain and slows down central nervous system activity.

Alcoholism Disease in which an individual loses control over drinking alcoholic-containing beverages.

Alveoli Air sacs in the lungs where gas exchange (oxygen and carbon dioxide) takes place.

Amenorrhea Cessation of regular menstrual flow.

Amino acids Chemical compounds that contain nitrogen, carbon, hydrogen, and oxygen. Amino acids are the basic building blocks that the body uses to build different types of protein.

Anabolic steroids Synthetic versions of the male sex hormone testosterone which promotes muscle development and hypertrophy.

Anabolism Process whereby simple substances are formed into more complex substances.

Anaerobic exercise Exercise which does not require oxygen to produce the necessary energy (ATP) to carry out the activity.

Aneurysm Weakness in the arterial wall allowing the formation of a balloon-like pouch.

Angina pectoris Chest pain.

Anorexia nervosa An eating disorder characterized by self-imposed starvation to lose and maintain very low body weight.

Antioxidants Compounds such as the vitamins C, E, beta-carotene (a precursor to vitamin A) and the mineral selenium which prevent oxygen from combining with other substances to which it may cause damage. Antioxidants are thought to play a key role in the prevention of heart disease and cancer.

Arteries Major vessels that carry blood away from the heart to bodily tissues.

Arteriosclerosis Hardening of the arteries.

Atherosclerosis Type of arteriosclerosis characterized by plaque formation or the buildup of fatty tissue in the inner layers of the wall of the arteries.

ATP See adenosine triphosphate.

Atrophy A decrease in the size of a cell.

Autogenic training Stress management technique. It is a form of self-suggestion where an individual is able to place him/herself in an autohypnotic state by repeating and concentrating on feelings of heaviness and warmth in the extremities.

B

Ballistic or dynamic stretching (flexibility) Stretching exercises that are performed using jerky, rapid, and bouncy movements.

Basal cell carcinoma Type of skin cancer that occurs primarily on the face. It grows slow and rarely spreads to other parts of the body.

Basal metabolic rate The lowest level of oxygen consumption (uptake) necessary to sustain life.

Behavior modification A process to permanently change destructive or negative behaviors for positive behaviors that will lead to better health and well-being.

Benign Noncancerous.

Beta-carotene A precursor to vitamin A.

Bioelectrical impedance Technique to assess body composition, including percent body fat, by running a weak electrical current (totally painless) through the body.

Biofeedback Stress management technique. A process in which a person learns to reliably influence physiological responses of two kinds: either responses which are not ordinarily under voluntary control or responses which ordinarily are easily regulated but for which regulation has broken down due to trauma or disease.

Blood pressure The pressure of the blood exerted against the walls of the arteries.

BMI See body mass index.

Body composition Term used in reference to the fat and nonfat components of the human body. Body composition is important in the assessment of recommended or "ideal" body weight.

Body density The weight of the body per unit volume.

Body mass index (BMI)   Ratio of weight to height, usually expressed in kg/(mts)2.

Breathing techniques for relaxation   Stress management technique where the individual concentrates on "breathing away" the tension and inhaling fresh air to the entire body.

Brown fat cells   Cells that produce body heat by burning fat.

Bulimia   An eating disorder characterized by a pattern of binge eating and purging to attempt to lose and maintain low body weight.

C

CAD   Coronary artery disease, see coronary heart disease.

Caffeine   A central nervous system stimulating drug most frequently found in coffee, tea, and colas.

Calorie   A unit to measure heat energy. A calorie (also referred to as small calorie) is the amount of heat necessary to raise the temperature of one gram of water one degree Centigrade. Short term for kilocalorie and it is used to measure the energy value of food and cost of physical activity.

Calorimeter   Equipment used to measure the caloric value of food or heat production of animals and humans.

Cancer   Group of diseases characterized by uncontrolled growth and spread of abnormal cells into malignant tumors.

Capillary   Smallest blood vessels carrying oxygenated blood in the body.

Carbohydrates   Compounds containing carbon, hydrogen, and oxygen. Carbohydrates are the major source of energy for the human body.

Carcinogens   Substances that contribute to the formation of cancers.

Cardiac output   Amount of blood ejected by the heart in one minute.

Cardiovascular diseases   Diseases that affects the heart and the circulatory system (blood vessels). Examples of cardiovascular diseases are coronary heart disease, peripheral vascular disease, congenital heart disease, rheumatic heart disease, atherosclerosis, strokes, high blood pressure, and congestive heart failure.

Cardiovascular endurance   The ability of the lungs, heart, and blood vessels to deliver adequate amounts of oxygen to the cells to meet the demands of prolonged (aerobic) physical activity.

Catabolism   Process whereby complex substances are broken down into more simple substances.

Catecholamines   Hormones, includes epinephrine and norepinephrine.

Cellulite   Term frequently used in reference to fat deposits that "bulge out." These deposits are nothing but enlarged fat cells due to excessive accumulation of body fat.

CHD   See coronary heart disease.

Chlamydia   A sexually transmitted disease caused by a bacterial infection that can cause significant damage to the reproductive system and may occur without symptoms.

Cholesterol   A waxy substance that is technically a steroid alcohol found only in animal fats and oil.

Chronic diseases   Diseases that develop over a prolonged period of time, usually associated to unhealthy lifestyle factors (hypertension, atherosclerosis, coronary disease, strokes, diabetes, and cancer).

Chronic obstructive pulmonary disease (COPD)   An air flow limiting disease that includes diseases such as chronic bronchitis and emphysema.

Chronological age   Actual age of the individual (also see functional age).

Cocaine   2-beta-carbomethoxy-3-betabenozoxytropane the primary psychoactive ingredient derived from coca plant leaves. Also referred to as coke, C, snow, blow, toot, flake, Peruvian lady, white girl, and happy dust.

Coenzyme   Nonprotein molecule required in enzyme reactions.

Complex carbohydrates   Carbohydrates formed by three or more simple sugar molecules linked together, also referred to as polysaccharides. Commonly used to designate foods high in starch.

Compound fats   A combination of simple fats with other chemicals. Examples of compound fats are phospholipids, glucolipids, and lipoproteins.   Concentric muscle contraction

Shortening of fibers during muscle contraction.

Congenital heart disease   Heart defects present at birth.

Coronary arteries   Arteries that supply the myocardium or heart muscle with oxygen and nutrients.

Coronary heart disease   Disease caused by the obstruction of the coronary arteries by plaque formation (also see atherosclerosis).

Cruciferous vegetables   Plants that produce cross-shaped leaves (cauliflower, broccoli, cabbage, Brussels sprouts, and kohlrabi). These vegetables seem to have a protective effect against cancer.

D

Dehydration   A loss of body water below normal volume.

Deoxyribonucleic acid (DNA)   Genetic material, substance of which genes are made.

Derived fats   A combination of simple and compound fats.

Diabetes mellitus   Condition where the blood glucose is unable to enter the cells because the pancreas either totally stops producing insulin or produces an insufficient amount for the body's needs.

Diastolic blood pressure   Pressure exerted by the blood against the walls of the arteries during the relaxation phase (diastole) of the heart.

Dietary fiber   Fiber in plant foods that cannot be digested by the human body.

Dietary induced thermogenesis (DIT)   Extra amount of heat production caused by the metabolism of food.

Disaccharides   Simple carbohydrates formed by two monosaccharide units linked together, one of which is glucose. The major disaccharides are sucrose, lactose, and maltose.

Distress   Negative stress. Refers to unpleasant or harmful stress under which health and performance begin to deteriorate.

DIT   See dietary induced thermogenesis.

DNA   See deoxyribonucleic acid.

Dysmenorrhea   Painful menstruation.

E

Eccentric muscle contraction Lengthening of fibers during muscle contraction.

ECG See electrocardiogram.

EKG See electrocardiogram.

Elastic elongation (flexibility) Refers to an elastic or temporary lengthening of soft tissue (muscles, tendons, and ligaments).

Electrocardiogram (ECG or EKG) A recording of the electrical activity of the heart.

Emphysema Pulmonary disease caused by distention (overinflation) of the alveoli.

Endorphines Morphine-like substances released from the pituitary gland in the brain during prolonged aerobic exercise. They are thought to induce feelings of euphoria and natural well-being.

Endurance See cardiovascular endurance and muscular endurance.

Energy The ability to do work.

Enzyme A catalyst that facilitates chemical reactions.

Epidemiology Science that studies the relationship between diverse factors (lifestyle and environmental) and the occurrence of disease.

Essential amino acids Amino acids that must be obtained in the diet because they cannot be produced in the body.

Essential fat Minimal amount of body fat needed for normal physiological functions. It constitutes about 3 percent of the total fat in men and 12 percent in women.

Estrogen Female sex hormone. Essential for bone formation and bone density conservation.

Eumenorrhea Normal menstrual cycle.

Eustress Positive stress: health and performance continue to improve, even as stress increases.

Exercise adherence Initiating and participating in an exercise program for life.

Exercise electrocardiogram An exercise test during which the workload is gradually increased (until the subject reaches maximal fatigue) with blood pressure and twelve-lead electrocardiographic monitoring throughout the test.

Exercise intolerance Exercise conducted at intensity levels well beyond a person functional capacity leading to symptoms such as very rapid or irregular heart rate, labored breathing, nausea, vomiting, light-headedness, headaches, dizziness, pale skin, flushness, excessive weakness, lack of energy, shakiness, sore muscles, cramps, and tightness in the chest.

Exercise tolerance test See exercise electrocardiogram.

F

Fatigue The inability to maintain a given workload.

Fats Compounds made by a combination of triglycerides.

Fiber A form of complex carbohydrate made up of plant material that cannot be digested by the human body.

Fight or flight mechanism Physiological response of the body to stress which prepares the individual to take action by stimulating the vital defense systems.

Flexibility The ability of a joint to move freely through its full range of motion.

Fraud See quackery.

Free fatty acids (FFA) Fatty acids released by the breakdown of triglycerides.

Free radicals See oxygen free radicals.

Functional age Physiological age of the individual. Usually lower than the chronological (actual) age in fit people and vice versa in unfit people.

G

Genetics Science that studies genetic or hereditary conditions.

Genital warts A sexually transmitted disease caused by a viral infection. Genital warts increase the risk of cervical cancer. Enlargement and spread of the warts leads to obstruction of the urethra, vagina, and anus.

Girth measurements technique Technique to assess body composition, including percent body fat, by measuring circumferences at various body sites.

Glucose Blood sugar, type of carbohydrate (monosaccharide), a primary source of energy for the human body.

Glucose intolerance Inability to properly metabolize glucose.

Glycogen Form of carbohydrate (polysaccharide) storage in muscle.

Glycolysis Breakdown of glucose to pyruvic or lactic acid.

Gonorrhea A sexually transmitted disease caused by a bacterial infection that can lead to pelvic inflammation in women, infertility, widespread bacterial infection, heart damage, arthritis in men and women, and blindness in children born to infected women.

H

HDL See high density lipoprotein.

Health promotion Programs aimed at helping people develop healthy lifestyle behaviors that will lead to a higher state of wellness.

Health-related fitness Refers to fitness components that when enhanced lead to better health (cardiovascular endurance, body composition, muscular strength and endurance, and muscular flexibility).

Heart attack See myocardial infarct

Heart rate reserve The difference between the maximal heart rate and the resting heart rate.

Heat cramps Muscle cramps caused by heat-induced changes in electrolyte balance in muscle cells.

Heat exhaustion Heat-related condition; symptoms include fainting, dizziness, profuse sweating, cold clammy skin, headaches and a rapid, weak pulse.

Heat stroke Heat-related emergency; symptoms include serious disorientation, warm dry skin, no sweating, rapid full pulse, vomiting, diarrhea, unconsciousness, and high body temperature.

Hemoglobin Protein-iron compound in red blood cells that transports oxygen in the blood.

Herpes A sexually transmitted disease caused by a viral infection (herpes simplex virus types I and II). No known cure is available for the disease. The disease is characterized by the appearance of sores on the mouth, genitals, rectum, or other parts of the body.

Hidden fat Fat in food that can not be readily observed (lean meats contain about 30 to 40 percent fat calories).

High density lipoprotein (HDL) Cholesterol-transporting molecules in the blood. High HDL-cholesterol (good cholesterol) seems to offer protection against some forms of cardiovascular disease.

HIV   See human immunodeficiency virus.

Human immunodeficiency virus (HIV)   Virus that causes acquired immunodeficiency syndrome (AIDS).

Hydrostatic weighing   Underwater weighing technique to assess body composition, including percent body fat.

Hyperglycemia   Elevated blood sugar (glucose).

Hyperlipidemia   Elevated blood fats or lipids.

Hyperplasia   An increase in the number of cells.

Hypertension   Chronically elevated blood pressure.

Hypertrophy   An increase in the size of the cell (for example, muscle hypertrophy).

Hypoglycemia   Low blood sugar (glucose).

Hypokinetic disease   Diseases associated with a lack of physical activity (for example, hypertension, coronary heart disease, obesity, and diabetes).

I

Insulin   Hormone secreted by the pancreas that increases the absorption and utilization of glucose by the body.

Interval training   Training method with repeated bouts of exercise with rest intervals between each exercise bout.

Ischemia   Lack of blood flow.

Isokinetic contraction   Muscular contraction at a constant velocity.

Isokinetic training   Strength-training method where the speed of the muscle contraction is kept constant because the equipment (machine) provides an accommodating resistance to match the user's force (maximal) through the range of motion.

Isometric training   Strength-training method that refers to a muscle contraction producing little or no movement, such as pushing or pulling against immovable objects.

Isotonic training   Strength-training method that refers to a muscle contraction with movement, such as lifting an object over the head.

K

Kilocalorie   A unit to measure heat energy. A kilocalorie (kcal) or large calorie is the amount of heat necessary to raise the temperature of one kilogram of water one degree Centigrade. One kcal equals 1,000 calories.

L

Lactic acid   Strong acid, end product of anaerobic glycolysis (metabolism).

Lactovegetarians   Vegetarians who also eat foods from the milk group.

LDL   See low density lipoprotein.

Lean body mass   Body weight without body fat.

Life experiences survey   Questionnaire used to assess sources of stress in life.

Low density lipoprotein (LDL)   Cholesterol-transporting molecules in the blood. High LDL-cholesterol (bad cholesterol) seems to increase the risk for some forms of cardiovascular disease.

M

Malignant melanoma   Deadliest of all types of skin cancer. Tumors grow at a rapid rate and readily spread to other parts of the body if not treated at an early stage.

Marijuana   A psychoactive drug prepared from a mixture of crushed leaves, flowers, small branches, stems, and seeds from the hemp plant cannabis sativa. Also referred to as pot and grass.

Max VO$_2$ See maximal oxygen uptake

Maximal oxygen uptake (Max VO$_2$)   The maximal amount of oxygen that the body is able to utilize per minute of physical activity, commonly expressed in ml/kg/min. The best indicator of cardiovascular or aerobic fitness.

Meditation   Stress management technique used to gain control over one's attention, clearing the mind and blocking out the stressor(s) responsible for the increased tension.

Megadose (of vitamins)   Large amount of vitamin(s) intake. For most vitamins, a megadose is ten times the RDA or more.

Metabolism   All energy and material transformations that occur within living cells necessary to sustain life.

METS (metabolic equivalents)   A measurement unit of resting energy expenditure. One MET is the equivalent of 3.5 ml/kg/min.

Minerals   Inorganic elements found in the body and in food which are essential for normal body functions.

Mitochondria   Structures within the cells where energy transformations take place.

Monosaccharides   The simplest carbohydrates (sugars) formed by five- or six-carbon skeletons. The three most common monosaccharides are glucose, fructose, and galactose.

Monounsaturated fat   Fatty acids with only one double bond found along the carbon atom chain.

Motor skill-related fitness   Refers to fitness components that when improved lead to enhanced athletic performance (agility, balance, coordination, power, reaction time, and speed).

Motor unit   The combination of a motor neuron and the muscle fibers that it innervates.

Muscle fiber   A muscle cell.

Muscular endurance (localized muscular endurance)   The ability of a muscle to exert submaximal force repeatedly over a period of time (for example, 30 repetitions on a bench press exercise). It usually implies a specific muscle group (chest, thighs, abdominals).

Muscular strength   The ability of a muscle to exert maximum force against resistance (for example, 1 repetition maximum or 1 RM on the bench press exercise).

Myocardial infarct   Death of part of the myocardium.

Myocardium   Heart muscle.

Myoglobin   Iron-containing compound that holds oxygen in muscle tissue.

N

Neuron   A nerve cell.

Nicotine   Poisonous compound found in tobacco leaves.

Nonessential amino acids   Amino acids that can be manufactured in the body, therefore, the do not have to be obtained in the diet.

Nulliparity   Never having had a child.

Nutrient density   Ratio of nutrients to calories in food.

Nutrient   Substance found in food that provide energy, regulate metabolism, and help with growth and repair of body tissues.

Nutrition   Science that studies the relationship of foods to optimal health and performance.

O

Obesity   Refers to an excessive accumulation of body fat, usually about 30 percent above recommended body weight according to body size.

Oligomenorrhea   Irregular menstrual cycles.

Omega-3 fatty acids   Polyunsaturated fatty acids found primarily in cold water seafood and are thought to be effective in lowering blood cholesterol and triglycerides.

One repetition maximum (1 RM)   The maximal amount of resistance (weight) that an individual is able to lift in a single effort.

Osteoporosis   Softening, deterioration, or loss of total body bone.

Overload principle   Key training concept which states that the demands placed on a system (cardiovascular, muscular) must be systematically and progressively increased over a period of time to cause physiologic adaptation (development or improvement).

Ovolactovegetarians   Vegetarians who include egg and milk products in their diet.

Ovovegetarians   Vegetarians who allow eggs in their diet.

Oxygen free radicals   Substances formed during metabolism which attack and damage proteins and lipids, in particular the cell membrane and DNA; leading to the development of diseases such as heart disease, cancer, and emphysema. Antioxidants are believed to exert a protective effect by absorbing free radicals before they can cause damage and also by interrupting the sequence of reactions once damage has begun.

P

Percent body fat   Term used in body composition assessment. It represents the total amount of fat in the body based on the person's weight. It includes both essential and storage fat.

Peripheral vascular disease   Narrowing of the peripheral blood vessels (it excludes the cerebral and coronary arteries).

Physical fitness (health-related)   The general capacity to adapt and respond favorably to physical effort, implying that individuals are physically fit when they can meet the ordinary as well as the unusual demands of daily life safely and effectively without being overly fatigued, and still have energy left for leisure and recreational activities.

Plastic elongation (flexibility)   Refers to a permanent lengthening of soft tissue (capsules, tendons, and ligaments).

PNF   See proprioceptive neuromuscular facilitation.

Polyunsaturated fat   Fatty acids with two or more double bonds along the carbon atom chain.

Prevention index   An annual measure of the effort Americans are making to prevent disease and accidents and to promote good health and longevity. The index is based on the 21 most significant health-promoting behaviors in the United States.

Progressive muscle relaxation   Stress management technique. It involves progressive contraction and relaxation of muscle groups throughout the body.

Proprioceptive neuromuscular facilitation (PNF for flexibility development)   Stretching technique where muscles are progressively stretched out with intermittent isometric contractions.

Protein   Complex organic compounds containing nitrogen and formed by combinations of amino acids. Proteins are the main substances used in the body to build and repair tissues such as muscles, blood, internal organs, skin, hair, nails, and bones. They are also part of hormones, antibodies, and enzymes.

Q

Quackery (fraud)   The conscious promotion of unproven claims for profit.

R

Rate of perceived exertion (RPE)   A perception scale to monitor or interpret the intensity of aerobic exercise.

RDA   See recommended dietary allowances.

Recommended dietary allowances (RDA)   Daily recommended intakes of nutrients for normal, healthy people in the United States.

Red muscle fibers (slow-twitch or type I)   Muscle fibers with greater aerobic potential and slow speed of contraction.

Repetition (in strength training)   The number of times that a given resistance is performed (for example, 12 repetitions on the bench press exercise).

Repetition maximum (in strength training)   The maximum number of repetitions (RM) that can be performed with a specific resistance or weight (for example, 10 RM with 150 pounds).

Residual volume   Volume of air left in the lungs following complete exhalation.

Resistance (in strength training)   The amount of weight that is lifted.

Ribonucleic acid (RNA)   Genetic material involved in the formation of cell proteins.

Risk factors   Lifestyle and genetic factors that may lead to disease.

RNA   See ribonucleic acid.

RPE   See rate of perceived exertion.

S

Saturated fat   Fatty acids with carbon atoms fully saturated with hydrogens, therefore only single bonds link the carbon atoms on the chain. High intake of saturated fats increases the risk for coronary heart disease.

Serum cholesterol   Blood cholesterol level.

Set (in strength training)   A number of repetitions (1 set of 12 repetitions).

Setpoint theory   The weight control theory that indicates that the body has an established weight and strongly attempts to maintain that weight.

Sexually transmitted diseases (STDs)   Diseases spread through sexual contact.

Shin Splints   Injury to the lower leg characterized by pain and irritation in the shin region or front of the leg.

Simple carbohydrates   Carbohydrates formed by simple or double sugar units with little nutritive value (for example, candy, pop, cakes, etc.), frequently denoted as sugars. Simple carbohydrates are divided into monosaccharides and disaccharides.

Simple fats   A glyceride molecule linked to one, two, or three units of fatty acids (monoglycerides, diglycerides, and triglycerides).

Skinfold thickness   Technique to assess body composition, including percent body fat, by measuring the thickness of a double fold of skin at different body sites.

Slow-sustained or static stretching (flexibility)   Stretching technique where the muscles are gradually lengthened through a joint's complete range of motion and the final position is held for a few seconds.

Specificity of training   Training programs must be specifically aimed at the desired outcome. This is accomplished by training with the specific activity that the person is attempting to improve (aerobic, anaerobic, strength, flexibility).

Sphygmomanometer   Equipment used to measure blood pressure. Consists of an inflatable bladder contained within a cuff and a mercury gravity manometer or an aneroid manometer from which the pressure is read.

Spiritual well-being   An affirmation of life in a relationship with God, self, community, and environment that nurtures and celebrates wholeness.

Spot reducing   Theory that claims that exercising a specific body part (for example, abdominal or midsection of the body) will result in significant fat reduction in that area. It does not work! (See Chapter 7 — Exercise: The Key to Successful Weight Loss and Weight Maintenance).

Squamous cell carcinoma   Type of skin cancer that grows at a faster rate that basal cell carcinomas and seems to grow on sun-damaged areas. Squamous cell tumors spread to other parts of the body if not treated at an early stage.

STDs   See sexually transmitted diseases

Storage fat   Body fat in excess of the essential fat. It is stored in adipose tissue.

Strength   See muscular strength.

Strength training   A conditioning program that requires the use of weights to help increase muscular strength, endurance, power, and/or body size.

Stress test   See exercise electrocardiogram.

Stress   The nonspecific response of the human organism to any demand that is placed upon it.

Stress Vulnerability Scale   Questionnaire used to identify a number of factors that can help people decrease their vulnerability to stress.

Stressor   Reaction of the organism to a stress-causing event.

Stroke volume   Amount of blood ejected by the heart in one beat.

Structured Interview   Assessment tool used in determining behavioral patterns (Type A and B personality).

Syphilis   A sexually transmitted disease caused by a bacterial infection. During the last stage of the disease, some people will suffer from paralysis, crippling, blindness, heart disease, brain damage, insanity, and even death.

Systolic blood pressure   Pressure exerted by the blood against the walls of the arteries during the forceful contraction (systole) of the heart.

T

Tar   Chemical compound that forms during the burning of tobacco leaves.

Testosterone   Male sex hormone.

Triglycerides   Fats formed by glycerol and three fatty acids.

Type A (personality)   Behavior pattern characteristic of a hard-driving, overambitious, aggressive, at times hostile, and overly competitive person.

Type B (personality)   Behavior pattern characteristic of a calmed, casual, relaxed, and easy-going individual.

Type C (personality)   Behavior pattern of individuals who are just as highly stressed as the Type A but do not seem to be at higher risk for disease than the Type B.

U

U.S. RDA   The United States recommended daily allowances. Derived from the RDA and developed as a standard for nutrition labeling.

V

Vasoconstriction   Narrowing or clamping down of blood vessels.

Vasodilation   Widening or opening up of blood vessels.

Vegans   Vegetarians who eat no animal products at all.

Vegetarian   Individuals whose diet is of vegetable or plant origin.

Veins   Major vessels that carry blood back to the heart.

Very low density lipoprotein (VLDL)   Triglyceride, cholesterol and phospholipid-transporting molecules in the blood. Only a small amount of cholesterol is carried by the VLDL molecules.

Vitamins   Organic substances essential for normal metabolism, growth, and development of the body.

VLDL   See very low density lipoprotein.

W

Waist-to-Hip Ratio   Test designed by a panel of scientists appointed by the National Academy of Sciences and the Dietary Guidelines Advisory Council for the U.S. Departments of Agriculture and Health and Human Services to assess potential risk for diseases associated with obesity.

Weight training   A conditioning program that requires the use of weights to help increase muscular strength, endurance, power, and/or body size.

Weight-regulating mechanism   Mechanism located in the hypothalamus of the brain that regulates how much the body should weigh (also see setpoint theory).

Wellness   The constant and deliberate effort to stay healthy and achieve the highest potential for well-being. Implies the adoption of healthy lifestyle factors that will decrease the risk for disease and enhance well-being.

White muscle fibers (fast-twitch or type II)   Muscle fibers with greater anaerobic potential and fast speed of contraction.

Work   The ability to utilize energy.

Workload   A given level of exercise intensity or physical performance.

Y

Yellow fat cells   Cells used for fat storage (stores of energy in the form of fat).